Nerve Transfers for Brachial Plexus Reconstruction after Trauma

Fernando Guedes • Christian Heinen
Lukas Rasulic • Alexander Y. Shin
Mariano Socolovsky
Editors

Nerve Transfers for Brachial Plexus Reconstruction after Trauma

Springer

Editors
Fernando Guedes
Division of Neurosurgery
Gaffree and Guinle University Hospital, Federal University of the State of Rio de Janeiro
Rio de Janeiro, Rio de Janeiro, Brazil

Lukas Rasulic
Faculty of Medicine, University of Belgrade, Neurosurgical Clinic
University Clinical Center of Serbia
Belgrade, Serbia

Mariano Socolovsky
Division of Neurosurgery, Hospital de Clínicas
University of Buenos Aires School of Medicine
Buenos Aires, Argentina

Christian Heinen
Neuro-, Spine and Nerve Surgery
Christliches Krankenhaus Quakenbrück
Quakenbrück, Germany

Alexander Y. Shin
Department of Orthopedic Surgery
Mayo Clinic
Rochester, MN, USA

ISBN 978-3-031-92444-6 ISBN 978-3-031-92445-3 (eBook)
https://doi.org/10.1007/978-3-031-92445-3

This Springer imprint is published by the registered company Springer Nature Switzerland AG
The registered company address is: Gewerbestrasse 11, 6330 Cham, Switzerland

To my lovely wife Elizabeth, my dear son Thiago and his wife Maria Eduarda, and our little treasure Gabriel, my grandson
Also to all my patients
-Fernando Guedes

To Elisa, Matthias, Daniela, and Giuliana
-Christian Heinen

To my driving force, my family: my wife, Katarina; our children, Milica and Mihailo; my late parents, Grujica and Dušanka; my sister, Katarina. To my mentor, Prof. Dr. Miroslav Samardžić; my colleagues, collaborators, and team; and, last but not least, my patients who suffer from injuries and diseases of the peripheral nervous system
-Lukas Rasulic

To Patricia, Alexandra, Delaney, Nathaniel, and Andrew
-Alexander Y. Shin

To Verónica, Federico, Valentina, and Francisco
-Mariano Socolovsky

Foreword 1

The treatment of traumatic lesions of the brachial plexus is very complex. The situation becomes more problematic when nerve root avulsions are present. In recent decades, nerve transfers, either intraplexual or extraplexual, have greatly helped patients. The results are best when not all the nerve roots have been avulsed, allowing many functions to be restored. Even with complete root avulsions, surprisingly good results can be achieved with the help of ipsilateral nerves that do not belong to the brachial plexus or the contralateral C7 root.

Fernando Guedes, Christian Heinen, Lukas Rasulic, Mariano Socolovsky, and Alexander Shin, the five editors from Europe and North and South America with great experience in the field of brachial plexus surgery, have been able to involve contributions from experts in different specialities from all around the world.

This book consists of six sections: The first contains contributions on brachial plexus anatomy, intraoperative monitoring, cortical plasticity, and surgical indications. Of particular importance from my perspective is the indication for nerve transfers, which has been explained very clearly and in great detail, only being indicated if there is no possibility of autologous nerve grafting. The remaining sections cover all nerve transfers for shoulder function, as well as flexion and extension at the elbow, the hand, including the contralateral C7 nerve transfer. All chapters contain clear diagrams, tables, and intraoperative images.

I have been intensively involved in brachial plexus surgery for over 40 years and have witnessed first-hand the entire development of treatment options. I am delighted that for the first time a comprehensive work is now available that addresses patients with brachial plexus injuries and nerve root avulsions while illuminating this topic from all sides.

I would like to congratulate all the authors on this very successful work and wish it a wide distribution among all those involved in the surgery of traumatic brachial plexus lesions. The knowledge imparted here will be just as useful to them as will be the opportunity to recognize their own limitations. Furthermore, it is also suitable for all medical colleagues so that affected patients can be diagnosed promptly and referred to experienced plexus surgeons for treatment.

Division Peripheral Nerve Surgery
University of Ulm
Ulm, Baden-Württemberg, Germany

Gregor Antoniadis

Foreword 2

It is both an honor and a privilege to contribute the preface to this remarkable and timely volume on nerve transfers. This book represents the collective work of an extraordinary group of international leaders who have pushed the boundaries of what is possible in peripheral nerve surgery. Their efforts have resulted in a comprehensive and sophisticated guide to one of the most dynamic and evolving fields in nerve surgery, with broad implications for surgeons (neurosurgeons, orthopedists, and hand surgeons), physicians (neurologists, physiatrists, radiologists, and internists), therapists, anatomists, neuroscientists, and of course, patients.

Nerve transfers are not new—their history spans well over a century. One of the earliest pioneers was Harvey Cushing, whose work in the early twentieth century laid the foundation for modern neurosurgery. As with so many aspects of neurosurgery, he was prescient: his meticulous approach to brain and spinal cord lesions paved the way for greater exploration of connections between the central and peripheral nervous systems.

In early eras, nerve transfers were reserved almost exclusively for select upper extremity or facial nerve reconstructions. A major turning point came in 1969, when Japanese surgeon Katsuro Tsuyama and colleagues demonstrated the reliable use of intercostal nerves to restore elbow flexion by transferring them to the musculocutaneous nerve. This seminal contribution showcased the power of using non-limb nerves as donors and reinforced the foundational principles that continue to guide modern nerve transfer strategies. Over the past two to three decades, the field has undergone a renaissance, led by pioneers such as Christophe Oberlin and Susan Mackinnon, who popularized not only fascicular transfers but also distal nerve transfers for brachial plexus and upper limb injuries; these techniques have resulted in improved outcomes and more rapid recovery time and subsequently have led to a paradigm shift in our way of tackling complex problems in all nerves throughout the body. Once a niche technique, nerve transfer is now a cornerstone of reconstructive peripheral nerve surgery—driven by innovations in microsurgical technique, more detailed (macro and micro)-anatomical understanding, and broader clinical applications. In tandem, rehabilitation strategies have evolved to enhance functional outcomes.

Modern nerve transfers have expanded well beyond the upper limb. They are now applied to the lower extremities, complex head and neck cases, and even central lesions involving the spinal cord and brain. For instance, nerve transfers are being used to bypass spinal cord injuries and reanimate paralyzed limbs by connecting functional proximal nerves to distal targets. Similarly, in stroke, peripheral nerve transfers can harness intact motor pathways to promote cortical reorganization and recovery.

One of the most exciting frontiers is not surgical, but neurological: how the brain adapts to new neural circuits following transfer. As we deepen our understanding of neural plasticity and sensorimotor relearning, we now see nerve transfers not merely as structural repairs but as invitations for the nervous system to reinvent itself. Rehabilitation is no longer passive—it is an active, essential partner in recovery. This brain-driven model may well define the future of the field.

Looking ahead, progress will be shaped by interdisciplinary collaboration. Advances in neuroimaging, neuromodulation, brain–computer interfaces, and targeted rehabilitation will play central roles in optimizing outcomes. Individualized algorithms, real-time assessments, and AI-guided planning will further refine care. As access grows globally, our commitment to equity must match our pursuit of excellence.

This book is a tribute to the ingenuity, rigor, and dedication of the surgeons who contributed to its pages. I offer my deepest congratulations to my colleagues and friends around the world for this outstanding achievement. May this work serve not only as a reference but also as a source of inspiration for both the second edition of this book and the next generation of innovators in nerve surgery.

Mayo Clinic, Brachial Plexus Clinic
Departments of Orthopedics and Neurosurgery
Rochester, MN, USA

Robert J. Spinner

Foreword 3

By definition, nerve transfer is a surgical technique in which a nearby healthy nerve is sacrificed to serve as a donor for an injured, more important recipient nerve. Historically, credit should be given to Harris and Low (1903), who first proposed this technique. Many others have contributed with new methods or modifications of the original approach. Names such as Tuttle (1913), Vulpian and Stoffel (1920), Foerster (1929), and Lurje (1948) should also be remembered as pioneers in the field of nerve transfers.

In more recent years, increasing knowledge in nerve anatomy, microsurgical techniques, and nerve regeneration—as well as the remarkable publications of Narakas, Gu, Oberlin, Leechavengvongs, Mackinnon, and Samardzic—has significantly advanced the acceptance and use of nerve transfer procedures in many types of nerve injuries.

Peripheral nerve transfers have been performed primarily in cases of brachial plexus injuries and, in recent years, have become the preferred method of treatment for many specialists—even without surgical exploration of the plexus. In many cases, the functional outcomes achieved with nerve transfers surpass those obtained through traditional nerve repair or tendon transfers.

The editors—Fernando Guedes, Christian Heinen, Lukas Rasulic, Alexander Shin, and Mariano Socolovsky—have brought together a distinguished group of authors from various specialties, all experts in peripheral nerve surgery from around the world, to create this important book *Nerve Transfers for Brachial Plexus Reconstruction after Trauma*.

The editors, as well as all contributing authors, should be congratulated for publishing such an outstanding book. It will undoubtedly become an indispensable resource for all specialists interested in the surgical treatment of brachial plexus injuries.

It is an honor to have been invited to write this foreword.

Mario G. Siqueira, MD, PhD

Peripheral Nerve Surgery Unit,
Department of Neurosurgery
University of São Paulo Medical School
São Paulo, SP, Brazil

Contents

The original version of the book has been revised. A correction to this book can be found at https://doi.org/10.1007/978-3-031-92445-3_31

Part I

General Considerations

1 Introduction to Nerve Transfer

Heather Rossong, Suganth Suppiah, and Rajiv Midha

Brachial plexus injuries affect at least 1% of multi-trauma patients [1]. The evolution of surgical management for brachial plexus trauma has evolved over the past century from surgical nihilism, amputations, nerve exploration with grafting, and, over the past 25 years, increasingly to use of nerve transfers [2]. Nerve transfers have now become common practice for the repair of brachial plexus injuries after trauma and have been gaining increasing use throughout peripheral nerve surgery centers globally. The primary principle of peripheral nerve repair is to preserve the continuity of the nerve without tension to support nerve regeneration [3]. There are different approaches to repairing a nerve. First, primary end-to-end neurorrhaphy is used when the gap between two ends of an injured nerve is relatively small (typically under 2 cm) and involves joining the two ends together. In brachial plexus trauma, this is only feasible for the rare sharp laceration injury. Direct end-end repair however is not usually feasible in the majority of plexal injuries, so nerve grafts or nerve transfers are often used. Nerve grafts utilize a donor nerve that joins the two ends of an injured nerve and acts as a nonimmunologic scaffold that provides Schwann cells and other neurotrophic factors to aid in axonal regeneration. Based on the pioneering work of Millesi, initially on major injuries to limb nerves, autologous grafts are the gold standard [4].

Nerve transfers are often used for proximal nerve injuries and will be discussed herein regarding brachial plexus injuries. The principle of nerve transfers is to transfer a donor "expendable" nerve to a recipient outside the proximal zone of injury and ideally near the target muscle. Nerve transfers have multiple benefits that include decreasing the distance required for axonal regeneration, reinnervation of the entire musculotendinous unit, and dissecting through healthy, non-scarred tissue [3, 5, 6]. Furthermore, the existing evidence suggests good functional outcomes in patients who undergo nerve transfers for traumatic brachial plexus injuries [7, 8].

To fully understand the concept of nerve transfers, it is also important to delve into the relevant history. The first report of a nerve transfer dates back to 1903 by Charles Balance, who reported the transfer of the spinal accessory nerve to the facial nerve [9]. Following that, in 1913, Howard

H. Rossong
Division of Neurosurgery, University of Calgary Cumming School of Medicine, Calgary, AB, Canada
e-mail: heather.rossong1@ucalgary.ca

S. Suppiah
Division of Neurosurgery, University Health Network, University of Toronto, Toronto, ON, Canada
e-mail: suganth.suppiah@uhnresearch.ca

R. Midha (✉)
Department of Clinical Neurosciences, Hotchkiss Brain Institute, Cumming School of Medicine, University of Calgary, Calgary, AB, Canada
e-mail: rajiv.midha@albertahealthservices.ca

F. Guedes et al. (eds.), *Nerve Transfers for Brachial Plexus Reconstruction after Trauma*,
https://doi.org/10.1007/978-3-031-92445-3_1

Tuttle was the first to describe a nerve transfer for a brachial plexus injury [10]. The battlefield and resulting causalities were often a place of medical discoveries and in World War I, Harris reported a transfer of the radial nerve to the median nerve [11]. Regardless of the emerging techniques reported in the literature, nerve grafts were still the primary method for repairing brachial plexus injuries until the 1960–1970s. In 1972, Algimantas Otanas Narakas and Yves Alieu, at the XIIIth National Spanish Congress, considered the use of nerve transfers and interfascicular nerve grafts in brachial plexus injuries. It was after this that extraplexal nerve transfers started gaining more attention [12]. Surgeons in South-East Asian countries quickly began to utilize this technique and have contributed to many advancements in this field [13–15]. It was then brought to North America by Allan Friedman at Duke University who was one of the first neurosurgeons to employ this technique in his country [16]. Intra-plexal nerve transfers have now gained increasing popularity, with contributions to the field by multiple pioneering surgeons [17–20].

After all these remarkable contributions, nerve transfers are now a common practice used for brachial plexus injuries and this practice continues to evolve over time. Many indigenous different nerve transfers have since been described. The technique of nerve transfers has far surpassed other nerve repair techniques in terms of functional outcome [21, 22], and they have the potential to be applied to a broad array of pathologies such as lower limbs injuries, strokes, and spinal cord injuries [23].

As mentioned, the basic concept of a nerve transfer is to convert a proximal injury into a distal injury and decrease the amount of time it takes to reinnervate the target muscle. Skeletal muscle becomes refractory to reinnervation after 15–18 months; therefore, time is of the essence. The choice of the donor nerve is an important concept. The donor nerve should be one that will not produce much of a deficit after harvesting and is redundant. Furthermore, a strong donor (at least British MRC grade 4+) that is close to the recipient in physical distance is ideal to avoid the need for an interposed nerve graft. When possible, the donor and recipient should be synergistic in action and modality. For example, a motor donor should be transferred to a motor recipient. The donor nerve is often identified first using electrical stimulation and the repair should not be under any tension. Postoperatively, the patient's limb is often immobilized for 7–21 days, depending on the location and tension expected on the repair. It usually takes months for clinical evidence of target muscle reinnervation, but this depends on the distance required for the nerve to grow. Typically, the rate of nerve regeneration is between 1 and 1.5 mm per day, but clinical recovery often starts several weeks after axons first arrive at the target muscle. Physical therapy is key and patient selection should take into account their capacity to undergo the extensive rehabilitation and relearning process required [24].

References

1. Midha R. Epidemiology of brachial plexus injuries in a multitrauma population. Neurosurgery. 1997;40(6):1182–9.
2. Midha R, Grochmal J. Surgery for nerve injury: current and future perspectives. J Neurosurg. 2019;130:675–85.
3. Ray WZ, Mackinnon SE. Management of nerve gaps: autografts, allografts, nerve transfers, and end-to-side neurorrhaphy. Exp Neurol. 2010;223(1):77–85.
4. Millesi H, Meissl G, Berger A. The interfascicular nerve-grafting of the median and ulnar nerves. J Bone Joint Surg Am. 1972;54:727–50.
5. Dvali L, Mackinnon S. Nerve repair, grafting, and nerve transfers. Clin Plast Surg. 2003;30(2):203–2.
6. Nath RK, Mackinnon SE. Nerve transfers in the upper extremity. Hand Clin. 2000 Feb;16(1):131–9.
7. Merrell GA, Barrie KA, Katz DL, Wolfe SW. Results of nerve transfer techniques for restoration of shoulder and elbow function in the context of a meta-analysis of the English literature. J Hand Surg. 2001;26(2):303–14.
8. Yang LJ, Chang KW, Chung KC. A systematic review of nerve transfer and nerve repair for the treatment of adult upper brachial plexus injury. Neurosurgery. 2012;71:417–29.
9. Ballance CA, Ballance HA, Stewart P. Remarks on the operative treatment of chronic facial palsy of peripheral origin. Br Med J. 1903;1(2209):1009–13.
10. Tuttle HK. Exposure of the brachial plexus with nerve-transplantation. JAMA. 1913;61(1):15–7.
11. Harris RI. The treatment of irreparable nerve injuries. Can Med Assoc J. 1921;11:833–41.

12. Taleb C, Nectoux E, Awada T, Liverneaux P. The destiny of an ace: Algimantas Otanas Narakas (1927-1993). J Brachial Plex Peripher Nerve Inj. 2013;8(1):e1.
13. Ogino T, Naito T. Intercostal nerve crossing to restore elbow flexion and sensibility of the hand for a root avulsion type of brachial plexus injury. Microsurgery. 1995;16:571–7.
14. Gu YD, Wu MM, Zhen YL, Zhao JA, Zhang GM, Chen DS, Yan JQ, Cheng XM. Phrenic nerve transfer for treatment of root avulsion of the brachial plexus. Chin Med J. 1990 Apr;103(4):267–70.
15. Nagano A, Yamamoto S, Mikami Y. Intercostal nerve transfer to restore upper extremity functions after brachial plexus injury. Ann Acad Med. 1995;24:42–5.
16. Friedman AH, Nunley JA 2nd, Goldner RD, Oakes WJ, Goldner JL, Urbaniak JR. Nerve transposition for the restoration of elbow flexion following brachial plexus avulsion injuries. J Neurosurg. 1990 Jan;72(1):59–64.
17. Bertelli JA, Ghizoni MF. Nerve root grafting and distal nerve transfers for C5-C6 brachial plexus injuries. J Hand Surg Am. 2010;35:769–75.
18. Leechavengvongs S, Witoonchart K, Uerpairojkit C, Thuvasethakul P, Malungpaishrope K. Combined nerve transfers for C5 and C6 brachial plexus avulsion injury. J Hand Surg Am. 2006;31:183–9.
19. Mackinnon SE, Novak CB, Myckatyn TM, Tung TH. Results of reinnervation of the biceps and brachialis muscles with a double fascicular transfer for elbow flexion. J Hand Surg Am. 2005;30:978–85.
20. Oberlin C, Beal D, Leechavengvongs S, Salon A, Dauge MC, Sarcy JJ. Nerve transfer to biceps muscle using a part of ulnar nerve for C5-C6 avulsion of the brachial plexus: anatomical study and report of four cases. J Hand Surg Am. 1996;19:232–7.
21. Estrella EP. Functional outcome of nerve transfers for upper-type brachial plexus injuries. J Plast Reconstr Aesthet Surg. 2011;64:1007–13.
22. Weber RA, Mackinnon SE. Nerve transfers in the upper extremity. J Am Soc Surg Hand. 2004;4:200–13.
23. Vanaclocha-Vanaclocha V, Ortiz-Criado JM, Sáiz-Sapena N, Vanaclocha N. Nerve transfers in the treatment of peripheral nerve injuries. In: Peripheral nerve regeneration—from surgery to new therapeutic approaches including biomaterials and cell-based therapies development. InTech; 2017.
24. Novak CB, Mackinnon SE, Tung TH. Patient outcome following a thoracodorsal to musculocutaneous nerve transfer for reconstruction of elbow flexion. Br J Plast Surg. 2002;55:416–9.

2 Surgical Anatomy of the Brachial Plexus

Fernando Martínez

2.1 Introduction

Brachial plexus is formed by the anterior rami of C5 to T1 spinal nerves. By means of its collateral and terminal branches, this nerves innervates the shoulder and superior limb with motor, sensory, and vegetative information [1–7].

In the classic form of description, brachial plexus is formed by C5 to T1 spinal nerves, but another spinal nerves can constitute the brachial plexus: C4 and T2 (prefixed and postfixed plexus, respectively) [1–7].

The brachial plexus (BP) is a very important *site of organization* of sensory, motor, and vegetative innervation for muscles, skin, bones, and vessels of the superior limb [4]. So, the understanding of its basic anatomy is of paramount importance for the peripheral nerve surgeon. But it is also important to understand its surgical anatomy (location and relationships) and its internal anatomy, in order to plan the surgical approaches and reconstruction strategies in BP injuries.

In this chap. I will try to review the classical anatomy of brachial plexus, the main variations in the formation of the trunks and cords, the functional aspects of the trunks and cords, the intraneural topography of the main motor information inside the spinal nerve roots and trunks, and the topographic and the surgical anatomy of supraclavicular and infraclavicular plexus. Finally, I will try to analyze some key points of clinical anatomy of the brachial plexus.

2.2 Basic Composition of Brachial Plexus and a Brief Functional Insight

The classic description of the brachial plexus is the following: C5 to T1 nerve roots combining to form three trunks (superior, middle, and inferior), and trunks originate six divisions (three anterior and three posterior) that combine to form three cords (posterior, lateral, and medial) [1–15]. Cords give rise to five main terminal motor/sensory branches to the upper extremity (radial, axillary, median, musculocutaneous, and ulnar nerves) (Fig. 2.1). But it is a simplification to some degree, because many variants of the brachial plexus exists, with none representing a majority of patients. But we must describe the classical anatomy pattern to understand the basic anatomy, and after that, we can discuss the most frequent variations of BP.

First, anterior rami of C5 and C6 unite to form the superior trunk, C7 forms the middle trunk, and C8-T1 unite to form the inferior trunk. Trunks of the brachial plexus are located in the

F. Martínez (✉)
Department of Anatomy, Facultad de Medicina UCLAEH, Maldonado, Uruguay

Department of Neurosurgery, Hospital de Clínicas de Montevideo, Montevideo, Uruguay

F. Guedes et al. (eds.), *Nerve Transfers for Brachial Plexus Reconstruction after Trauma*, https://doi.org/10.1007/978-3-031-92445-3_2

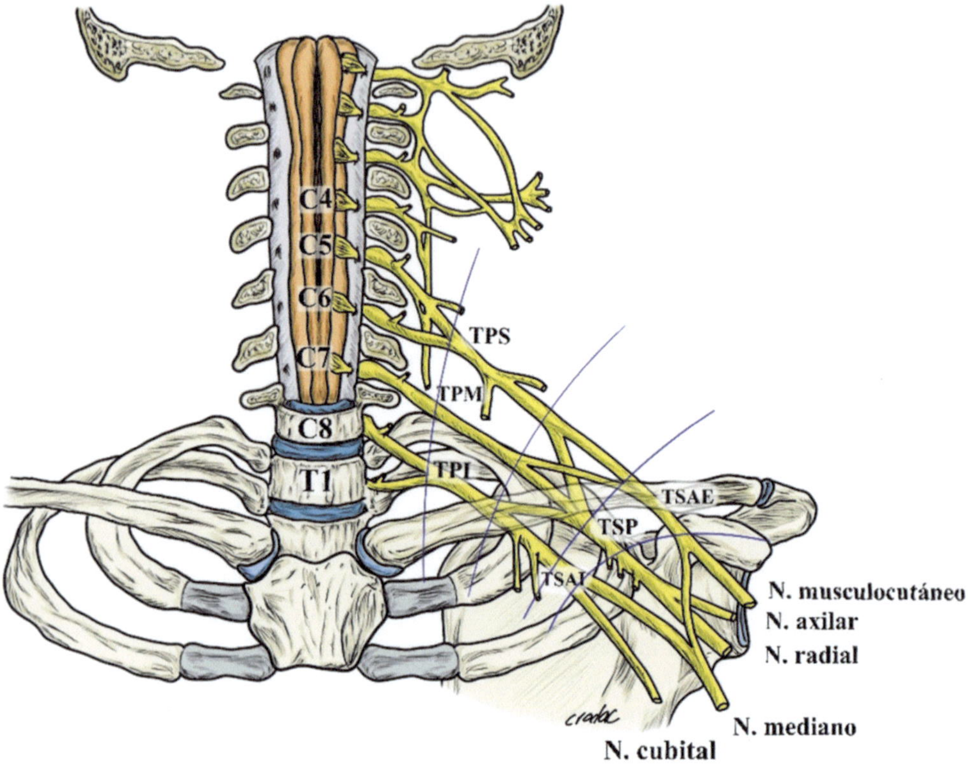

Fig. 2.1 Brachial plexus anatomy. TPS, superior trunk; TPM, middle trunk; TPI, inferior trunk; TSAE, lateral cord; TSP, posterior cord; TSAI, medial cord; N. musculocutaneo, musculocutaneous nerve; N. axilar, axillary nerve; N. radial, radial nerve; N. mediano, median nerve; N. cubital, ulnar nerve. (From: Corderi F, Rodríguez CA, Martínez F. Plexo braquial. In: Martinez F (Ed): Cuadernos de Anatomía. Tomo 1. Bibliomédica, Montevideo, 2023. With authorization)

supraclavicular region. Each trunk gives rise to two divisions: anterior and posterior. Six divisions combine to form the cords: All of the three posterior divisions form the posterior cord, anterior divisions of the superior and middle trunk form the lateral cord, and anterior division of inferior trunk forms the medial cord.

Terminal branches of brachial plexus (that means: axillary, radial, musculocutaneous, median, and ulnar nerves) are originated from the cords (Fig. 2.1).

2.2.1 Terminal Branches

Some authors stated that BP originate seven branches and others stated that the terminal branches are five [2, 4, 8, 10].

Actually, the most important terminal branches according to function of the superior limb are five: axillary, radial, musculocutaneous, median, and ulnar nerve. The other two branches are sensitive: medial cutaneous brachial and antebrachial nerves.

If we consider seven branches, it can be organized on two groups: anterior and posterior depending on whether they arise from the external or internal cords or from the posterior cord. As we have seen, these groups have different functions: The anterior cords belongs to the flexor plane, and the posterior cord to the extensor plane.

The information in the brachial plexus is not randomly distributed in every nerve, trunk, division, or cord: As we will see, the information in the brachial plexus *is segregated in a functional way*.

The fifth spinal nerve goes mainly to shoulder movements (abduction), C6 to flex the elbow, C7 to extend the elbow and wrist, and C8 to flex the fingers and wrist, and T1 innervates the intrinsic muscles of the hand. The posterior cord is mainly extensor, and medial and lateral cords are mainly flexors. Musculocutaneous, median, and ulnar nerves form the flexor system and radial and axillary nerve forms the extensor system [4, 9].

To reach this goal, fibers mix between them, but obviously, not in a random way.

2.3 Functional Anatomy and Topographic Aspects of the Radicular and Trunk Composition in Brachial Plexus

The nerve roots of the plexus, as they exit the intervertebral foramina, are typically comprised of a single large fascicle, surrounded by epineurium [3]. But if we dissect and study the intraneural topography of the nerve, we can see fascicles arranged in a functional way to reach the distal targets (muscles and skin). The greater nerves then divide and recombine along the length of the plexus until, eventually, most fascicles have been segregated into largely motor, sensory, or mixed fascicles, bound for a particular area or structure. The number of fascicles increases and their cross-sectional area decreases, from proximal to distal in the plexus. At the same time, the amount of connective tissue of the epineurium progressively increases from proximal to distal.

It's important to review some aspects of functional anatomy BP anatomy:

The nerves that make up the brachial plexus carry motor and sensory information, but when they begin to divide and combine with each other, they do not necessarily contribute both types of information to the resulting trunk. For example, the lateral and medial cords will originate among other nerves, the median nerve. The lateral cord supplies the median nerve with primarily sensory fibers, while the medial cord supplies primarily motor fibers. This organization of information occurs in various peripheral nerves. Therefore, when we say that the median nerve is made up of information from C6, C7, and C8, it is not necessarily the same type of information. C6 and C7 provide fundamentally sensitive information and C8 provides fundamentally motor information [14].

(a) Conceptually we can recognize that the brachial plexus has the shape of an hourglass or two triangles that touch at their vertices. The first triangle is based on the cervical spine and the vertex faces the clavicle. It corresponds to the sector where the roots C5 to T1 begin to meet to form the three trunks, going from five to three nerve structures. The second triangle has its vertex at the clavicle and its base faces the armpit. It corresponds to the sector where the trunks begin to divide, meet to form cords, and then diverge into their terminal branches [8, 11, 13, 14].
(b) The upper triangle is approached in the supraclavicular region, and the lower triangle generally requires the opening of the armpit to be reached.

2.4 Intraneural Topography in the Brachial Plexus

As we said previously, the information is not randomly located in the spinal nerves and trunks of brachial plexus. Brachial plexus itself is a point of *organization* of the neural information. If we can locate, for example, the location of fibers of C5 going to the suprascapular nerve, we can choose the specific site of reconstruction of this nerve. For that reason, the knowledge of intraneural location of fascicles with specific functions is very important for the surgeon of peripheral nerves. The cords show the largest number of fascicles, the trunks intermediate number of fascicles, and the spinal nerves being oligo-or monofascicular. Although the fascicular topography roots are complex, a few general observations can be made [3, 16–19].

If we look at a section of a nerve and we divide it in four quadrants (as a clock with four areas located between 12 and 3, 3 and 6, 6 and 9, and 9 and 12), we can find a relatively constant location of the fibers inside a specific nerve.

C5: In a cross section of C5 nerve, the fibers of the suprascapular nerve are located cranially (between 12 and 3 o'clock), fibers to musculocutaneous nerve in front (between 3 and 6 o'clock), fibers to axillary nerve are posterior (between 9 and 12 o'clock), and fibers to posterior and lateral cords are located caudally (between 6 and 9 o'clock).

C6: Fibers of musculocutaneous nerve are located anteriorly, fibers to axillary and radial nerve posteriorly, and fibers to median and pectoral nerves inferiorly.

C7: Fibers to radial nerve are located superior and posteriorly (between 9 and 12 o'clock), fibers to median nerve between 12 and 3, and fibers to ulnar and pectoral nerves inferiorly (ulnar fibers in the posterior aspect and pectoral fibers in the anterior aspect).

C8: Fibers to median nerve occupies the entire aspect of anterior surface of the nerve (from 12 to 6 o'clock), fibers to posterior chord are located between 9 and 12, and ulnar and sensitive fibers for cutaneous antebrachial nerve are located between 6 and 9 o'clock).

T1: The anterior aspect of the nerve (from 12 to 6 o'clock) contents fibers to medial cord, and the posterior aspect of the nerve, from cranial to caudal, contents fibers to posterior cord, ulnar nerve and again, posterior cord.

2.5 Anatomical Variations of Trunks

More than 50% of humans have variations in the formation or distribution of brachial plexus [2, 6, 7, 20–35]. Ten to 65% of the specimens were of the "prefixed" type, in which the C4 root joins the plexus (C5) and contribute to form the superior trunk, while 1–4% were of the "postfixed" type, with a contribution from T2 root to the inferior trunk [7].

Very rarely, some specimens can have two or four trunks [20, 30].

In specimens with two trunks (2–10%), the less frequent pattern is the union of C5, C6, and C7 to form a single trunk (superior trunk C5 to C7 and inferior trunk C8 and T1). The other possibility (more frequent) is the union of C7 to T1 to form an inferior trunk [20].

In cases with four trunks, the most frequent pattern is the nonunion of C5 and C6. In this cases, superior trunk doesn't exist. In cases with no superior trunk, we can find two patterns: C5 and C6 remains independent (and each nerve originates and anterior and posterior divisions) or they just change fibers with absence of a real trunk [2, 20, 30]. It also can be found a nonunion of C8 and T1 with no inferior trunk formation, but it is more infrequent [20].

2.6 Anatomy of Divisions and Cords

The branches of the plexus follow the same pattern: They all divide into two branches or divisions. Both divisions have sensory and motor information and combine to form the fascicles. The anterior division of the upper trunk joins the anterior division of the middle trunk to form the lateral fascicle (due to its relationship with the axillary artery). The anterior division of the lower trunk forms, on its own, the medial fascicle. The posterior divisions of the three trunks unite to form the posterior fascicle.

2.7 Terminal Branches

They originate from the divisions of the plexus.

The lateral fascicle gives rise to the musculocutaneous nerve and the lateral root of the median nerve.

The medial fascicle originates the medial cutaneous nerves of the forearm, ulnar nerve, and medial root of the median nerve.

The posterior fascicle originates the axillary and radial nerves.

As mentioned earlier, the information from the roots and divisions does not randomly "mix" in the plexus.

Anterior group of terminal branches: is mainly a flexor group and is composed by three motor and sensory nerves and two sensory nerves.

Musculocutaneous nerve: Its main function is elbow flexion and hand supination.

Median nerve: Its main function is hand pronation, finger flexion, and wrist flexion. From a sensory perspective, it innervates the palmar surface of the hand along with the ulnar nerve.

Medial cutaneous nerves of forearm and arm: They innervate the inner surface of the arm and forearm.

Ulnar nerve: Its main function is wrist flection and innervation of the intrinsic muscles of the hand.

Posterior group of terminal branches: is mainly extensor and is composed of two mixed nerves.

Axillary nerve: Its main function is arm abduction and it innervates the skin of the shoulder region.

Radial nerve: Its main function is elbow, wrist, and finger extension. From a sensory perspective, it innervates the back of the hand.

In this way, we can recognize the following anatomo-functional facts in the organization of the brachial plexus:

(a) The anterior cords (lateral and medial) give rise to the musculocutaneous, median, and ulnar nerves. All are flexor nerves.
(b) The posterior fascicle gives rise to the radial nerve, which is the major extensor nerve of the upper limb.
(c) The C5 root primarily composes the axillary nerve. When it is said primarily, it means primarily. There are other roots that contribute to it, but C5 is the primary one in terms of its motor role.
(d) The C6 root to the musculocutaneous nerve.
(e) The C7 root to the radial nerve.
(f) The C8 root to the median nerve.
(g) The T1 root to the ulnar nerve.
(h) The medial root of the median nerve primarily provides motor information, while the lateral root provides primarily sensory information.

2.8 Some Anatomical Variations of Cords and Terminal Branches

2.8.1 Cord Variations

Posterior cord can be formed by posterior division of upper and middle trunk only [31].

Lower trunk can continue as medial cord without dividing into anterior and posterior divisions. Lateral cord can be formed only by anterior division of superior trunk.

It is reported also a common trunk formed by the three anterior divisions of superior, middle, and inferior trunk, but no existence of lateral and medial cords [26, 27].

The terminal nerves with more variations in its origin are median and musculocutaneous nerves [29, 32–34].

Median nerve: It is originated from two branches from medial and lateral cords, but origins from one to four branches are reported.

In cases of origin from one branch (4.5%), it originates in medial cord. In cases with three branches of origin (22–36.4% of cases), the third branch takes it origin from musculocutaneous nerve. Finally, in 2 to 7.1% of cases, the median nerve originates from four branches. In 3.6 to 8.3% of cases, the union of the branches is not located in the axilla, but in the proximal third of the arm [23, 24].

Musculocutaneous nerve: It can be absent in 10–11% of cases. In this cases, median nerve innervates the muscles of anterior compartment of the arm [25, 26, 29].

2.9 Surgical Anatomy and Approaches of the Brachial Plexus (Figs. 2.2, 2.3, 2.4, 2.5 and 2.6)

The brachial plexus is located at the base of the neck (trunks) and the armpit (divisions, fascicles, and the beginning of the terminal branches).

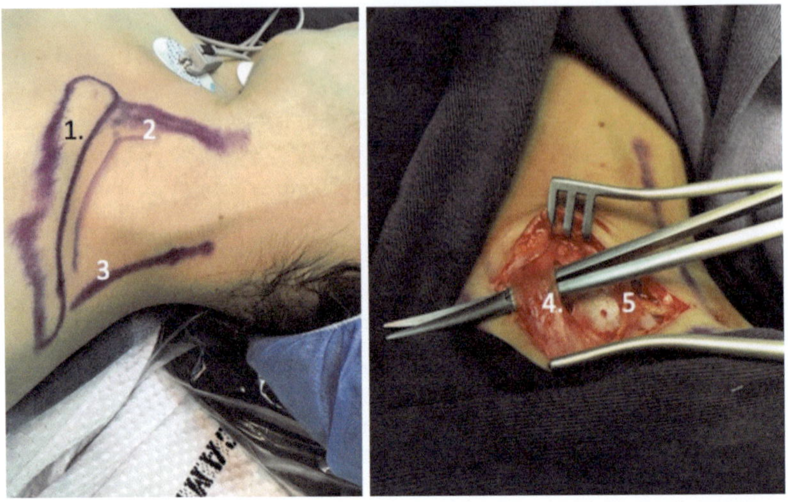

Fig. 2.2 Surgical approach to the supraclavicular brachial plexus. On the left, the cutaneous planes with the topography of the clavicle (1), sternocleidomastoid muscle (2), and trapezius muscle (3). On the right, the incision has already been made, and the platysma muscle (4) and branches of the superficial cervical plexus (5) are recognized

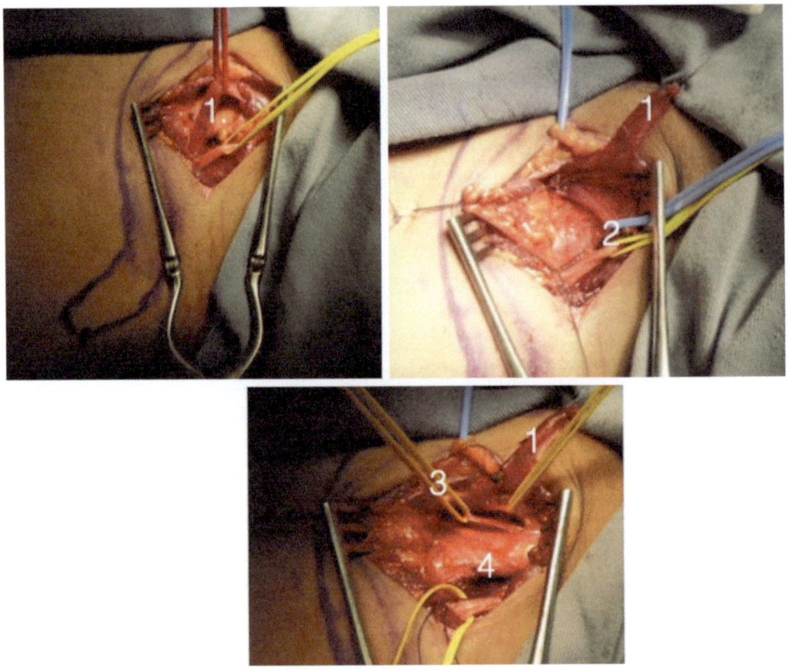

Fig. 2.3 Supraclavicular approach to a BP injury. Superior left: The skin is opened, and the omohyoid muscle is seen (1). Superior right: the omohyoid muscle was cut and retracted. 2: transverse cervical vessels. Inferior: superior trunk (4) (with a continuity neuroma) is exposed. 3: frenic nerve retracted with a vessel loop

2.9.1 Relationships

Neck: The brachial plexus is situated in the lateral cervical region, covered by the skin, the platysma muscle, and the deep cervical fascia.

The roots exit through the intervertebral foramina and are located between the anterior and middle scalene muscles (interscalene groove). The subclavian artery runs through the same groove, over the first rib, in front of the lower trunk. The subclavian vein is even more anterior (passes in front of the anterior scalene muscle). There are anatomical variations of the scalenic muscles, such as supernumerary muscles or tendinous bands [35].

2.9.2 Supraclavicular Region

The trunks and the beginning of the divisions are located in this region [5, 36–42].

The anatomical landmarks to locate the brachial plexus are the sternocleidomastoid muscle in front, the prominence of the trapezius muscle behind, and the clavicle below.

A triangle is formed here where we find the superficial cervical plexus and the brachial plexus.

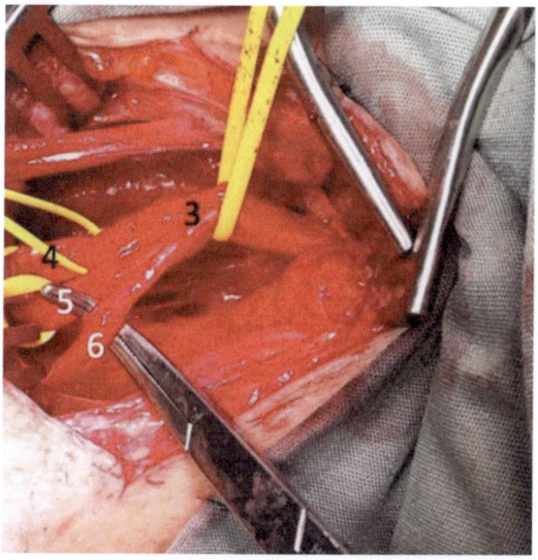

Fig. 2.4 Supraclavicular approach to the brachial plexus. Upper trunk (3) with its anterior and posterior divisions (4 and 5), as well as the suprascapular nerve (6)

If an incision is made 1 cm above the clavicle, the planes separating the surgeon from the plexus are:

(a) Skin.
(b) Platysma muscle of the neck and superficial aponeurosis.
(c) The omohyoid muscle, which superficially crosses the upper trunk and therefore serves as a reference to locate it.
(d) The next structure is the transverse cervical vascular bundle, which also crosses in front of the upper trunk.
(e) After these structures, the upper trunk can be visualized (Fig. 2.3).
(f) Dissecting proximally, the interscalene groove and the C5 and C6 roots can be located. On the anterior surface of the anterior scalene muscle, the phrenic nerve is an important reference because if the upper trunk is not easily located, the phrenic nerve will guide us to C4 and C5.
(g) Once the upper trunk is located, dissection will allow us to recognize the rest of the components of the brachial plexus, remembering that the subclavian vein lies anterior and slightly below, while the subclavian artery lies in front of the lower trunk (Figs. 2.4, 2.5 and 2.6).
(h) The upper trunk generally ends in an anatomy that resembles a tripod, giving rise to the suprascapular nerve, anterior division, and posterior division. Neto [21] emphasizes

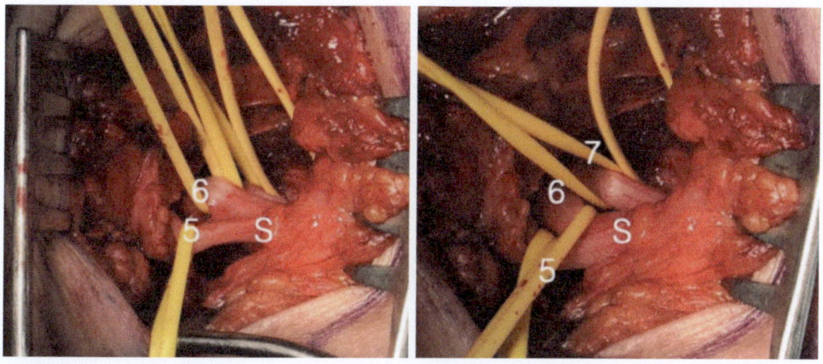

Fig. 2.5 Supraclavicular approach to BP. Left: C5, C6, and superior trunk are exposed (5: C5, 6: C6, S: superior trunk). Right: C5, C6, and C7 are exposed. (7: C7 retracted with a vessel loop, 5: C5 retracted with a vessel loop, 6: C6, S: superior trunk

that the arrangement of these three nerves is different from what is represented in most anatomical books. From cranial to caudal, the suprascapular nerve originates first, followed by the posterior division, and then the anterior division. In other words, the posterior division is posterior but cranial to the anterior division.

Axillary apex: The plexus is represented by the divisions.

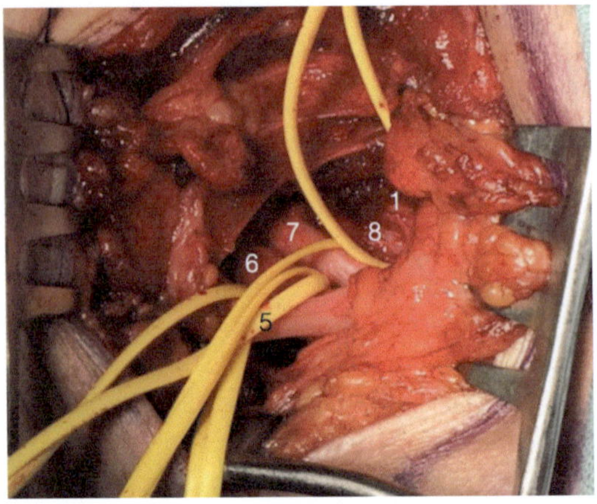

Fig. 2.6 Supraclavicular approach to BP. All of the roots are exposed: 5, 6, 7, 8, and 1: C5, C6, C7, C8 and T1, respectively

Axillary fossa:

- The lateral fascicle tends to be located laterally to the axillary artery.
- The medial fascicle crosses obliquely, from superior to inferior and from lateral to medial, the posterior surface of the arterial trunk, anteriorly to the posterior fascicle, and is positioned medially to it, between the artery and the vein.
- The posterior fascicle is located until its posterior termination to the axillary artery.

The three cords give rise to their terminal branches in the axillary fossa.

2.9.3 Infraclavicular Brachial Plexus Approach (Fig. 2.7)

Here, we find the union of the divisions, formation of the cords, and origin of the terminal branches.

The incision should be made in relation to the clavicle (above or below) and arched caudally in the region of the deltopectoral groove. The groove is opened, the cephalic vein is separated, and the tendon of the pectoralis major is sectioned.

Fig. 2.7 Infraclavicular approach to BP. An "N"-shaped incision is made in supra-and infraclaviclar region. Up: We can identify the clavicle (1), the deltoid (2), and the major pectoral muscle (3). Between the muscles, the deltopectoral groove (arrow)

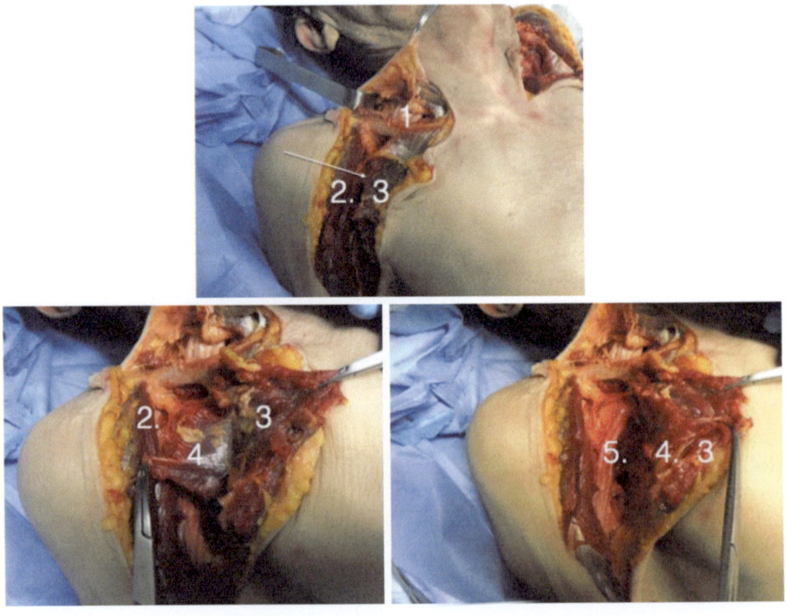

Then, the tendon of the pectoralis minor is sectioned, and wide access to the axillary region is obtained.

The anterior and posterior cords are located anteriorly to the axillary artery, while the posterior cord is located behind it.

Down left: The major pectoral muscle was incised (3) and the pectoral minor (4) is identified. Down right: Pectoral muscles are opened and retracted (3, 4) and the brachial plexus and axillary vessels are exposed (5).

2.10 Distribution of Collateral Branches of the Brachial Plexus

Collateral branches are distributed in the root of the upper limb and the shoulder girdle, providing motor innervation and, to a lesser extent, sensory innervation to this region. This is because the supraclavicular region and part of the root of the upper limb receive innervation from the cervical plexus.

The collateral branches of the brachial plexus are predominantly muscular branches that originate directly from the roots that form the plexus (C5 to T1), from the roots, trunks, or divisions. In other words, they arise in a staggered manner in the proximal portion of the plexus.

Although there are variations in the distribution of collateral branches of the plexus, only the C5 (the most important of all), C6, C7, and the superior trunk give rise to clinically significant collateral branches [6, 14].

1. Long thoracic nerve: It originates from the C5, C6, and C7 spinal nerves and innervates the serratus anterior muscle. This muscle stabilizes the scapula and allows its rotation and anterior displacement. Each functional sector of the serratus anterior receives innervation from a different root: C5 for the upper sector, C6 for the middle sector, and C7 for the lower sector. Injury to the long thoracic nerve or its component roots leads to winged scapula.
2. Dorsal scapular nerve: It originates from C5 and supplies the rhomboid muscles. These muscles allow approximation of the scapula to the midline.

The motor compromise of the described muscles in brachial plexus trauma is an indicator of a very proximal C5 lesion.

2.11 Clinical Examination

The serratus anterior stabilizes the scapula. The individual can be asked to push against a wall with the hand and observe if there is winging of the scapula.

The rhomboid muscles can be examined by asking the person to bring the scapulae closer to the midline.

1. Suprascapular nerve: It originates from the superior trunk (primarily C5, C6) and courses posteriorly to innervate the supraspinatus and infraspinatus muscles. This nerve passes through the suprascapular notch, below the superior transverse scapular ligament. This relationship explains the compressive neuropathy of the suprascapular nerve and the possibility of "double crush" (in the plexus and the notch) due to trauma [36]. The supraspinatus is a stabilizer of the humeral head and acts during the first 30 degrees of shoulder abduction. The infraspinatus is a stabilizer of the humeral head and an external rotator.

Clinical examination: The individual is asked to perform shoulder abduction and external rotation.

Nerves of the pectoral muscles: They originate in the infraclavicular portion of the plexus from the lateral and medial cords (lateral pectoral nerve and medial pectoral nerve, respectively). Medial pectoral nerve: C8-T1, lateral pectoral nerve: C5-C7

Clinical examination: The patient is asked to perform shoulder adduction and internal rotation

1. Thoracodorsal nerve (C6–C8): It arises from the posterior cord and is destined for the latissimus dorsi muscle.

Clinical examination: The individual is asked to perform shoulder abduction and internal rotation. The latissimus dorsi muscle allows reaching the hand to the back.

2.12 Sympathetic Anastomosis of the Brachial Plexus

The anterior branches of the spinal nerves that form the brachial plexus receive their sympathetic fibers in the form of gray communicating rami from the cervical sympathetic chain. The fifth cervical nerve receives fibers from the middle cervical ganglion; C6, C7, and C8 receive them from the inferior cervical or stellate ganglion; and T1 and T2 receive them from the stellate ganglion or the first and second dorsal ganglia.

These vegetative fibers provide the brachial plexus with information that it will carry to its destination through its branches.

They are responsible for the vasomotor tone of the muscles of the arteries of the upper limb (vasoconstriction and vasodilation), contraction of the muscles at the base of the hair (pilomotor response), and the muscles of the sweat glands, etc.

Characteristically, proximal brachial plexus root avulsion injuries.

References

1. Guday E, Bekele A, Muche A. Anatomical study of prefixed versus postfixed brachial plexuses in adult human cadaver. ANZ J Surg. 2017;87(5):399–403.
2. Hovelacque A. Anatomie des nerfs craniens et rachidiens et du systeme grand sympatique chez l'homme. Paris: Librarie Octave Doin, Gaston Doin et Cie Editeurs; 1927.
3. Johnson EO, Vekris M, Demesticha T, Soucacos PN. Neuroanatomy of the brachial plexus: normal and variant anatomy of its formation. Surg Radiol Anat. 2010;32(3):291–7.
4. Le LG. sistème nerveux pèriphérique. Paris: Masson et Cie Èditeurs; 1955.
5. Llusa M, Palazzi S, Valer A. Surgical anatomy of brachial plexus and peripheral nerves of superior limb. Panamericana: Buenos Aires; 2013. p. 5–91.
6. Pellerin M, Kimbal Z, Tubbs RS, Nguyen S, Matusz P, Cohen Gadol AA, Loukas M. The prefixed and postfixed brachial plexus: a review with surgical implications. Sur Radiol Anat. 2010;32:251–60.
7. Testut L. Tratado de anatomía humana. Sexta edición, Tomo III. Barcelona: Salvat; 1920. p. 188–9.
8. Martínez F, Pinazzo S. Anatomía del Sistema nervioso periférico: Parte 1: nervios del miembro superior. In: Socolovsky M, Siqueira M, Malessy M, editors. Introducción a la cirugía de los nervios periféricos. Bs As: Ediciones Journal; 2013. p. 1–19.
9. Corderi F, Rodríguez CA, Martínez F. Plexo braquial. In: Martinez F, editor. Cuadernos de Anatomía. Tomo 1. Montevideo: Bibliomédica; 2023.
10. Di Masi G, Bonilla GJH. Nerve anatomy of the upper limbs. In: Socolovsky M, Rasulic L, Midha R, Garozzo D, editors. Manual of peripheral nerve surgery. From the basics to the complex procedures. Stutgart: Thieme; 2018. p. 1–8.
11. Pro A. Anatomía Humana de Latarjet-Ruiz Liard. Buenos Aires: Editorial Panamericana; 2004.
12. Muset i Lara A, Dolz C, Rodriguez Baeza A. Anatomy of the brachial plexus. In: Gilbert A, editor. Brachial plexus injuries. London: Martin Dunitz; 2001. p. 3–16.
13. Siqueira MG, Martins RS, Pretto FL. Anatomia do plexo braquial. In: Siqueira MG, Martins RS, editors. Lesões do plexo braquial. Rio de Janeiro: Di Livros; 2011. p. 7–16.
14. Russell SM. Examination of peripherals nerve injuries. An anatomical approach. New York: Thieme; 2006. p. 1–107.
15. Rigoard P, Buffenoir-Billet K, Giot JP, Delmotte A, d'Houtaud S, Lapierre F. Bases anatomiques des voies d'abord chirurgicales des nerfs du membre superior : a l'usage des jeunes neurochirurgiens. Neurochirurgie. 2009;55:384–92.
16. Sinha S, Prasad GL, Lalwani SA. Cadaveric microanatomical study of the fascicular topography of the brachial plexus. J Neurosurg. 2016;125(2):355–62.
17. Siqueira MG, Foroni LHL, Martins RS, Chadi G, Malessy MJA. Fascicular topography of the suprascapular nerve in the C5 root and upper trunk of the brachial plexus: A microanatomic study from a nerve surgeon's perspective. Neurosurgery. 2010;67:ons402–6.
18. Yokoyama I. Study on the intraneural topography of the brachial plexus. Nihon Seikeigeka Gakkai Zasshi. 1989;63(9):1085–102. [Article in Japanese]
19. Brill NA, Tyler DJ. Quantification of human upper extremity nerves and fascicular anatomy. Muscle Nerve. 2017;56(3):463–71.
20. Natsis K, Piagkou M, Totlis T, Kapetanakis S. A prefix brachial plexus with two trunks and one anterior cord. Folia Morphol (Warsz). 2020;79(2):402–6.
21. Neto JHS, Neto BC, Eiras ABD, Botelho RHS, Carmo JMM, Passos MARF. The 2-dimensional and 3-dimensional anatomy of the adult brachial plexus divisions and cords. Hand (NY). 2022;17(1):50–4.
22. Orebaugh SL, Williams BA. Brachial plexus anatomy: normal and variant. Sci World J. 2009;9:300–12.
23. Akhtar J, Kumar S, Chandan BC, Kumnar B, Sinha RR, Akhtar K, Kumar A. Variations in the formation of the median nerve and its clinical correlation. Maedica (Bucur). 2022;17(4):878–84.
24. Bala A, Sinha P, Tamang BK, Sarda RK. Anatomical variation: median nerve formation: a case vignette. J Clin Diagn Res. 2014;8(6):AD03-4.

25. Bhanu PS, Sankar KD. Bilateral absence of musculocutaneous nerve with unusual branching pattern of lateral cord and median nerve of brachial plexus. Anat Cell Biol. 2012;45(3):207–10.
26. Budhiraja V, Rastogi R, Ashtana AK, Sinha P, Krishna A, Trivedi V. Concurrent variations of median and musculocutaneous nerves and their clinical correlation: a cadaveric study. Ital J Anat Embryol. 2011;116(2):67–72.
27. Chaudhary P, Singla R, Kalsey G, et al. A four trunked brachial plexus and a post fixed brachial plexus: a conjunction or a co-incidence? Report of three cases. Clin Anat. 2012;25(5):593–600.
28. Kimura S, Amatani H, Nakai R, et al. A novel case of multiple variations in the brachial plexus with the middle trunk originating from the C7 and C8. Anat Sci Int. 2020;95(4):559–63.
29. Martínez F, Ripoll G. Anatomical variants of the musculocutaneous nerve. Report of two cases. J Open Res Software. 2018;1(5):1.
30. Martínez Benia F, Rodríguez Aceves C, Robla CJ, Socolovsky M. Variante anatómica del tronco superior del plexo braquial. Reporte de caso Rev Arg Anat Onl. 2021;121:8–11.
31. Mohamed AMA, Grebballa A, Rizig S. Absence of upper trunk of the brachial plexus. Int J Appl Basic Med Res. 2001;1(2):123–4.
32. Singh R. Variations of cords of brachial plexus and branching pattern of nerves emanating from them. J Craniofac Surg. 2017;28(2):43–547.
33. Ramanujam V, Van Kirk P. Anatomy variation of brachial plexus trunks during supraclavicular nerve block: clinical image. Braz J Anesthesiol. 2022;72(6):834–5.
34. Emamhadi M, Chabok SY, Samini F, Behzadnia H, Firozabadi FA, Reihanian Z. Anatomical variations of brachial plexus in adult cadavers. A descriptive study. Arch Bone Jt Surg. 2016;4(3):253–8.
35. Martínez F, Salle F, Castelluccio G, Moragues R, Pinazzo S, Suárez E. Variante anatómica de los músculos escalenos y sus implicancias en ala cirugía del plexo braquial. Rev Arg Neuroc. 2013;27(2):76–8.
36. Martínez F. Technical note: spinal-accessory to suprascapular nerve transfer by posterior approach. Austin Neurosurg Open Access. 2017;4(1):1058.
37. Fazan VP, Amadeu AS, Caffi AL, Filho OA. Brachial plexus variation in its formation and main branches. Acta Cirurgica Brasi. 2003;18:14–8.
38. Singla RK, Sharma RK, Shree B. A two trunked brachial plexus: a case report. J Clin Diagn Res. 2013;7(4):704–5.
39. Unver Erdogan N, Uysal I, Seker M. The communications between the ulnar and median nerves in upper limb. Neuroanatomy. 2009;8:15–9.
40. Villamere J, Goodwin S, Hincke M, Jalali A. A brachial plexus variation characterized by the absence of the superior trunk. Neuroanatomy. 2009;8:4–6.
41. Won HS, Han SH, Oh CS, et al. Topographic relationship between the medial intermuscular septum and the ulnar nerve in the upper arm. J Neurosurg. 2011;114:1534–7.
42. Yildiz S, Comert A, Ozan H. A case of connected superior and middle trunks of the brachial plexus or with abnormal upper trunk. Romanian J Morphol Embryol. 2011;52(3 Suppl):1157–9.

Brain Plasticity After Nerve Transfers in Brachial Plexus Injuries

3

Martin Bourguet, Martijn J. A. Malessy, and Mariano Socolovsky

Abbreviations

BPI	Brachial plexus injury
CNS	Central nervous system
fMRI	Functional magnetic resonance imaging
ICN	Intercostal nerve
MCN	Musculocutaneous nerve
MRC	British Medical Council Motor Scale
NBPP	Neonatal brachial plexus palsy
NNBPI	Non-neonatal brachial plexus injury
PGS	Plasticity grading scale
RQS	Rehabilitation Quality Scale
SA	Spinal accessory nerve

3.1 Introduction

As nerve surgeons, in order to plan a goal when reinnervating certain muscle or group of muscles, it is important to be able to predict what we can expect from each patient, understanding that post-traumatic nerve repair is not just the reconnection of two wires that allow for the passage of current; it is the repair of a long dynamic path toward restimulation and relearning, through numerous changes in the nervous system called neuroplasticity and the influencing factors. In other words, this concept is the ability of the nervous system to adapt to external or internal stimuli in different situations, considering that it does not only occur in pathological scenarios. These take place not only in the brain but also at the level of the spinal cord and peripheral nerves.

Although nerve repair has been known for more than 100 years, throughout most of this time, emphasis has been placed on understanding the changes that occur at the peripheral level and what factors influence functional outcomes as age and time between trauma and repair. However, in the last two decades, we have begun to understand neurological adaptative changes that occur centrally, especially in the brain.

As we said before, neuroplasticity occurs always to a greater or lesser extent. As surgeons who seek to recover the functionality of a movement, we must understand that, in brachial plexus injuries, the whole process of brain plasticity in a pathological scenario is triggered by the lack of neural input to the central neural system produced due to the injury. Some of these plastic changes occur immediately after the trauma [1–3],, and many of them expand beyond the sensorimotor cortex. It should be noted that not all changes related to plasticity should be automati-

M. Bourguet (✉) · M. Socolovsky
Division of Neurosurgery, Hospital de Clínicas, University of Buenos Aires School of Medicine, Buenos Aires, Argentina

M. J. A. Malessy
Department of Neurosurgery, University of Leiden, Leiden, The Netherlands

F. Guedes et al. (eds.), *Nerve Transfers for Brachial Plexus Reconstruction after Trauma*,
https://doi.org/10.1007/978-3-031-92445-3_3

cally considered beneficial. For example, both deafferentation pain after severe brachial plexus injury (BPI) with radicular avulsions and phantom limb pain after amputation are related to plasticity-mediated maladaptive processes [4–6]. These stages of pain are linked to the creation of a "black hole" in sensory areas of the brain that are no longer receiving afferent information. To avoid these black holes, nerve repair, in terms of neuroplasticity, seeks to return most of the previously denervated areas to participate in motor control and perception.

In this dynamic route that includes neuroplasticity, it is important to know how many "kilometers" we have traveled to our goal. But how we can measure plasticity?

The objective of this chapter is to identify which brain changes occur after nerve transfer in brachial plexus injuries, to establish a semiological system for measuring this, and to find out what factors influence its development, including age.

3.2 How Does the Brain Change After a Nerve Transfer in a Brachial Plexus Injury?

3.2.1 Intercostal to the Musculocutaneous Nerve for Elbow Flexion

The intercostal (ICN) to musculocutaneous (MCN) nerve transfer is one of the most common techniques employed in the surgical reconstruction when all five roots are avulsed (Fig. 3.1a). The changes that occur in the brain after this nerve transfer have been studied most extensively.

At the beginning of axonal reinnervation, patients who have undergone this nerve transfer generally exhibit involuntary contraction of the biceps linked to breathing. After a short period of time, patients become aware that they can contract the biceps, but only by sustained inspiration or expiration (Fig. 3.1b). Ultimately, however,

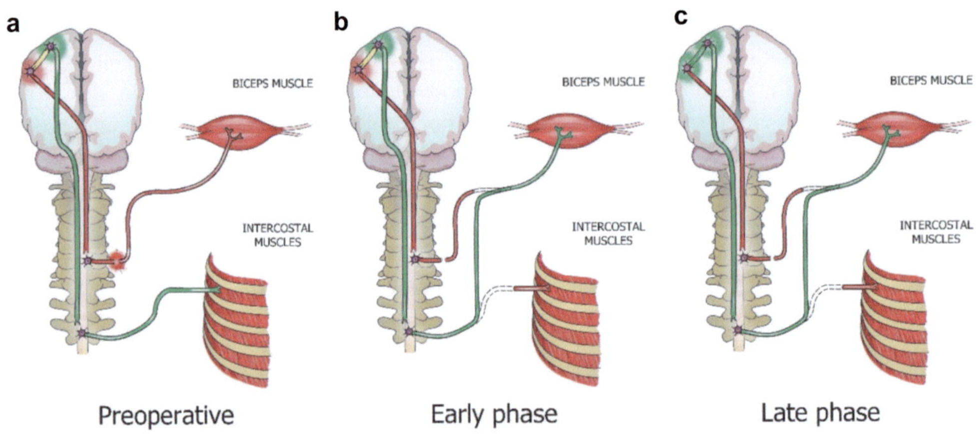

Fig. 3.1 Neuroplasticity after an intercostal to musculocutaneous nerve transfer for brachial plexus traction injury with root avulsions. (**a**) Preoperative. In red, the damaged original neural pathway for elbow flexion from the cortex to the cervical motor neuron pool via C6 to the musculocutaneous, which was injured during the trauma. In green, the pathway of innervation of the intercostal nerves. In the brain, in yellow, a preexisting connection between the biceps and the intercostals motor cortices are shown. (**b**) Early phase of recovery after a reconstructive surgery, where an intercostal to musculocutaneous nerve transfer was performed in order to recover elbow flexion. In green, the newly restored connection after transfer of intercostal nerves via the motor neuron pool at T3. In this early phase of recovery, biceps contraction is possible by sustained inspiration or expiration. These movements are mediated by the original intercostal nerve's primary motor cortex located in the midline. (**c**) Late phase of recovery. Some months later, patients learn to contract their biceps and thereby flexing the elbow independent of respiration as if normal. Cortical activation is located in the laterally located original biceps' primary motor cortex area; note the newly reactivated connection between the two cortexes (green arch). *(modified from Socolovsky, M. (2021). Brain changes after peripheral nerve repair: limitations of neuroplasticity. J Neurosurg Sci. 2021;65* (4)*:421–430)*

contraction (and the maintenance of elbow flexion) becomes independent of respiration. Flexion can then be maintained while breathing normally (Fig. 3.1c). Complete independence between the two functions is, however, rarely achieved [7].

These clinical findings correlate well with a physio-anatomical explanation: at the beginning of the elbow flexion recovery, the movement is initiated by the sagittal region of the primary motor cortex, which is related to the intercostal muscles that activate during respiration (Fig. 3.1b). After a few months, however, the more laterally located original area for voluntary biceps recovers voluntary control (Fig. 3.1c). This shift in cortical activity from medial to lateral is most likely based on activation of a preexisting interneuronal network with low active connections between the two involved cortical areas (yellow in Fig. 3.1a). Intercostal muscles contract simultaneously with the biceps, for instance, when a heavy object is lifted. This movement, after all, requires not only biceps contraction but also although less obvious, stabilization of the thorax and torso posture. From these studies it was concluded that in order to achieve successful voluntary control after nerve transfer, the donor and acceptor must have some previously existing connection between the two motor areas, prior to the nerve transfer (the so-called horizontal intrinsic connections) (Fig. 3.2) [8]. These central connections are activated by peripheral nerve transfers and specially by rehabilitation, thereby inducing plastic changes in the cortex.

3.2.2 Phrenic Nerve Transfer to the Musculocutaneous Nerve for Elbow Flexion

Similar changes from breathing-related control to voluntary flexion independent from breathing can be observed after a phrenic nerve–MCN transfer, with which the same clinical progression (starting with respiration-controlled arm movement, followed by voluntary control of elbow flexion) is seen. The reported results of phrenic nerve–MCN transfers are comparable to, and in some cases better than, those of ICN-MCN transfers [8, 9], which might have several explanations, including the greater number of axons that the phrenic nerve has relative to ICNs.

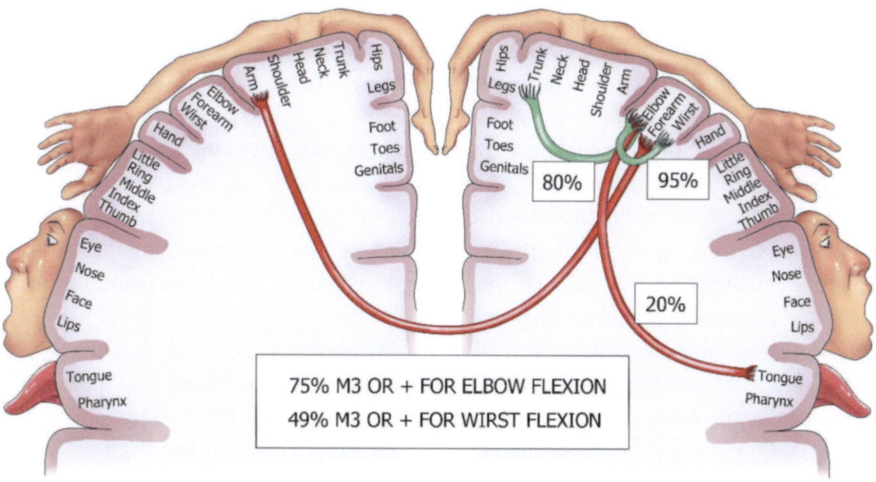

Fig. 3.2 Different nerve transfers achieve different grades of brain plasticity. The distance from the donor to the target nerve at the motor primary cortex has been related to the degree of independence of movement that is obtained after a long-term follow-up

3.2.3 Hypoglossal Nerve to the MCN or Facial Nerve

In contrast to the positive results obtained after a hypoglossal or trigeminal (masseter) nerve transfer to the facial nerve in facial palsy [10–13], a good recovery of elbow flexion is not the rule if the hypoglossal nerve fibers are used as axon donors in brachial plexus injuries [14] (Fig. 3.2). To control the biceps muscle to flex the elbow, the tongue has to be pushed against the hard palate. As soon as the tongue is relaxed, the biceps muscle also relaxes. Talking or chewing evokes involuntary biceps contractions, which cause the arm to move involuntarily. In this way, independent voluntary control over the reinnervated muscle is not restored, making the functional outcome poor. These findings can be easily explained in view of our knowledge of brain plasticity: the preexisting white matter connections between donor and receptor cortical motor areas slightly superpose between the tongue and the facial muscles areas, but not for elbow flexion. Therefore, when speaking, the motor cortex representing the tongue stimulates and moves the face in an apparently normal way. By contrast, after a hypoglossal to musculocutaneous nerve transfer, in order to control the biceps muscle to flex the elbow, the tongue must be pushed strongly against the hard palate. As soon as the tongue is relaxed, the biceps muscle also relaxes. Talking or chewing evokes involuntary biceps contractions, causing the arm to move unwantedly. The aforementioned good results for facial reanimation after a hypoglossal nerve transfer imply good symmetry at rest and normal talking, but if facial emotional movements are involved, like crying or laughing, asymmetry reappears, which is probably because there are not horizontal connections between emotional controlled movements—they are originated at different zones of the brain—and the hypoglossal cortex. In this case, as in many others, complete functional adaptation mediated by plastic changes has its limits.

3.2.4 Oberlin I and II and Triceps Branch to Axillary nerve

The transfer of a fascicle of the ulnar nerve to a biceps branch (the Oberlin procedure) was popularized in 1994 [15]. Afterward, a variation in the original technique, which increases the number of axons reaching the agonist target muscles (e.g., double transfers from ulnar to biceps and median to brachialis nerves) has generated even better results; between 95% and 99% of patients experience a good result. This technique changed brachial plexus surgery profoundly. The ulnar and/or median nerve transfer for elbow flexion can be used in severe BPI with root avulsions. This technique, the so-called Oberlin's procedure, represented a Copernican twist in brachial plexus surgery, because it brought about very good results (more than 90% of success rate), replacing the previously gold standard, which was elbow flexion reconstruction with grafts (Fig. 3.2) [2, 16–18]. Other distal nerve transfers based on this concept—like the triceps branch to axillary nerve (the so-called Somsak procedure) [19, 20] and wrist and finger extension branches for triceps branches [21]—have also been associated with very high success rates. The success of Oberlin's nerve transfer and the triceps branch to axillary nerve is based on the short distance that the outgrowing axon has to cross. In all these cases, the preexisting horizontal connections between the two motor cortices are short, sharing the two core principles of neuroplasticity that are necessary to achieve good results: (1) donor and acceptor cortical regions share the same motor control pathways and (2) there are previous connections between the two areas. It can be speculated that not only the short distance to the target muscles but also the good conditions for plasticity play a role in the high success rates of distal nerve transfers [22].

3.2.5 Contralateral C-7 Transfer

The opposite of ulnar and/or median nerve transfer, in terms of distance between donor and receptor cortical motor areas—and subcortical horizontal connections between them—is definitely the contralateral C7 root transfer. This technique can be used in severe BPI with root avulsions. In this procedure, the spinal nerve C7 from the healthy arm is transferred partially or completely to a target nerve in the affected upper limb. But according to the reviewed bibliography, the results are not as expected (Fig. 3.2). Recently, the literature on contralateral C7 transfers was reviewed [23, 24] and the results were not as excellent as formerly believed. The major concerns are that most patients never regain independent movement control. Indeed, in order to move the affected limb, they must flex their healthy arm to initiate muscle contraction in the reinnervated limb. Moreover, annoying involuntary movements in the reinnervated arm when moving the normal side forced those patients to express that they would have refused to accept the procedure if they had known how annoying the involuntary movements could be. Interestingly, a functional magnetic resonance imaging (fMRI) study showed that bilateral activation of the motor cortex occurred during movement of the reinnervated arm [25]. The original motor area for flexion of the arm, apparently, is reactivated, however now in concert with the ipsilateral cortex, which normally is not the case. This process is mediated by bilateral premotor and primary motor connections through the corpus callosum and provides an explanation for the main drawback of this technique: adult patients cannot regain motor control that is independent of their normal, unaffected side. This seems not to be the case in neonatal brachial plexus palsy (NBPP) or is at least less prominent. It might be that brain plasticity in newborns underlies the difference with adults in that it initiates completely new connections to develop. One case study focusing on the inter-hemispheric connections is of particular interest. A woman who suffered an amputation of her right arm above the elbow and who also had complete avulsion of the left brachial plexus underwent reconstructive surgery. The proximal right brachial plexus was connected to the distal left brachial plexus by interposing grafts. She recovered several movements in her left arm. In order to affect these movements, she had to think about flexing her phantom right arm. Interestingly, on fMRI, signals were detected bilaterally in the thalamus, caudate, insula, and sensorimotor cortex during any elbow flexion task [26].

3.2.6 Sensory Plasticity

In complete brachial plexus injuries, a sensory nerve that supplies sensation to the skin of the thoracic wall and axilla—the intercostobrachial nerve—was employed for transfer to the sensory component (lateral contribution) of the median nerve [27]. A couple of years after the procedure, stimulating the median nerve territory of the injured hand was perceived by the patient, but only in his axilla. This finding was predicted by one of the authors of this chapter (MJM) based on similar observations after ICN-MCN nerve transfer. If the area of the lateral antebrachial cutaneous nerve is touched or stroked, patients locate sensation on the thoracic wall, even years after the ICN-MCN transfer. So, although voluntary motor control over the biceps is restored, this does not account for localization of sensation. Finally, another example of the limitations of sensory plasticity is observed after corneal reinnervation. This procedure, described for recovery of corneal sensory innervation and consequently for ulcer prevention and ultimately sight preservation [28, 29], has shown good results as to improvement of corneal sensation and regaining of cornea transparency [30, 31]. Still, the patients reveal that they feel a cotton scrub touching their reinnervated cornea at the forehead (which represent the territory of the donor nerve, the supraorbital or supratrochear nerves). All these clinical findings demonstrate that sensitive and motor plasticity does not follow the same pathways, as would be logical to presume. These examples clearly demonstrate some of the limitations of neuroplasticity.

3.3 Is It Possible to Measure the Grade of Independence of a Regained Muscle from the Donor Nerve?

Routinely, the quality of volitional control over the acquired function is not even taken into consideration. The optimal outcome for regaining volitional control is that contraction of the target muscle occurs only in response to the command for the recipient nerve and not the donor (e.g., ICN-MCN, the elbow flexes in response to a command to flex the elbow, not when commanded to take a deep breath).

The process of central plasticity that underlies the restoration of volitional control can be divided into two steps: disconnection of the donor nerve's primary function and reconnection of the recipient nerve's primary function.

These two steps—of disconnection and reconnection—can be analyzed by looking at target muscle contractions when the donor nerve's motor program is activated.

In step 1, patients were asked to maximally activate their target muscle by using only the donor nerve program.

In step 2, patients were asked to maximally activate their target muscle while consciously trying to avoid using any donor nerve muscle.

Recently, one of the authors of this chapter (MS) developed a 4-point scale, plasticity grading scale (PGS), to rate the level of neuroplasticity that occurs and, hence, the extent of volitional control that is achieved following nerve transfers.

In this study, patients were assigned a PGS grade of 1 when British Medical Council Motor Scale (MRC) score 4 contraction of the target muscle only was obtainable during step 1, when the donor nerve was maximally activated (in response to the "donor muscle command"), with no response documented during step 2 when activation of the donor muscle was discouraged (the "target muscle command"). For example, a PGS score of 1 was assigned when the patient's biceps muscle achieved an MRC score of 4 for strength during deep inspiration (via activation of the phrenic nerve), and a minimum score (MRC score 0) when the patient was not breathing while just trying to flex the elbow. Meanwhile, whereas an MRC score of 4 was achieved for the target muscle in step 2 (with the target muscle command) for PGS grades 2–4, the donor muscle only exhibited MRC grades of two-, three-, or four-level strengths with the donor command for a PGS grade 2, only subtle contraction (MRC grade 1) with the donor command for PGS grade 3, and no noticeable contraction (MRS grade 0) with the donor muscle command for PGS grade 4. These definitions are summarized in Table 3.1. They also assessed patient compliance with the rehabilitation therapy by using our own 4-point Rehabilitation Quality Scale (RQS) [9, 32–35]. With this scale, any patient who failed to attend rehabilitation therapy at all or attended less than once a week was assigned an RQS score of 1; any patient who had rehabilitation therapy at a regular center more than once a week was assigned an RQS score of 2; any patient who exhibited good adherence to a rehabilitation program at a nonspecialized neurorehabilitation center with periodic assessments at a specialized neurorehabilitation center was assigned an RQS score of 3; and any patient who exhibited good adherence to a rehabilitation program at a specialized institution was assigned an RQS score of 4.

Table 3.1 PGS for nerve transfers

	Target muscle	MRC grade of target muscle contraction	
Grade	Contraction⟺Motor Program Activation	Donor command	Acceptor command
1	Exclusively donor (no plasticity)	4	0
2	Via donor and acceptor (poor plasticity)	2, 3, or 4	4
3	Subtle via donor, predominantly via acceptor (good plasticity)	1	4
4	Exclusively acceptor (excellent plasticity)	0	4

Socolovsky et al. JNS 2022

In total, 153 patients with a traumatic BPI were included (141 males, 92.2%). The PGS was grade 1 in 1 patient (0.6%), grade 2 in 21 patients (13.7%), grade 3 in 103 patients (67.3%), and grade 4 in 28 patients (18.3). For the phrenic nerve, the mean PGS grade was 2.57, with 11 patients having PGS grade 2 (25%) and 33 with PGS grade 3 (75%). The mean PGS grade for the spinal accessory (SA) nerve was 2.95, with 1 patient having PGS grade 1 (2.5%), 4 patients with PGS grade 2 (10%), 34 with PGS grade 3 (85%), and 1 patient with PGS grade 4 (2.5%). The mean PGS grade for the median and/or ulnar nerve fascicles was 3.27, with 4 patients with PGS grade 2 (9%), 20 with PGS grade 3 (45%), and 20 with PGS grade 4 (45%). The mean PGS grade for the triceps branch was 3.15, with 2 patients with PGS grade 2 (8%), 16 with PGS grade 3 (64%), and 7 with PGS grade 4 (28%).

Interestingly, the degree of plasticity achieved, when measured with the PGS scale, differed significantly when comparing extraplexual and intraplexual donors, the latter being better in terms of the aforementioned scale. There were no correlations between the PGS grade and a patient's age, time to surgery, length of follow-up, or extent of compliance with rehabilitation.

The development of central plasticity takes time and different phases can be discerned. At the beginning of reinnervation, the target muscle can be contracted only via a command linked to the donor nerve (e.g., if the surgeon connects the phrenic nerve, originally designed for inspiration by contracting the diaphragm, to elbow flexion muscles triggered by the MCN, then initially the patient flexes the elbow during inspiration). As time passes, usually over a couple of months, patients become increasingly able to activate their target muscle by focusing on the recipient nerve's primary function. Toward the end stages of reinnervation, the process of disconnection from the donor nerve may continue to the point that target muscle contractions may become possible solely based on acceptor muscle commands through changes that have been correlated with a shift in motor cortex activity [36–39].

The main and original finding of this study is that this independence is rarely complete and that a trace of the donor motor program (as in the above example of inspiration) remains when the patient flexes the elbow.

3.4 Do Children Have More Plasticity than Adults?

Neonatal brachial plexus palsy occurs during birth due to traction on the nerves running from the neck to the arm. Immediately after birth, patients have motor and sensory deficits of the upper limb. In those patients who did not recover spontaneously after few months, functional improvement can be obtained with reconstructive nerve surgery and/or secondary surgery in a selective group of NBPP patients.

As we saw, nerve transfer is widely used to restore function in patients with either neonatal brachial plexus palsy or non-neonatal traumatic brachial plexus injury (NNBPI) when roots are avulsed [40–45]. One of the main objectives of treatment is the restoration of biceps muscle function, and regaining volitional control of elbow flexion is essential. Neuroplasticity changes within the central nervous system (CNS) are critical to patients regaining such control.

Many factors can modulate cortical plasticity and influence motor function. One factor that is frequently mentioned is age. It has been stated that the potential for central plastic changes decreases with increasing age [46–48]. However, the evidence is generally inconsistent, and it is likely to depend on how plasticity in the primary motor cortex is measured. It was not until recent studies that it was possible to quantify this impact on plasticity terms and the recovery of volitional control of elbow flexion using the PGS described above.

We studied the differences in PGS scores between NBPP and NNBPI patients after those different nerve transfers that are most frequently used, namely, the ulnar and or median nerve fascicles to musculocutaneous nerve, spinal accessory nerve to nerves for elbow flexion, spinal accessory to suprascapular nerve, intercostal to musculocutaneous nerve, triceps branches to axillary nerve, and phrenic nerve to nerves for elbow flexion. To be included in the study, both NBPP and NNBPI had to have undergone an extra or intraplexual nerve transfer to regain a lost neurological function but not nerve grafting for the same function. The patients who underwent grafting were excluded because if a nerve root was reconstructed with grafts and subsequently a nerve transfer was performed to recover the same or a similar function, it is not possible to determine if the recovery was either due to the root repair or to the nerve transfer. The exclusion criteria were (1) patients who were lost to follow-up, (2) a clinical final result of the nerve transfer of MRC grade < 4, (3) surgical repair more than 12 months after the trauma, (4) NNBPI patients who had a concurrent brain contusion that might have affected their potential for brain plasticity, or (5) follow-up of less than 12 months. We also assessed patient compliance with rehabilitation therapy using our own 4-point Rehabilitation Quality Scale (RQS).

A total of 153 NNBPI patients and 35 NBPP babies met the inclusion criteria. They were examined in two steps as was explained above. When children younger than 3–4 years of age had to be examined, instead of a direct verbal order, another stimulus (e.g., candy) was used to elicit elbow flexion. Postoperative evaluations were performed independently every 6 months by at least two of the current authors to reduce ascertainment bias. At each evaluation, elbow flexion was tested three times, and the best PGS result was recorded.

The mean age at surgery of the NBPP group was 9 months (SD 5.42, range 4 to 23 months), and approximately half of them were male. The duration of follow-up and the compliance with the rehabilitation scale were not very different than NNBPI patients. The mean age of NNBPI patients was 22 years old (SD 12 years old, range 3 to 69). The mean time to surgery on the NBPP was 9.18 months (SD 5.06, range 3–23) and on the NNBPI group it was 6.37 months (SD 3.03, range 1–19) ($p < 0.001$).

All transfers performed in NBPP patients had a PGS score of 4. While all nerve transfers in NBPP group scored the maximum, this was not the case for the NNBPI population that reached a PGS score of 4 in less than one quarter of the cases. The difference in PGS scores of infants with NBPP and patients with NNBPI was statistically significant ($p < 0.001$).

Even though the time to surgery differed significantly between both groups, this time differed for reasons related to the different managements of each type of trauma. However, babies who have a NBPP may recover spontaneously in around 70–80% [49] probably due to the relatively low amount of kinetic energy involved, which is exerted over a period of minutes. Thus, unless a severe injury is diagnosed (i.e., a complete palsy with accompanying Horner sign or root avulsions determined by MRI), later surgeries are not uncommon. Notably, the statistically significant difference in interval between trauma and surgery, being longer in babies, did not affect the plasticity after a nerve transfer, a fact that again remarks the elevated plasticity shown by the NBPP group.

It is important to note that the compliance to rehabilitation measured employing the RQS [33, 34, 50–52] was not significantly different when comparing NBPP and NNBPI groups (2.76 versus 3.04, respectively).

Two fundamental differences exist between NBPP and NNBPI patients, which are both related to age and may underlie the age effect we observed. These differences concern the baseline status of the CNS prior to transfer, as well as the mechanisms underlying plasticity. First, the central motor program embedding of elbow flexion differs between NBPP and NNBPI patients at the moment the BPI occurs. In NBPP patients, the ability to flex the elbow disappears just after birth. At that time, the development of the central motor program for flexion comes to a halt within the mother's uterus. The program wiring at that time is at a level only sufficient for involuntary movements. These movements are not embedded in a sophisticated control program for directed patterns requiring various integrated muscle actions. In contrast, in NNBPI patients, the central programs for elbow flexion are completely developed, voluntary biceps contraction is possible following an elbow flexion command, and flexion movements are embedded in programs for patterns in which various muscles act. Second, the cellular mechanisms underlying plasticity—dendritic arborization and synaptogenesis—differ. Animal research has demonstrated that dendrite growth and remodeling are active processes for development that take place in childhood. After young adulthood, dendritic plasticity mechanisms are suppressed [53]. Comparably, synaptogenesis occurs with a peak of synapse density during the juvenile period with subsequent pruning through early adulthood [54, 55].

3.5 Summary

The ability of the central nervous system to change—neuroplasticity—is being increasingly recognized as one of the factors that determines the success of certain nerve transfer procedures, contributing to the effects of long-recognized influential factors such as the duration of time between the initial trauma and reparative surgery and the extent of the primary damage. Plasticity should be considered during surgical strategy planning in case of nerve injuries, because it determines volitional control over a reinnervated muscle following a nerve transfer, and the capacity of the CNS to reorganize is limited.

Considering that neuroplasticity is a dynamic process, developing a practical measurement system, it is important to know how far we are from our final goal. It also allows us to evaluate the impact of the factors and actions that influence it, in order to transmit and enhance the objectives of nerve surgery.

In adults, complete disconnection between the donor nerve's initial function and the reinnervated muscle restored function is achieved in less than 20% of patients, at least when the phrenic nerve, SA nerve, median nerve and/or ulnar fascicles, and a triceps branch are used as donors. This could be due to the fact that achieving successful voluntary control after a nerve transfer, the donor and acceptor must have some previously existing connection between the two motor areas, prior to the nerve transfer (the so-called horizontal intrinsic connections). These central connections are activated by peripheral nerve transfers and specially by rehabilitation, thereby inducing plastic changes in the cortex.

Babies with NBPP have a significantly greater capacity for plastic rewiring, using the same procedures, than adults with NNBPI. We must acknowledge that although the nerve surgical repair techniques are the same, the outcome regarding volitional control is not necessarily the same. The brain in the very young patient can process the changes induced by the peripheral nerve transfer better than in adults.

As nerve surgeons we must know that the level of plastic rewiring that occurs after distal nerve transfers at the level of the arm in older patients is not so poor that age should be an exclusion factor when considering using this transfer for reconstruction. Prior to planning ulnar and/or median nerve transfer surgery, NNBPI patients should be informed about the odds of regaining volitional control, so that their expectations can be realistic.

References

1. Qiu TM, Chen L, Mao Y, Wu JS, Tang WJ, Hu SN, et al. Sensorimotor cortical changes assessed with resting-state fMRI following total brachial plexus root avulsion. J Neurol Neurosurg Psychiatry. 2014;85:99–105.
2. Fraiman D, Miranda MF, Erthal F, Buur PF, Elschot M, Souza L, et al. Reduced functional connectivity within the primary motor cortex of patients with brachial plexus injury. Neuroimage Clin. 2016;12:277–84.
3. Yoshikawa T, Hayashi N, Tajiri Y, Satake Y, Ohtomo K. Brain reorganization in patients with brachial plexus injury: a longitudinal functional MRI study. ScientificWorldJournal. 2012;2012:501751.
4. Blom SM, Pfister JP, Santello M, Senn W, Nevian T. Nerve injury-induced neuropathic pain causes disinhibition of the anterior cingulate cortex. J Neurosci. 2014;34:5754–64.
5. Lundborg G, Richard P. Bunge memorial lecture. Nerve injury and repair—a challenge to the plastic brain. J Peripher Nerv Syst. 2003;8:209–26.
6. Simon NG, Franz CK, Gupta N, Alden T, Kliot M. Central adaptation following brachial plexus injury. World Neurosurg. 2016;85:325–32.
7. Malessy MJ, van Dijk JG, Thomeer RT. Respiration-related activity in the biceps brachii muscle after intercostal-musculocutaneous nerve transfer. Clin Neurol Neurosurg. 1993;95:S95–102.

8. Liu Y, Lao J, Zhao X. Comparative study of phrenic and intercostal nerve transfers for elbow flexion after global brachial plexus injury. Injury. 2015;46:671–5.
9. Socolovsky M, di Masi G, Bonilla G, Domínguez Paez M, Robla J, Calvache Cabrera C. The phrenic nerve as a donor for brachial plexus injuries: is it safe and effective? Case series and literature analysis. Acta Neurochir. 2015;157:1077–86.
10. Godefroy WP, Malessy MJ, Tromp AA, van der Mey AG. Intratemporal facial nerve transfer with direct coaptation to the hypoglossal nerve. Otol Neurotol. 2007;28:546–50.
11. Hayashi A, Nishida M, Seno H, Inoue M, Iwata H, Shirasawa T, et al. Hemihypoglossal nerve transfer for acute facial paralysis. J Neurosurg. 2013;118:160–6.
12. Rochkind S, Shafi M, Alon M, Salame K, Fliss DM. Facial nerve reconstruction using a split hypoglossal nerve with preservation of tongue function. J Reconstr Microsurg. 2008;24:469–74.
13. Socolovsky M, Martins RS, di Masi G, Bonilla G, Siqueira M. Treatment of complete facial palsy in adults: comparative study between direct hemihypoglossal-facial neurorrhaphy, hemihipoglossal-facial neurorrhaphy with grafts, and masseter to facial nerve transfer. Acta Neurochir. 2016;158:945–57. discussion 957
14. Malessy MJ, Hoffmann CF, Thomeer RT. Initial report on the limited value of hypoglossal nerve transfer to treat brachial plexus root avulsions. J Neurosurg. 1999;91:601–4.
15. Oberlin C, Béal D, Leechavengvongs S, Salon A, Dauge MC, Sarcy JJ. Nerve transfer to biceps muscle using a part of ulnar nerve for C5–C6 avulsion of the brachial plexus: anatomical study and report of four cases. J Hand Surg Am. 1994;19:232–7.
16. Noaman HH, Shiha AE, Bahm J. Oberlin's ulnar nerve transfer to the biceps motor nerve in obstetric brachial plexus palsy: indications, and good and bad results. Microsurgery. 2004;24:182–7.
17. Siqueira MG, Socolovsky M, Heise CO, Martins RS, Di Masi G. Efficacy and safety of Oberlin's procedure in the treatment of brachial plexus birth palsy. Neurosurgery. 2012;71:1156–60. discussion 1161
18. Tse R, Kozin SH, Malessy MJ, Clarke HM. International Federation of Societies for surgery of the hand committee report: the role of nerve transfers in the treatment of neonatal brachial plexus palsy. J Hand Surg Am. 2015;40:1246–59.
19. Leechavengvongs S, Witoonchart K, Uerpairojkit C, Thuvasethakul P. Nerve transfer to deltoid muscle using the nerve to the long head of the triceps, part II: a report of 7 cases. J Hand Surg Am. 2003;28:633–8.
20. Witoonchart K, Leechavengvongs S, Uerpairojkit C, Thuvasethakul P, Wongnopsuwan V. Nerve transfer to deltoid muscle using the nerve to the long head of the triceps, part I: an anatomic feasibility study. J Hand Surg Am. 2003;28:628–32.
21. Flores LP. The radio-radial nerve transfer for elbow extension restoration in C5 to C7 nerve root injury. Microsurgery. 2012;32:55–9.
22. de Sousa AC, Guedes-Corrêa JF. Post-Oberlin procedure cortical neuroplasticity in traumatic injury of the upper brachial plexus. Radiol Bras. 2016;49:201–2.
23. Yang G, Chang KW, Chung KC. A systematic review of contralateral C7 transfer for the treatment of traumatic brachial plexus injury: part 1. Overall Outcomes. Plast Reconstr Surg. 2015;136:794–809.
24. Yang G, Chang KW, Chung KC. A systematic review of outcomes of contralateral C7 transfer for the treatment of traumatic brachial plexus injury: part 2. Donor-site morbidity. Plast Reconstr Surg. 2015;136:480e–9e.
25. Beaulieu JY, Blustajn J, Teboul F, Baud P, De Schonen S, Thiebaud JB, Oberlin C. Cerebral plasticity in crossed C7 grafts of the brachial plexus: an fMRI study. Microsurgery. 2006;26:303–10.
26. Dimou S, Biggs M, Tonkin M, Hickie IB, Lagopoulos J. Motor cortex neuroplasticity following brachial plexus transfer. Front Hum Neurosci. 2013;7:500.
27. Foroni L, Siqueira MG, Martins RS, Heise CO, Sterman H, Imamura AY. Good sensory recovery of the hand in brachial plexus surgery using the intercostobrachial nerve as the donor. Arq Neuropsiquiatr. 2017;75:796–800.
28. Elbaz U, Bains R, Zuker RM, Borschel GH, Ali A. Restoration of corneal sensation with regional nerve transfers and nerve grafts: a new approach to a difficult problem. JAMA Ophthalmol. 2014;132:1289–95.
29. Catapano J, Antonyshyn K, Zhang JJ, Gordon T, Borschel GH. Corneal neurotization improves ocular surface health in a novel rat model of neurotrophic keratopathy and corneal neurotization. Invest Ophthalmol Vis Sci. 2018;59:4345–54.
30. Catapano J, Fung SS, Halliday W, Jobst C, Cheyne D, Ho ES, et al. Treatment of neurotrophic keratopathy with minimally invasive corneal neurotisation: long-term clinical outcomes and evidence of corneal reinnervation. Br J Ophthalmol. 2019;103:1724–31.
31. Ebner R, Fridrich G, Socolovsky M, Luna A, Croxatto JO. In vivo corneal confocal microscopy: pre-and post-operative evaluation in a case of corneal Neurotization. Neuroophthalmology. 2019;44:193–6.
32. Socolovsky M, Di Masi G, Battaglia D. Use of long autologous nerve grafts in brachial plexus reconstruction: factors that affect the outcome. Acta Neurochir. 2011;153(11):2231–40.
33. Socolovsky M, Malessy M, Bonilla G, Di Masi G, Conti ME, Lovaglio A. Phrenic to musculocutaneous nerve transfer for traumatic brachial plexus injuries: analyzing respiratory effects on elbow flexion control. J Neurosurg. 2018;131(1):165–74. https://doi.org/10.3171/2018.4.JNS173248.
34. Flores LP, Socolovsky M. Phrenic nerve transfer for reconstruction of elbow extension in severe brachial plexus injuries. J Reconstr Microsurg. 2016;32(7):546–50.
35. Havton LA, Carlstedt T. Repair and rehabilitation of plexus and root avulsions in animal models and patients. Curr Opin Neurol. 2009;22(6):570–4.

36. Kwee RM, Chhabra A, Wang KC, Marker DR, Carrino JA. Accuracy of MRI in diagnosing peripheral nerve disease: a systematic review of the literature. AJR Am J Roentgenol. 2014;203(6):1303–9.
37. Iwase Y, Mashiko T, Ochiai N, Kurosawa H. Postoperative changes on functional mapping of the motor cortex in patients with brachial plexus injury: comparative study of magnetoencephalography and functional magnetic resonance imaging. J Orthop Sci. 2001;6(5):397–402.
38. Malessy MJ, Bakker D, Dekker AJ, Van Duk JG, Thomeer RT. Functional magnetic resonance imaging and control over the biceps muscle after intercostal-musculocutaneous nerve transfer. J Neurosurg. 2003;98(2):261–8.
39. Dai TH, Liu JZ, Sahgal V, Brown RW, Yue GH. Relationship between muscle output and functional MRI-measured brain activation. Exp Brain Res. 2001;140(3):290–300.
40. Oberlin C, Béal D, Leechavengvongs S, Salon A, Dauge MC, Sarcy JJ. Nerve transfer to biceps muscle using a part of ulnar nerve for C5-C6 avulsion of the brachial plexus: anatomical study and report of four cases. J Hand Surg Am. 1994;19(2):232–7.
41. Mackinnon SE, Novak CB, Myckatyn TM, Tung TH. Results of reinnervation of the biceps and brachialis muscles with a double fascicular transfer for elbow flexion. J Hand Surg Am. 2005;30(5):978–85.
42. Yang LJ, Chang KW, Chung KC. A systematic review of nerve transfer and nerve repair for the treatment of adult upper brachial plexus injury. Neurosurgery. 2012;71(2):417–29.
43. Ali ZS, Heuer GG, Faught RW, et al. Upper brachial plexus injury in adults: comparative effectiveness of different repair techniques. J Neurosurg. 2015;122(1):195–201.
44. Chang KWC, Wilson TJ, Popadich M, Brown SH, Chung KC, Yang LJS. Oberlin transfer compared with nerve grafting for improving early supination in neonatal brachial plexus palsy. J Neurosurg Pediatr. 2018;21(2):178–84.
45. Heise CO, Siqueira MG, Martins RS, Foroni LH, StermanNeto H. Distal nerve transfer versus supraclavicular nerve grafting: comparison of elbow flexion outcome in neonatal brachial plexus palsy with C5-C7 involvement. Childs Nerv Syst. 2017;33(9):1571–4.
46. Mohamed Khalifa Gawi E. The effects of age factor on learning English: a case study of learning English in Saudi schools, Saudi Arabia. Engl Lang Teach. 2012;5(1):127–39.
47. Auer T, Pinter S, Kovacs N, et al. Does obstetric brachial plexus injury influence speech dominance? Ann Neurol. 2009;65(1):57–66.
48. Anastakis DJ, Malessy MJ, Chen R, Davis KD, Mikulis D. Cortical plasticity following nerve transfer in the upper extremity. Hand Clin. 2008;24(4):425–444, vi-vii.
49. Pondaag W, Malessy MJ. The evidence for nerve repair in obstetric brachial plexus palsy revisited. Biomed Res Int. 2014;2014:434619. https://doi.org/10.1155/2014/434619.
50. Socolovsky M, Barillaro K, Bonilla G, Di Masi G, Malessy M. Use of long autologous nerve grafts in brachial plexus reconstruction. J Neurosurg. 2022;138(5):1419–25. https://doi.org/10.3171/2022.7.JNS22887.
51. Socolovsky M, Lovaglio A, Bonilla G, Di Masi G, Barillaro K, Malessy M. Brain plasticity and age after restoration of elbow flexion with distal nerve transfers in neonatal brachial plexus palsy and traumatic brachial plexus injury using the plasticity grading scale, vol. 139. J Neurosurg In press; 2023. p. 1568.
52. Socolovsky M, Di Masi G, Bonilla G, Lovaglio A, Krishnan KG. Nerve graft length and recovery of elbow flexion muscle strength in patients with traumatic brachial plexus injuries: case series. Oper Neurosurg (Hagerstown). 2021;20(6):521–8. https://doi.org/10.1093/ons/opab007.
53. Prigge CL, Kay JN. Dendrite morphogenesis from birth to adulthood. Curr Opin Neurobiol. 2018;53:139–45.
54. Bianchi S, Stimpson CD, Duka T, et al. Synaptogenesis and development of pyramidal neuron dendritic morphology in the chimpanzee neocortex resembles humans. In: National Academy of Sciences, Cela-Conde CJ, Lombardo RG, Avise JC, et al., editors. In the light of evolution: Volume VII: the human mental machinery. National Academies Press; 2014.
55. Feng JT, Liu HQ, Xu JG, Gu YD, Shen YD. Differences in brain adaptive functional reorganization in right and left total brachial plexus injury patients. World Neurosurg. 2015;84(3):702–8.

4 Surgical Indications

Stephen P. Miranda, Zarina S. Ali, and Eric L. Zager

4.1 Introduction

The primary aim of any nerve reconstruction surgery is to maximize overall functional outcome while minimizing morbidity [1]. The traditional surgical options for traumatic brachial plexus palsies, including primary repair, neurolysis, and nerve grafting, have long been used but frequently are unable to fully restore meaningful function, prompting surgeons to explore other approaches in recent decades [2]. Through advancement in microsurgical techniques and a greater understanding of the internal topography of peripheral nerves, nerve transfer has evolved to become an integral component of the reconstruction strategy for brachial plexus injuries [3, 4].

Although there are no definitive guidelines for when nerve transfers should be used, general indications include delayed presentation, prior injury, dense scar tissue, segmental loss of nerve function, and long distances to target motor end plates [1]. Patients with brachial plexus trauma meet many of these criteria and therefore are prime candidates for nerve transfer, due to their proximal lesions and broad zones of injury, which can be bypassed through nerve transfer. During nerve transfer, or neurotization, an intact and redundant nerve or nerve fascicle is redirected to a distal, undamaged portion of an injured nerve that has lost proximal innervation [5]. This strategy has distinct advantages. Donor nerves are often selected for transfer nearby the target motor end plates, improving the potential for earlier reinnervation, by converting a "high-level" injury into a "low-level" one [1, 5, 6]. The morbidity associated with harvesting autograft can be avoided, along with the need for an interposition nerve graft, which can increase the likelihood of axonal loss or misdirection at each microsuture repair site [6]. However, there are disadvantages to nerve transfer, including the need for central reeducation (via cortical plasticity) to achieve recovery, and the possibility of loss of function at the donor nerve, which may mean that donor muscles are downgraded or unavailable for future muscle/tendon transfer [6].

In this chapter, we will review the indications and objectives for nerve transfer during surgical reconstruction of traumatic brachial plexus injuries in adults. As always, each patient's reconstruction must be tailored to his or her individual pattern of injury. However, there are several domains that must be considered carefully when preparing for nerve transfer, including a thorough

S. P. Miranda
Department of Neurosurgery, University of Pennsylvania, Philadelphia, PA, USA

Department of Neurosurgery, Icahn School of Medicine at Mount Sinai, New York, NY, USA
e-mail: Stephen.Miranda@mountsinai.org

Z. S. Ali · E. L. Zager (✉)
Department of Neurosurgery, University of Pennsylvania, Philadelphia, PA, USA
e-mail: Zarina.Ali@pennmedicine.upenn.edu

F. Guedes et al. (eds.), *Nerve Transfers for Brachial Plexus Reconstruction after Trauma*,
https://doi.org/10.1007/978-3-031-92445-3_4

preoperative evaluation of the injury, timing of reconstruction, suitability of donor nerves, and priorities for functional restoration.

4.2 Preoperative Considerations for Nerve Transfer

Many adult patients with brachial plexus trauma present in delayed fashion after closed traction injuries and therefore their injury pattern must be thoroughly assessed using clinical, radiologic, and electrodiagnostic examinations [7].

For motor nerve transfers, a viable muscle recipient is a prerequisite. Using electromyography (EMG), fibrillation potentials can be seen as early as 3 weeks after injury and are an acceptable indication of denervated but viable muscle [8, 9]. Thereafter, serial EMG should be performed to evaluate the likelihood of recovery for axonotmetic (Sunderland grade II–IV) injuries and to exclude neurapraxic (Sunderland grade I) injuries, which typically recover spontaneously by 4 months [7]. As the muscle recovers, fibrillation potentials decrease and motor unit action potentials (MUAPs) appear on EMG, signifying collateral sprouting from adjacent uninjured axons; nascent units may also be seen, representing end plate reinnervation [10, 11]. If either is present at 3 or 4 months after injury, spontaneous recovery of function is possible and observation with ongoing physical therapy is acceptable [8]. Electrodiagnostic studies can be performed periodically (e.g., every 8 to 12 weeks) and conservative management can be continued if the patient continues to show improvement [7, 12].

Deciding when to perform a nerve transfer can be challenging. For patients with preganglionic injuries, such as those with nerve root avulsions, nerve transfer can be considered as soon as feasible because there is no potential for spontaneous recovery [9, 13]. However, for postganglionic injuries, it is prudent to observe these patients for at least 3 months in case of spontaneous functional recovery [7]. It is also critical to evaluate whether motor recovery is proceeding in an anatomical sequence from proximal to distal [14]. If some distal muscles recover before proximal ones, there may be a mixed pattern of injury; nerve transfer could be warranted to reinnervate the muscles showing no evidence of recovery, as early as 4 months post-injury [7, 14].

The absolute length of time by which reinnervation is no longer possible remains unknown, although there is general agreement that earlier intervention leads to better outcomes [7, 9]. The first few months post-injury is a privileged period for functional recovery, before motor endplates are lost to degeneration and fibrosis [12]. Prolonged denervation beyond 6 months can reduce the number of regenerating axons by as much as two-thirds, and the rate of axonal regeneration can degrade exponentially as Schwann cells undergo apoptosis [5, 12, 15]. Beyond 6 months after axotomy, there is a progressive decline in the nerve's regenerative capacity, as regeneration-associated genes are downregulated and Schwann cells are lost in the distal nerve stump [16]. After 2 years, muscle fibers fragment, disintegrate, or are replaced by fat cells and can no longer be reinnervated [8, 12]. Optimal muscle reinnervation depends on a critical number of motor axons reaching target neuromuscular junctions within 12 months of injury [7]. Given that nerves regenerate at a rate of 1.0–1.5 mm per day [17], decision-making about nerve transfer is therefore encouraged as early as 3 or 4 months post-injury, to consider options that could shorten the distance (and time) for reinnervation of target motor end plates within this 12-month timeframe [7, 18].

4.3 Donor Nerve Selection

Several criteria should be considered when selecting donor nerves [6, 7, 19]. Ideally, for motor nerve transfers, fascicles with high numbers of motor fibers or "pure" motor nerves should be selected as donors [20]. Donor nerves should also be redundant or expendable, meaning that any function sacrificed at donor muscles is outweighed by the utility of the reinnervated neuromuscular element. Similarly, sensory donors should be pure sensory nerves that are also expendable, supplying a noncritical sensory distribution. Donor nerves should be selected in close proximity to their recipients to avoid the need for interposition nerve grafts (and additional neurorrhaphy sites). Although not required, selecting donor motor nerves that innervate synergistic muscles can facilitate postoperative motor reeducation, as reported outcomes are less favorable when nerves to non-synergistic or antagonistic muscles have been used [21]. Similarly, the donor nerve should ideally be uninjured or fully functional, so that the recipient nerve receives a maximal number of healthy motor fibers and some function can be retained at donor sites. However, recovering nerves can be considered for transfer if there is limited donor availability [14].

4.4 Indications for Nerve Transfer

Although there are no absolute guidelines for when nerve transfer should be used, the following criteria are strong indications for incorporating nerve transfers into the reconstruction scheme after brachial plexus trauma: (1) nerve root avulsion or intra-foraminal injury with limited or no nerve stump available for nerve grafting; (2) high-level or proximal injury with long distances for regeneration to target muscles; (3) concomitant trauma to vascular or bony structures surrounding the brachial plexus, creating scarred areas that would increase the risk of surgical exploration; (4) major limb trauma in which long segments of nerve are lost or damaged; (5) delayed presentation (e.g., >6 months), when time to reconstruction may be too long for proximal repair or nerve grafting to be successful; and (6) previously failed attempts at brachial plexus or primary nerve repairs [5–7, 22].

Relative contraindications to use of nerve transfer include (1) availability of a superior reconstruction option that could provide equivalent outcomes with shorter recovery time or less morbidity, (2) excessive time between injury and reconstruction (e.g., >18 months), and (3) inadequate donor nerve potential for functional restoration (e.g., donor nerve motor strength less than British Medical Research Council grade M4) [5, 23].

The following principles should be applied to optimize functional outcomes after nerve transfer [9, 19, 22]: (1) nerve transfer should be performed as early as possible; (2) the recipient nerve should be reinnervated as close as possible to the target organ; (3) direct repairs are preferred over interposition nerve grafts; (4) transfers of similarly behaving neuromuscular units are preferred; and (5) intraplexal nerve transfers may perform better than extraplexal transfers due to greater cortical readaptation. End-to-end coaptation is preferable, if possible, for all nerve transfers, although end-to-side transfers have demonstrated efficacy for sensory nerves [5, 7, 24].

4.5 Reconstruction Priorities and Strategies

As discussed, surgical management is dictated by the patient's specific injury pattern, and electrodiagnostic studies are critical for identifying viable roots and potential donor nerves, as well as evaluating which components of the plexus are injured (and to what degree). Nerve transfers can be categorized as proximal or distal based on their proximity to the terminal units of the target muscle or sensory territory [25, 26]. Proximal nerve transfers can be subdivided further based on whether origin of the donor nerve is intraplexal or extraplexal [6, 14, 23]. Intraplexal donors include medial pectoral nerve (MPN), ulnar nerve, median nerve, triceps branch of radial nerve, thoracodorsal nerve, long thoracic nerve (LTN), dorsal scapular nerve, subscapular nerve, brachialis branch of the musculocutaneous nerve (MCN), and the pectoral fascicle from the middle trunk of C7. Extraplexal donors include cervical plexus, spinal accessory nerve (SAN), phrenic nerve, contralateral C7 nerve root, and intercostal nerves (ICN) [23].

While there is no consensus on the exact hierarchy of upper extremity functions, and the order in which they should be restored, generally the main objectives for brachial plexus reconstruction in adults are shoulder abduction, external rotation, elbow flexion, and forearm supination, as these movements are critical for activities of daily living [6]. Initial neurotization procedures therefore usually focus on either the shoulder muscles or the biceps (or both), and the reconstruction approach taken depends on the exact injury pattern of the patient [13, 14].

Although not an exhaustive list, potential strategies for nerve transfers are briefly described below, based on the type of injury to the brachial plexus:

For C5–6 (upper trunk) palsies, shoulder abduction can be restored by transferring the distal SAN to the suprascapular nerve (SSN) and the triceps branch of the radial nerve to the anterior division of the axillary nerve [27–29]. An alternative donor nerve to the axillary is the thoracodorsal nerve, although more rehabilitation may be needed as the latissimus dorsi is antagonistic to the deltoid [14]. If an upper brachial plexus injury involves C7 and there is triceps weakness, the thoracodorsal nerve may be preferred over the radial nerve, to avoid downgrading the triceps muscle any further [6]. The MPN and ICN may also be transferred to the axillary if they are not being used to restore elbow flexion [13, 30]. Though less common, the serratus anterior muscle can be reinnervated to provide additional shoulder stabilization and improve scapular rotation; donor options for the LTN include ICN, thoracodorsal nerve, as well as pectoral fascicles of the middle trunk [13, 23, 31]. If possible, reinnervation of the teres minor branch of the axillary nerve can also allow for improved external rotation [23].

Elbow flexion can typically be restored through a single- or double-fascicular transfer from the ulnar and/or median nerves to the biceps and/or brachialis branches of the MCN [32–34]. Alternative donor nerves include MPN, thoracodorsal nerve, distal SAN, medial cord, and ICN [14, 23]. Elbow extension is usually given less priority, but if C7 involvement is evident, the triceps can be reinnervated using the MPN or ICN (though many other intra- and extraplexal donors have also been reported, including ICN, thoracodorsal nerve, phrenic nerve, ulnar nerve, axillary nerve, and contralateral C7 nerve root) [6, 23, 35, 36].

It should be noted that traumatic avulsion of C5 is relatively uncommon, even among pan-plexus injuries, and supraclavicular exploration often confirms the presence of a viable C5 nerve root stump, which can be used as a source of axons for plexo-plexal reconstruction with interposed nerve autografts, usually to the anterior and/or posterior divisions of the upper trunk [6, 13]. In this situation, some authors advocate for graft reconstruction in tandem with nerve transfers, claiming that this strategy permits additional reinnervation to downstream targets, including the pectoral muscles and sensory organs in the median nerve distribution [13].

For C8–T1 (lower trunk) palsies, patients with partial injury or partial recovery may be candidates for distal nerve transfers to restore hand function. Median nerve deficits can be addressed by transferring expendable branches of the radial nerve or the brachialis branch of the MCN to the anterior interosseous nerve (AIN), to restore finger flexion and pronation [37–39]. If C7 is involved, posterior interosseous nerve (PIN) function and wrist extension can be restored through transfer of median nerve branches (from either the supinator, flexor digitorum superficialis, pronator, or flexor carpi radialis) [40]. Hand intrinsic weakness can be addressed through transfer of the distal AIN to the ulnar nerve, although other donor options are also available, including LTN, thoracodorsal, subscapular, PIN, and transverse cervical nerve [23, 41].

For C5–T1 (total plexus) palsies, elbow flexion and shoulder function (stabilization, abduction, and external rotation) are typically prioritized for reconstruction, leaving few remaining donors to restore distal function [6, 13, 14]. Because only extraplexal donors are available for these injuries, elbow flexion can be restored via ICN-MCN transfer and shoulder abduction via SAN-SSN transfer [6]. Contralateral C7 root and phrenic nerve are also potential donors, although the former usually requires a long nerve graft (and a more involved rehabilitation process for both upper extremities), while the latter has the potential to compromise diaphragmatic function [14, 42–44]. Overall, reported outcomes after nerve transfers for pan-plexus injuries have historically been worse than those for upper plexus injuries, possibly due to the use of extraplexal donors [13, 45]. Therefore, if there is no meaningful recovery by 2 years after reconstruction, patients should undergo evaluation for tendon transfers, joint fusions, or free functional muscle transfers to improve the position and function of the upper limb [23].

Although restoration of motor function is usually the priority for brachial plexus reconstruction, sensory nerve transfers should not be overlooked, as many of the available donor sensory nerves are accessible through the same exposures used for motor nerve transfers [6, 14]. Recovering sensation in the hand and forearm is protective and can also decrease neuropathic pain and facilitate postoperative motor reeducation after reconstruction [14, 24]. Several sensory nerve donors are available depending on which operative approach is being taken for motor nerve harvest, such as intercostal sensory nerves on the chest wall and the intercostobrachial nerve in the axilla [14]. Based on the distance to the sensory distribution of interest, the following nerves can also be dissected for sensory transfer: superficial radial nerve, digital nerves, lateral antebrachial cutaneous nerve, and dorsal cutaneous branch of ulnar nerve [23, 46, 47].

Lastly, it is worth mentioning that, despite the expanding indications and improved outcomes of nerve transfers, surgical exploration of the plexus and graft reconstruction should not be abandoned until high-quality evidence exists demonstrating that this approach is inferior or unneeded. Meta-analyses conducted to date have reported conflicting results on the optimal timing and components of complex nerve reconstruction (e.g., donor nerve selection, nerve grafting vs. transfer) for brachial plexus injuries [48–55]. As long as this uncertainty remains, surgeons must rely on their expertise, experience, and detailed knowledge of the patient's injury pattern and patho-anatomy to devise the most appropriate surgical plan.

4.6 Conclusion

In summary, nerve transfer is an essential procedure in the nerve surgeon's repertoire that can significantly enhance the recovery potential for adult patients with traumatic brachial plexus injuries. Surgeons must be aware of the requirements for successful nerve transfers and should conduct a thorough evaluation of the patient's injury pattern to develop a tailored reconstruction strategy. As the indications for nerve transfer continue to grow, it is critical for surgeons to be knowledgeable of the various motor and sensory nerves available for transfer, including their prior applications and expected outcomes, so that patients have access to the full breadth of complex nerve reconstruction before the window of opportunity for recovery closes.

References

1. Ray WZ, Mackinnon SE. Management of nerve gaps: autografts, allografts, nerve transfers, and end-to-side neurorrhaphy. Exp Neurol. 2010;223(1):77–85. https://doi.org/10.1016/j.expneurol.2009.03.031.
2. Rohde RS, Wolfe SW. Nerve transfers for adult traumatic brachial plexus palsy (brachial plexus nerve transfer). HSS J. 2007;3(1):77–82. https://doi.org/10.1007/s11420-006-9027-y.
3. Dvali L, Mackinnon S. The role of microsurgery in nerve repair and nerve grafting. Hand Clin. 2007;23(1):73–81. https://doi.org/10.1016/j.hcl.2007.02.003.
4. Moore AM, Novak CB. Advances in nerve transfer surgery. J Hand Ther. 2014;27(2):96–104; quiz 105. https://doi.org/10.1016/j.jht.2013.12.007.
5. Tung TH, Mackinnon SE. Nerve transfers: indications, techniques, and outcomes. J Hand Surg Am. 2010;35(2):332–41. https://doi.org/10.1016/j.jhsa.2009.12.002.
6. Addas BM, Midha R. Nerve transfers for severe nerve injury. Neurosurg Clin N Am. 2009;20(1):27–38., vi. https://doi.org/10.1016/j.nec.2008.07.018.

7. Weber RV, Davidge KM. Nerve transfer for the forearm and hand. In: Mackinnon SE, editor. Nerve surgery. 1st ed. Thieme Medical Publishers, Inc.; 2015.
8. Ferrante MA. Electrodiagnostic assessment of the brachial plexus. Neurol Clin. 2012;30(2):551–80. https://doi.org/10.1016/j.ncl.2011.12.005.
9. Sinha S, Khani M, Mansoori N, Midha R. Adult brachial plexus injuries: surgical strategies and approaches. Neurol India. 2016;64(2):289–96. https://doi.org/10.4103/0028-3886.177597.
10. Leffert RD. Clinical diagnosis, testing, and electromyographic study in brachial plexus traction injuries. Clin Orthop Relat Res. 1988;237:24–31.
11. Parry CB. Thoughts on the rehabilitation of patients with brachial plexus lesions. Hand Clin. 1995;11(4):657–75.
12. Ferrante MA, Wilbourn AJ. The Electrodiagnostic examination with peripheral nerve injuries. In: Mackinnon SE, editor. Nerve surgery. 1st Edition ed. Thieme Medical Publishers, Inc.; 2015.
13. Garozzo D. Traumatic brachial plexus injuries: surgical techniques and strategies. In: Socolovsky M, Rasulic L, Midha R, Garozzo D, editors. Manual of peripheral nerve surgery: from the basics to complex procedures. 1st ed. Georg Thieme Verlag KG; 2017.
14. Tung TH, Moore AM. Brachial plexus injuries. In: Mackinnon SE, editor. Nerve surgery. 1st Edition ed. Thieme Medical Publishers, Inc.; 2015.
15. Fu SY, Gordon T. Contributing factors to poor functional recovery after delayed nerve repair: prolonged denervation. J Neurosci. 1995;15(5 Pt 2):3886–95. https://doi.org/10.1523/jneurosci.15-05-03886.1995.
16. Sulaiman W, Gordon T. Neurobiology of peripheral nerve injury, regeneration, and functional recovery: from bench top research to bedside application. Ochsner J Spring. 2013;13(1):100–8.
17. Seddon HJ, Medawar PB, Smith H. Rate of regeneration of peripheral nerves in man. J Physiol. 1943;102(2):191–215. https://doi.org/10.1113/jphysiol.1943.sp004027.
18. Martin E, Senders JT, DiRisio AC, Smith TR, Broekman MLD. Timing of surgery in traumatic brachial plexus injury: a systematic review. J Neurosurg. 2019;130(4):1333–45. https://doi.org/10.3171/2018.1.Jns172068.
19. Midha R. Nerve transfers for severe brachial plexus injuries: a review. Neurosurg Focus. 2004;16(5):E5. https://doi.org/10.3171/foc.2004.16.5.6.
20. Narakas AO, Hentz VR. Neurotization in brachial plexus injuries. Indication and results. Clin Orthop Relat Res. 1988;237:43–56.
21. Dvali L, Mackinnon S. Nerve repair, grafting, and nerve transfers. Clin Plast Surg. 2003;30(2):203–21. https://doi.org/10.1016/s0094-1298(02)00096-2.
22. Sun G, Wu Z, Wang X, Tan X, Gu Y. Nerve transfer helps repair brachial plexus injury by increasing cerebral cortical plasticity. Neural Regen Res. 2014;9(23):2111–4. https://doi.org/10.4103/1673-5374.147939.
23. Lee SK, Wolfe SW. Nerve transfers for the upper extremity: new horizons in nerve reconstruction. J Am Acad Orthop Surg. 2012;20(8):506–17. https://doi.org/10.5435/jaaos-20-08-506.
24. Leechavengvongs S, Ngamlamiat K, Malungpaishrope K, Uerpairotkit C, Witoonchart K, Kulkittiya S. End-to-side radial sensory to median nerve transfer to restore sensation and relieve pain in C5 and C6 nerve root avulsion. J Hand Surg Am. 2011;36(2):209–15. https://doi.org/10.1016/j.jhsa.2010.10.009.
25. Chuang DC. Distal nerve transfers: a perspective on the future of reconstructive microsurgery. J Reconstr Microsurg. 2018;34(9):669–71. https://doi.org/10.1055/s-0038-1656719.
26. Doi K. Distal nerve transfer: perspective of reconstructive microsurgery. J Reconstr Microsurg. 2018;34(9):675–7. https://doi.org/10.1055/s-0038-1639369.
27. Bertelli JA, Ghizoni MF. Reconstruction of C5 and C6 brachial plexus avulsion injury by multiple nerve transfers: spinal accessory to suprascapular, ulnar fascicles to biceps branch, and triceps long or lateral head branch to axillary nerve. J Hand Surg Am. 2004;29(1):131–9. https://doi.org/10.1016/j.jhsa.2003.10.013.
28. Leechavengvongs S, Witoonchart K, Uerpairojkit C, Thuvasethakul P. Nerve transfer to deltoid muscle using the nerve to the long head of the triceps, part II: a report of 7 cases. J Hand Surg Am. 2003;28(4):633–8. https://doi.org/10.1016/s0363-5023(03)00199-0.
29. Colbert SH, Mackinnon S. Posterior approach for double nerve transfer for restoration of shoulder function in upper brachial plexus palsy. Hand (N Y). 2006;1(2):71–7. https://doi.org/10.1007/s11552-006-9004-4.
30. Ray WZ, Murphy RK, Santosa K, Johnson PJ, Mackinnon SE. Medial pectoral nerve to axillary nerve neurotization following traumatic brachial plexus injuries: indications and clinical outcomes. Hand (N Y). 2012;7(1):59–65. https://doi.org/10.1007/s11552-011-9378-9.
31. Ray WZ, Pet MA, Nicoson MC, Yee A, Kahn LC, Mackinnon SE. Two-level motor nerve transfer for the treatment of long thoracic nerve palsy. J Neurosurg. 2011;115(4):858–64. https://doi.org/10.3171/2011.5.Jns101615.
32. Brandt KE, Mackinnon SE. A technique for maximizing biceps recovery in brachial plexus reconstruction. J Hand Surg Am. 1993;18(4):726–33. https://doi.org/10.1016/0363-5023(93)90328-z.
33. Mackinnon SE, Novak CB, Myckatyn TM, Tung TH. Results of reinnervation of the biceps and brachialis muscles with a double fascicular transfer for elbow flexion. J Hand Surg Am. 2005;30(5):978–85. https://doi.org/10.1016/j.jhsa.2005.05.014.
34. Oberlin C, Béal D, Leechavengvongs S, Salon A, Dauge MC, Sarcy JJ. Nerve transfer to biceps muscle using a part of ulnar nerve for C5-C6 avulsion of the brachial plexus: anatomical study and report of four

cases. J Hand Surg Am. 1994;19(2):232–7. https://doi.org/10.1016/0363-5023(94)90011-6.
35. Gao K, Lao J, Zhao X, Gu Y. Outcome after transfer of intercostal nerves to the nerve of triceps long head in 25 adult patients with total brachial plexus root avulsion injury. J Neurosurg. 2013;118(3):606–10. https://doi.org/10.3171/2012.10.Jns12637.
36. Pet MA, Ray WZ, Yee A, Mackinnon SE. Nerve transfer to the triceps after brachial plexus injury: report of four cases. J Hand Surg Am. 2011;36(3):398–405. https://doi.org/10.1016/j.jhsa.2010.11.024.
37. Palazzi S, Palazzi JL, Caceres JP. Neurotization with the brachialis muscle motor nerve. Microsurgery. 2006;26(4):330–3. https://doi.org/10.1002/micr.20247.
38. Hsiao EC, Fox IK, Tung TH, Mackinnon SE. Motor nerve transfers to restore extrinsic median nerve function: case report. Hand (N Y). 2009;4(1):92–7. https://doi.org/10.1007/s11552-008-9128-9.
39. Mackinnon SE, Yee A, Ray WZ. Nerve transfers for the restoration of hand function after spinal cord injury. J Neurosurg. 2012;117(1):176–85. https://doi.org/10.3171/2012.3.Jns12328.
40. Ray WZ, Mackinnon SE. Clinical outcomes following median to radial nerve transfers. J Hand Surg Am. 2011;36(2):201–8. https://doi.org/10.1016/j.jhsa.2010.09.034.
41. Brown JM, Yee A, Mackinnon SE. Distal median to ulnar nerve transfers to restore ulnar motor and sensory function within the hand: technical nuances. Neurosurgery. 2009;65(5):966–77; discussion 977–8. https://doi.org/10.1227/01.Neu.0000358951.64043.73.
42. Gu Y, Xu J, Chen L, Wang H, Hu S. Long term outcome of contralateral C7 transfer: a report of 32 cases. Chin Med J. 2002;115(6):866–8.
43. Gu YD, Ma MK. Use of the phrenic nerve for brachial plexus reconstruction. Clin Orthop Relat Res. 1996;323:119–21. https://doi.org/10.1097/00003086-199602000-00016.
44. Hou Z, Xu Z. Nerve transfer for treatment of brachial plexus injury: comparison study between the transfer of partial median and ulnar nerves and that of phrenic and spinal accessary nerves. Chin J Traumatol. 2002;5(5):263–6.
45. Samardzić M, Rasulić L, Grujicić D, Milicić B. Results of nerve transfers to the musculocutaneous and axillary nerves. Neurosurgery. 2000;46(1):93–101; discussion 101–3.
46. Bertelli JA, Ghizoni MF. Very distal sensory nerve transfers in high median nerve lesions. J Hand Surg Am. 2011;36(3):387–93. https://doi.org/10.1016/j.jhsa.2010.11.049.
47. Ducic I, Dellon AL, Bogue DP. Radial sensory neurotization of the thumb and index finger for prehension after proximal median and ulnar nerve injuries. J Reconstr Microsurg. 2006;22(2):73–8. https://doi.org/10.1055/s-2006-932500.
48. Kim RB, Bounajem M, Hamrick F, Mahan MA. Optimal donor nerve to restore elbow flexion after traumatic brachial plexus injury: a systematic review and meta-analysis. Neurosurgery. 2022;90(1):39–50. https://doi.org/10.1227/neu.0000000000001737.
49. Li WJ, He LY, Chen SL, et al. Contralateral C7 nerve root transfer for function recovery in adults: a meta-analysis. Chin Med J (Engl). 2017;130(24):2960–8. https://doi.org/10.4103/0366-6999.220316.
50. Yang LJ, Chang KW, Chung KC. A systematic review of nerve transfer and nerve repair for the treatment of adult upper brachial plexus injury. Neurosurgery. 2012;71(2):417–29; discussion 429. https://doi.org/10.1227/NEU.0b013e318257be98.
51. Ali ZS, Heuer GG, Faught RW, et al. Upper brachial plexus injury in adults: comparative effectiveness of different repair techniques. J Neurosurg. 2015;122(1):195–201. https://doi.org/10.3171/2014.9.Jns132823.
52. Hoang D, Chen VW, Seruya M. Recovery of elbow flexion after nerve reconstruction versus free functional muscle transfer for late, traumatic brachial plexus palsy: a systematic review. Plast Reconstr Surg. 2018;141(4):949–59. https://doi.org/10.1097/prs.0000000000004229.
53. Sneiders D, Bulstra LF, Hundepool CA, Treling WJ, Hovius SER, Shin AY. Outcomes of single versus double fascicular nerve transfers for restoration of elbow flexion in patients with brachial plexus injuries: a systematic review and meta-analysis. Plast Reconstr Surg. 2019;144(1):155–66. https://doi.org/10.1097/prs.0000000000005720.
54. Vernon Lee CY, Cochrane E, Chew M, Bains RD, Bourke G, Wade RG. The effectiveness of different nerve transfers in the restoration of elbow flexion in adults following brachial plexus injury: a systematic review and meta-analysis. J Hand Surg Am. 2023;48(3):236–44. https://doi.org/10.1016/j.jhsa.2022.11.013.
55. Texakalidis P, Hardcastle N, Tora MS, Boulis NM. Functional restoration of elbow flexion in nonobstetric brachial plexus injuries: a meta-analysis of nerve transfers versus grafts. Microsurgery. 2020;40(2):261–7. https://doi.org/10.1002/micr.30510.

Intraoperative Monitoring in Brachial Plexus Surgery: Fundamentals and Applications

5

Carlos Alberto Rodríguez-Aceves,
María Elena Córdoba-Mosqueda,
Pablo Calvo-Calleja, and Miguel Domínguez-Páez

Abbreviations

BP	Brachial plexus
cEMG	Continuous electromyography
cMAP	Compound motor action potential
DRG	Dorsal root ganglion
eEMG	Evoked electromyography
MEP	Motor evoked potential
MIOM	Multimodal intraoperative monitoring
NAP	Nerve action potential
sNAP	Sensory nerve action potential
SSEP	Somatosensory evoked potential

5.1 Introduction

Surgical pathology of the brachial plexus (BP) may include traumatic injuries, compressive syndromes, and extra-or intraneural tumors. Surgical management is demanding owing to its complex internal anatomy, its relationship with surrounding non-neural structures, the localization within a narrow space, scarring, and the limited disposal components when reconstruction is necessary or anatomy deformation because of any kind of space-occupying lesions [1].

Multimodal intraoperative monitoring (MIOM) refers to those intraoperative neurophysiologic techniques used for the continuous monitoring, identification, and quantification of various parameters that serve in revealing the functional status of nerve structures during surgical procedures. In such a way, they allow to reveal viable and nonviable nerves for microsurgical reconstruction, protect functional fascicles and nerves during microsurgical decompression or resection of tumors, and select nonfunctional fascicles for biopsies [1–3].

5.2 Applied Anatomy

Topographic and organizational anatomy of BP have been exposed in previous chapters, but some considerations regarding the anatomy of proximal roots contributing to form the BP need to be remarked for the correct understanding and interpretation of MIOM, mostly in traumatic injuries.

A spinal nerve is formed within the intervertebral foramen by the joining of both ventral and dorsal roots, which conduct motor and sensory information, respectively. Motor cell bodies of

C. A. Rodríguez-Aceves (✉)
Peripheral Nerve Clinic, Neurological Center, The American British Cowdray Medical Center, Mexico City, Mexico

M. E. Córdoba-Mosqueda
Neurosurgery, Hospital Ángeles Pedregal, Mexico City, Mexico

P. Calvo-Calleja
Hospital de Cabueñes, Gijón, Spain

M. Domínguez-Páez
Neurosurgery Division, Hospital Regional Universitario de Málaga, Málaga, Spain

F. Guedes et al. (eds.), *Nerve Transfers for Brachial Plexus Reconstruction after Trauma*,
https://doi.org/10.1007/978-3-031-92445-3_5

ventral roots are in the anterior horn of the spinal cord, and sensory cell bodies of dorsal roots are within the dorsal root ganglion (DRG).

After exiting the intervertebral foramen, the spinal nerve branches off in a posterior ramus, which innervates paraspinal muscles, the skin of the dorsal region, bone, and joint segmentary structures. A ventral ramus contributes to the origin of the BP. The other branches arising from the spinal nerve are the recurrent meningeal branch and the communicating rami. So, all the spinal nerves conduce mixed information (sensory, motor, and autonomic).

Sensory fibers have a segmentary distribution (dermatomes) over the skin, and all ventral rami are associated with the ventral rami of other spinal nerves; so, they contribute to more than one myotome [4–6].

Any injury between the spinal cord and the DRG is defined as a preganglionic injury. On the other hand, an injury distal to the DRG is called a postganglionic injury.

Thus, after a BP injury, identification of the level of lesion is paramount; since in preganglionic injuries, a reconstruction using the proximal stump of the injured root is not possible (Fig. 5.1).

Many clinical, radiologic, and neurophysiologic signs assist the surgeon in preoperatively identifying when the level of injury is preganglionic or not.

The following signs are highly suggestive of preganglionic injuries: [1] clinically, compromise of the very proximal branches of the BP (e.g., phrenic, dorsal scapular and long thoracic nerves), sensory and motor impairment, and Horner's syndrome (sympathetic dysfunction in T1 root injury) and [2] electrically, paraspinal muscles denervation, positive recording of sensory nerve action potential (sNAP), absence of both compound motor action potential

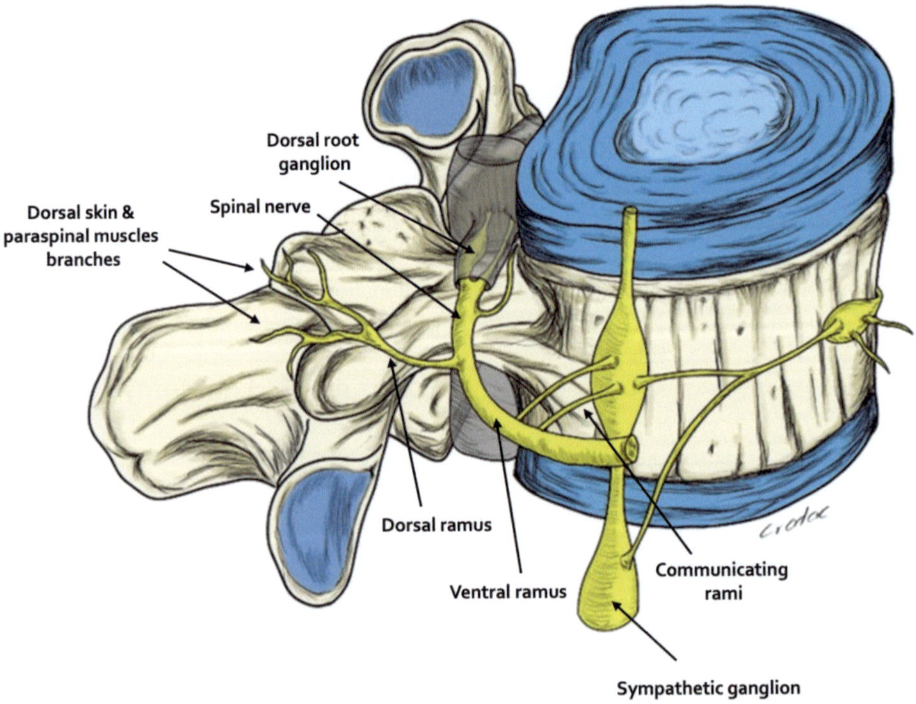

Fig. 5.1 Spinal nerve anatomy. Dorsal and ventral roots forming spinal nerve distal to the dorsal root ganglion. The spinal nerve branches off in a meningeal, dorsal, ventral, and communicating rami after exiting the intervertebral foramen

(cMAP), and somatosensory evoked potential (SSEP) [7–9].

The surgical team should be aware of anatomic variations and multilevel contribution of spinal nerves in the presence of unexpected muscle denervation or in the absence of expected muscle denervation patterns, being that these findings may reflect not only the irregular nature of the injury but also anatomical variations.

In addition, registry optimization by proper selection of the studied structures (i.e., muscles) is essential, because of the multiple contributions of the roots to innervate the same myotomes [9].

5.3 Neurophysiologic Intraoperative Monitoring Techniques

Recording techniques in MIOM are divided according to the type of elicited bioelectrical signals in spontaneous and evoked responses.

In the first group, continuous electromyography (cEMG) is used to follow and guard the electrical activity of functional neural structures during surgical manipulation. In the second group, techniques that evoke responses from different sources are SSEP, motor evoked potentials (MEP), evoked electromyography (eEMG), and nerve action potential (NAP) recording; and these are used to evaluate, reveal, and demonstrate abnormal conduction, define the anatomical distribution, and also monitor worseness of function during handling neural structures [3, 10, 11].

5.3.1 Continuous Electromyography

cEMG consists of the uninterrupted recording of the electrical activity of the studied muscles, which provides the real-time neurophysiologic status of the motor circuit at risk. After anesthetic induction and positioning, multiple needle electrodes are placed on the muscles of interest. The signals are analogically and digitally processed to reduce artifacts because of the use of many electronic devices in the operating room [12].

This technique is used to prevent nerve trunk or fascicular injury during surgical manipulation of non-damaged nerves. In such a way, monitoring BP components during decompressive surgery (i.e., thoracic outlet syndrome) or tumor resection (intraneural or extraneural) are the main indications.

If mechanical (e.g., stretching and compression), thermal (i.e., bipolar coagulation), or ischemic insult exists, nerve irritation is developed and muscle activity increases in the way of rapid and irregular bursts of short-lasting or long-lasting (prolonged trains) neurotonic discharges, displayed on a digital screen and as an audible signal to provide visual and auditory feedback to the surgical team [2, 3, 11–14] (Fig. 5.2).

5.3.2 Evoked Electromyography

Stimulus-triggered or eEMG comprises the brief and low-intensity electrical stimulation of a nerve, with the subsequent recording of a cMAP. For recording, the same electrodes are used as in cEMG, and the stimulator electrode handled by the surgeon may be a monopolar or bipolar device, and the second one is preferable to reduce current spreading to nearby neural structures, preferentially in a dry surgical field [2, 13].

This technique is useful for identifying and mapping nerves or fascicles, providing quantitative information about their localization and functional integrity through the registry of cMAP. Thus, it is used in surgical procedures oriented to microsurgical repair of BP, such as in traumatic injuries (e.g., nerve transfers), and for tumor resection.

A cMAP also can be obtained by supramaximal stimulation of the motor or mixed nerve, and its size is correlated with the number of functional axons. An absent cMAP correlates with nonfunctional nerves, and its reduction or increased stimulation threshold during manipulation of the nerve correlates with intraoperative injury, so eEMG may dictate the surgical proceed [2, 3, 13] (Fig. 5.3).

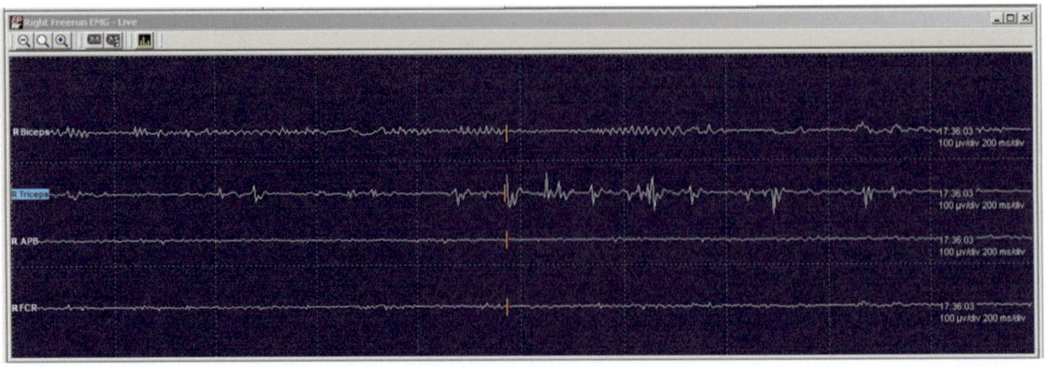

Fig. 5.2 Continuous electromyography. Continuous electromyography during infraclavicular neurolysis after shoulder dislocation. Neurotonic discharges are observed due to mechanical irritation by manipulation. *Source: Neurophysiology archives, The American Cowdray Medical Center*

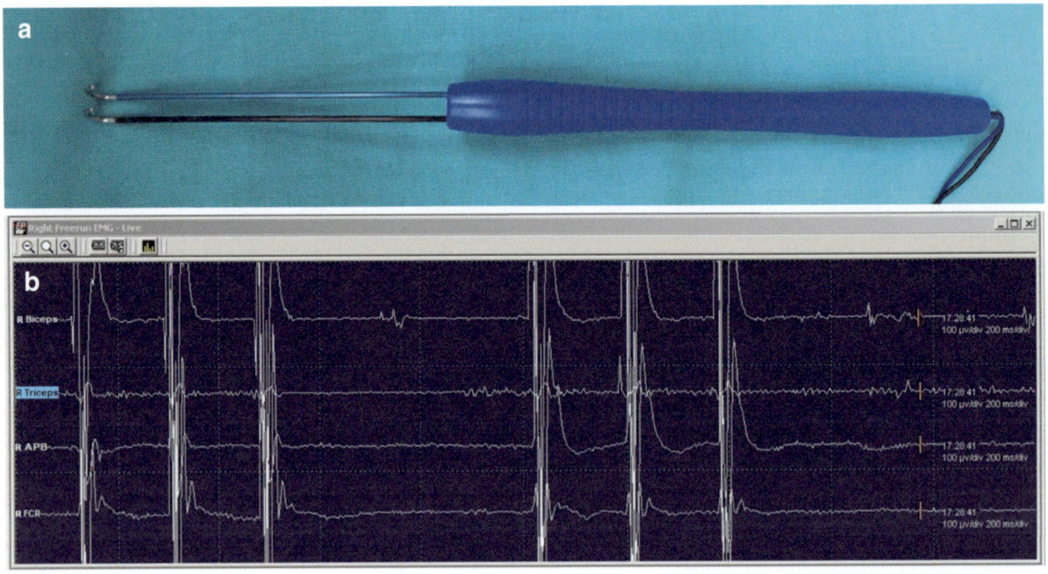

Fig. 5.3 Evoked electromyography. (**a**) Stainless bipolar hook electrodes. (**b**) Evoked electromyography during brachial plexus tumor resection. *Source: Neurophysiology archives, The American Cowdray Medical Center*

5.3.3 Nerve Action Potential

A NAP is an intraoperative nerve conduction study acquired by direct supramaximal stimulation of a determined segment of a nerve trunk or fascicles proximal to the site of injury and the simultaneous recording distal to the site of injury.

This parameter represents the summation of all the potentials of the individual fibers within a nerve, requiring at least 3000 to 4000 fibers to be elicited [15].

Bipolar electrodes are used for stimulus delivery, and tripolar electrodes for the registry, preferentially. Both consist of stainless-steel hooks of different sizes, to suspend the nerve away from neighboring tissues and fluids, preventing artifact formation and dispersion of the current. The tips of the electrode should be separated by at least 3 mm in smaller nerves and 5–7 mm in larger nerves. The distance between the stimulating and recording electrodes should be at least 4 cm to avoid masking of NAP by shock artifact. For this reason, measuring NAP in proximal injuries could be challenging.

Evoked NAP assesses the motor pathway and can show a lack of conduction across the fascicles involved in tumors. Its main indication is to evaluate in-continuity neuromas seen in postganglionic traumatic injuries to determine if axonal conduction exists or if axonal regeneration is ongoing before reaching its target muscle. So, this tool also guides intraoperative decisions when correctly applied [15–20] (Fig. 5.4).

5.3.4 Somatosensory Evoked Potentials

SSEP can be evoked after applying multiple pulses over the somatosensory pathway. The response is recorded in the upper relay stations (e.g., Erb's point, cervical spine) and cerebral cortex, through subcutaneous needle electrodes. It can be elicited by superficial stimulation of the peripheral pathway or by direct bipolar electrode stimulation of the root, as it exits the intervertebral foramen.

This modality assesses the integrity of the root by stimulating the dorsal column-lemniscal sensory pathway.

An intraoperative baseline record is suggested before surgical manipulation when tumor resection or decompressive surgery is conducted to avoid inadvertent nerve trunk injury. In these cases, intraoperative recording is compared with reference values, and changes in amplitude (<50% decrease) and/or latency (>10% increase) may reflect nerve damage by stretching or compression.

Furthermore, it allows the identification of preganglionic lesions in traumatic injuries. When microsurgical reconstruction is considered, absent SSEP and positive sNAP confirm root avulsion; therefore, root grafting is not possible, and another surgical strategy is needed [3, 21–24] (Fig. 5.5).

5.3.5 Motor Evoked Potentials

A MEP is elicited by high-voltage, short-duration, and repetitive transcranial stimulation delivered via scalp needle electrodes, and is recorded either at the nerve root level, near the intervertebral foramen, using a bipolar hook stimulator, or in the target muscles innervated by the studied nerve with a needle electrode.

This technique asesses evaluates the functional continuity of motor fibers and, like SSEP, allows evaluation of proximal root integrity in the context of traumatic BP injuries. A detectable and reproducible MEP indicates preserved motor root continuity, while the abscence of a MEP is strongly suggestive of nerve root avulsion [16, 21, 25, 26] (Fig. 5.6).

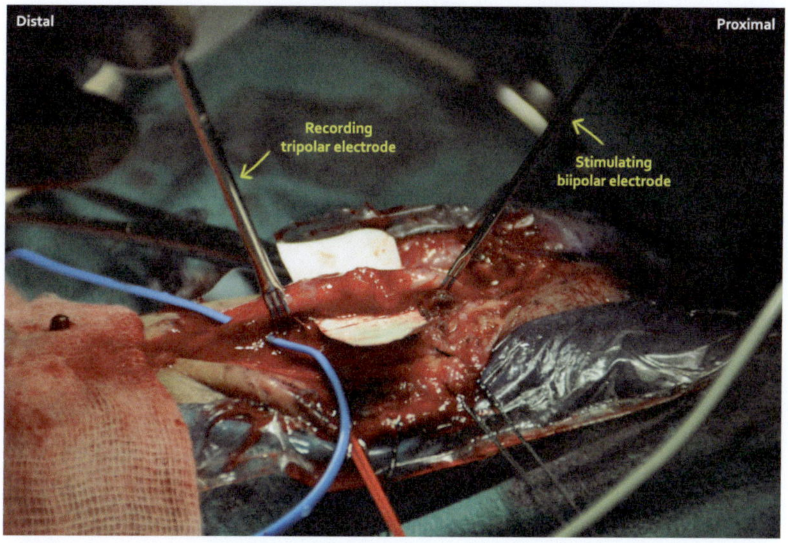

Fig. 5.4 Nerve action potential. Nerve action potential assessment of in-continuity neuroma

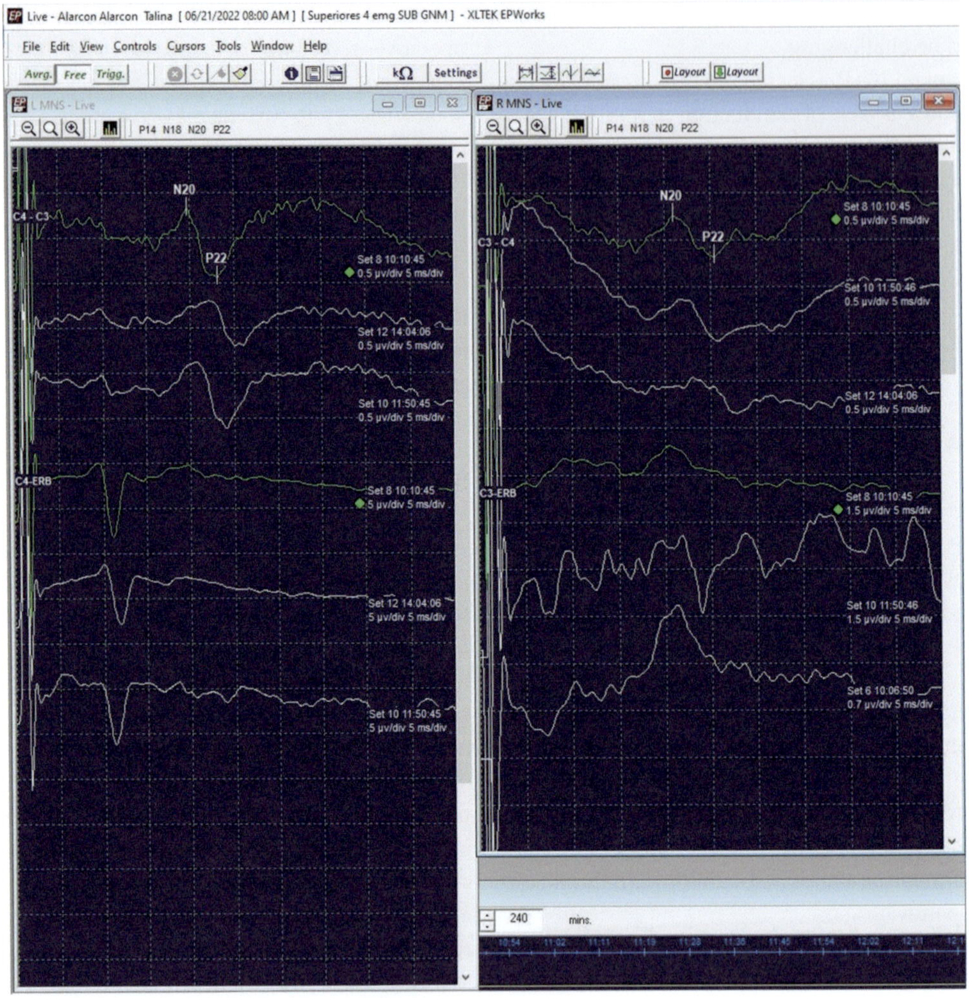

Fig. 5.5 Somatosensory evoked potential. Somatosensory evoked potentials recording during supraclavicular brachial plexus decompression from surrounding fibrosis after shoulder dislocation. *Source: Neurophysiology archives, The American Cowdray Medical Center*

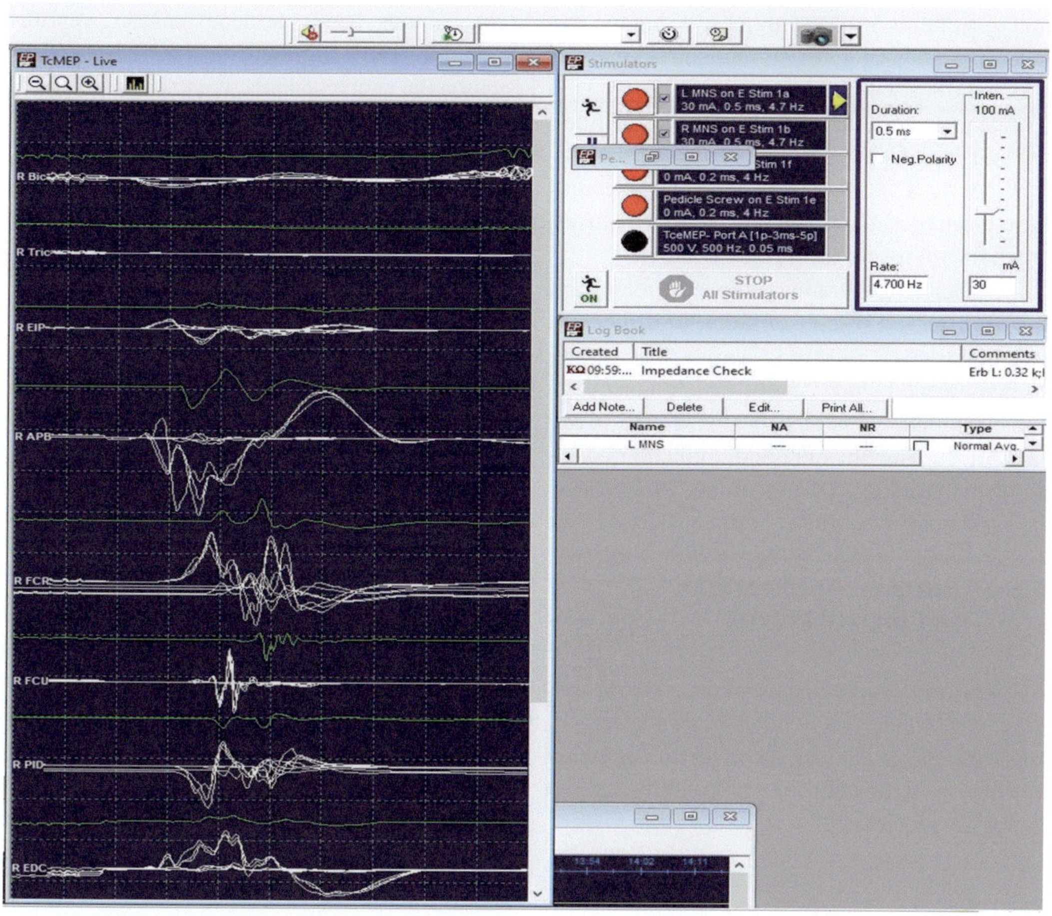

Fig. 5.6 Motor evoked potential. Motor evoked potentials improvement after infraclavicular brachial plexus external neurolysis in a patient with history of shoulder osteosynthesis. *Source: Neurophysiology archives, The American Cowdray Medical Center*

5.4 Technical Considerations for Optimal Registry and Avoidance of Pitfalls

MIOM follows the same principles as in preoperative evaluation, and all electrodes for stimulation and recording within the surgical field must be sterile.

Assembling electrodes outside the surgical field should be planned carefully by both the surgeon and neurophysiologist. It is performed after the anesthetic induction and patient positioning.

Anesthetic induction is conducted with short-acting muscle relaxants and total intravenous anesthesia with propofol is recommended, because inhalational agents may suppress excitability at the cortical level, impeding the stimulation and recording of cerebral cortex in MEP and SEEP, respectively.

Short-acting muscle relaxants are preferable to long-acting ones, to avoid flawless recordings over muscles. Anytime, avoid the use of any drug bolus, as they affect the electrical responses.

Proper positioning and holding of electrodes in the muscles or studied nerves is an important issue. Malpositioning, inadequate contact, or insulation of electrodes on nerves over humid surgical fields may lead to the erroneous application of stimulus or recording, dispersing the current to neighboring nerves and masking NAP within the studied segment.

Adequate amplification and the use of filters will aid in reducing artifacts generated by electronic devices and reduce the risk of generating false-positive or false-negative recordings, using grounding to reduce artifact generation.

Regulation of operating room temperature and avoiding the use of cold solution to irrigate are recommended [2, 3, 15, 21, 27–32].

Equipment failure cannot be eliminated for complete. Thus, qualified personnel are necessary for the identification and correction of any problem in setting up the recording equipment.

5.5 Surgical Applications in Brachial Plexus

As mentioned in previous sections, MIOM may have several purposes in brachial plexus surgery, and these are guided by the surgical pathology, whether a traumatic injury, compression, or tumor is being treated.

5.5.1 Compressive Syndromes

Thoracic outlet syndrome is a compressive syndrome, in which various anatomical structures (e.g., fibrous bands, scalene muscles, cervical ribs) may cause different degrees of compression on the supraclavicular components of BP.

Given this pathophysiology, the primary goal of decompressive surgery is to relieve pressure on the neural elements while preserving their functional integrity. To achieve this, MIOM is essential and typically includes cEMG, SSEPs, MEPs, and direct electrical stimulation of the nerve trunks to assess real-time function and ensure protection of the BP during dissection. After decompression, also eEMG testing can corroborate the functional integrity of the motor pathway [1, 21, 30, 33] (Fig. 5.7).

5.5.2 Tumor Resection

MIOM application for tumor removal includes surveillance and preservation of functional fascicles in intraneural or extraneural tumors.

In the first case, before the resection is started, mapping of the tumor surface with direct electrical stimulation or cMAP recording is conducted to identify safe zones to approach the tumor. Nonfunctional fascicles contributing to the origin of the tumor can be identified by the lack of recording of NAPs and being sacrificed. The same strategy is used for selecting nonfunctional tissue in open biopsies.

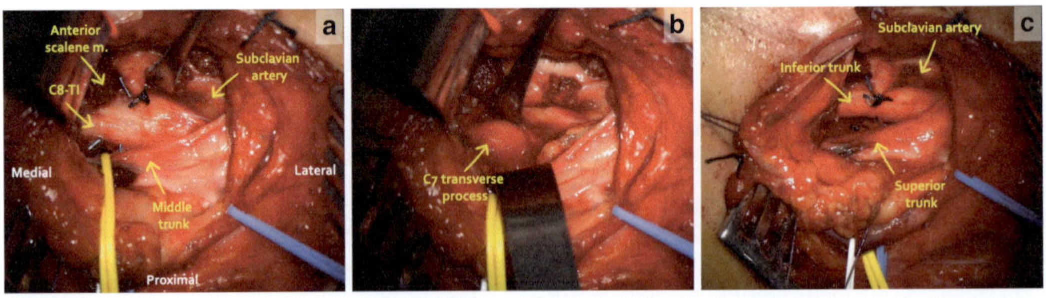

Fig. 5.7 Thoracic outlet syndrome. Supraclavicular microsurgical decompression in a left-sided thoracic outlet syndrome: (**a**) Anterior scalenectomy and exposure of subclavian artery, C8 and T1 roots, and the inferior trunk. They look displaced laterally and dorsally from below by a large C7 transverse process. (**b**) Neural elements are retracted gently to expose the large C7 transverse process. (**c**) Brachial plexus appearance after decompression by anterior scalenectomy, and resection of large C7 transverse process

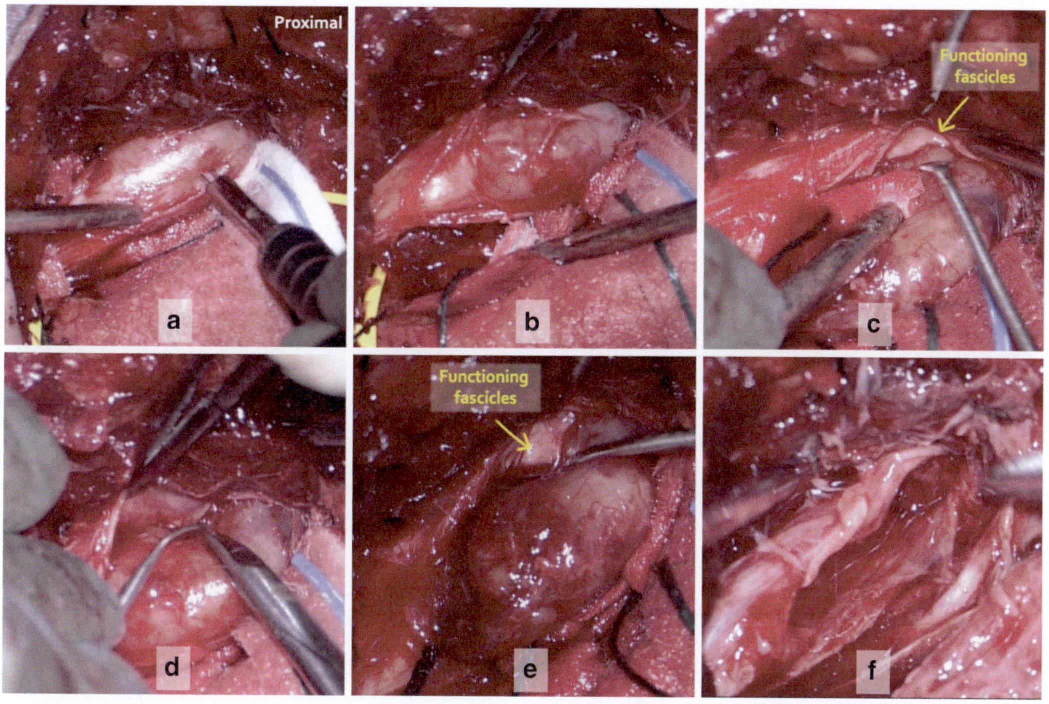

Fig. 5.8 C7 Schwannoma. A left-sided C7 Schwannoma microsurgical resection: (**a**) Mapping tumor surface, (**b**) Epineurotomy, (**c**, **d**) Intraneural dissection of functional fascicles, (**e**) tumor enucleation, and (**f**) complete resection preserving functional integrity

In extraneural tumors, BP may be displaced or hidden by the lesion, so in these cases, direct electrical stimulation, eEMG, and deterioration of SSEP and MEP may help clarify the localization of neural structures [1, 2, 21, 31] (Fig. 5.8).

5.5.3 Traumatic Injuries

The surgical management of traumatic injuries is by far the most complex scenario in BP surgery, since altered anatomical configuration, fibrosis, and scar formation make difficult the manipulation and visual identification of structures.

Three situations are emphasized regarding the use of MIOM in traumatic injuries: recognizing the level of injury (preganglionic vs postganglionic), assessing in-continuity neuromas in postganglionic injuries, and selecting functional donors to perform nerve transfers.

Differentiation between preganglionic and postganglionic injuries is of particular importance, especially in total BP injury, because the surgical strategy is determined by the level of the injury, and recognizing viable roots for grafting adds a complimentary useful option, given the limited availability of donors to perform a reconstruction.

Intraoperatively, the absence of SSEP and MEP with positive sNAP correlates with preganglionic injuries. So, in these cases, grafting is not possible and nerve transfers are the only available option to reconstruct.

In-continuity neuromas should be electrically evaluated in all cases since visual inspection alone does not determine whether conduction exists or not, and its treatment relies on this information. Conduction assessment is achieved with NAP recording. If a NAP is registered through the site of injury, then the surgeon can expect a recovery of function after neurolysis. If conduction does not exist, the injured segment should be resected and reconstructed with grafts.

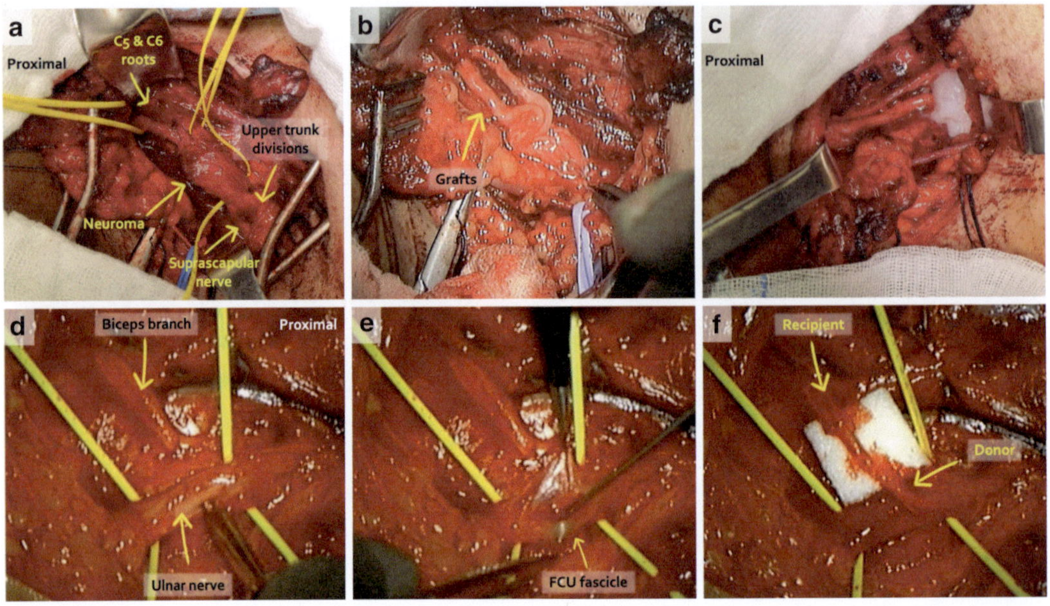

Fig. 5.9 Traumatic injury. MIOM may help to identify and properly select viable elements for microsurgical reconstruction in different strategies: (**a**) Upper trunk in-continuity neuroma, (**b**) sural nerve grafts positioned between the stumps, and (**c**) C5-C6 roots grafting to the posterior and anterior divisions of the upper trunk. (**d**) Ulnar nerve mapping by direct electrical stimulation, (**e**) internal neurolysis to isolate the flexor carpi ulnaris fascicle for an (**f**) Oberlin nerve transfer

A nerve transfer consists of taking a healthy, expendable, functioning, and nearby nerve or fascicle (donor) to be rerouted and connected with a damaged nerve (recipient).

To avoid the development of a new significant deficit, MIOM may aid in the careful selection of donors for this purpose, through direct electrical stimulation, or cMAP recording [1, 8, 21, 31] (Fig. 5.9).

5.6 Summary

In recent years, clinical outcomes following BP surgery have improved significantly due to several factors, including advances in surgical equipment, microsurgical techniques, imaging modalities, and intraoperative neurophysiological monitoring. The latter has proven especially valuable in guiding real-time intraoperative decision-making, thereby enhancing the safety and precision of surgical interventions.

Knowledge of anatomical, physiological, and technical basis, besides communication between the surgical team (surgeon, anesthesiologist, and neurophysiologist), is fundamental for the proper interpretation and utilization of MIOM.

Many intraoperative goals can be achieved with the use of MIOM in BP surgery: identification and monitoring of the functional status of healthy peripheral nerves obscured by tumors or scarring to prevent their damage, localization of the level and extension of the injury, as well as typification of preganglionic lesions, to determine if a root can be grafted, assessment of functional continuity across the site of injury, identification of potential donors for nerve transfers, and proper targets for nerve biopsy.

Whenever possible, MIOM should be considered a routine tool for BP surgical procedures.

References

1. Wang H, Bishop AT, Shin AY, Spinner RJ. Intraoperative testing and monitoring during brachial plexus surgery. In: Handbook of clinical neurophysiology [internet]. Elsevier; 2008. p. 720–30. https://linkinghub.elsevier.com/retrieve/pii/S1567423107080513.
2. Rodríguez-Aceves CA, Tello VA. Neurophysiological monitoring during surgery. In: Guedes F, Zager EL, Garozzo D, Rasulic L, Socolovsky M, editors. Diagnostic assessment and treatment of peripheral nerve tumors [Internet]. Cham: Springer International Publishing; 2021. p. 115–23. https://doi.org/10.1007/978-3-030-77633-6_11.
3. Rodríguez-Aceves CA, Domínguez-Páez M, Fernández-Sánchez VE. Electrodiagnostic pre-, intra-, and postoperative evaluations. In: Manual of peripheral nerve surgery: from the basics to complex procedures [internet]. Stuttgart: Georg Thieme Verlag; 2018. p. b-006–149755. https://doi.org/10.1055/b-006-149755.
4. Smith BE. Anatomy and histology of peripheral nerve. In: Handbook of clinical neurophysiology [internet]. Elsevier; 2006. p. 3–22. https://linkinghub.elsevier.com/retrieve/pii/S1567423109700620.
5. Catala M, Kubis N. Gross anatomy and development of the peripheral nervous system. In: Handbook of clinical neurology [internet]. Elsevier; 2013. p. 29–41. https://linkinghub.elsevier.com/retrieve/pii/B9780444529022000035.
6. Johnson EO, Vekris M, Demesticha T, Soucacos PN. Neuroanatomy of the brachial plexus: normal and variant anatomy of its formation. Surg Radiol Anat. 2010;32(3):291–7.
7. Russell SM. Examination of peripheral nerve injuries: an anatomical approach. 2nd ed. New York: Thieme; 2015. p. 229.
8. Goldstein B. Applied anatomy and Electrodiagnosis of brachial Plexopathies. Phys Med Rehabil Clin N Am. 1994;5(3):477–93.
9. Simmons Z. Electrodiagnosis of brachial Plexopathies and proximal upper extremity neuropathies. Phys Med Rehabil Clin N Am. 2013;24(1):13–32.
10. Walsh P. The clinical role of evoked potentials. J Neurol Neurosurg Psychiatry. 2005;76(suppl_2):ii16–22.
11. Kim SM, Kim SH, Seo DW, Lee KW. Intraoperative neurophysiologic monitoring: basic principles and recent update. J Korean Med Sci. 2013;28(9):1261.
12. Kobylarz EJ, Randhawa J, Mason S, Lawson VH. Preoperative electrodiagnostic studies and intraoperative neurophysiologic monitoring: power and pitfalls. Plast Aesthet Res. 2023;10(1):2.
13. Holland NR. Intraoperative electromyography. J Clin Neurophysiol. 2002;19(5):444–53.
14. Strommen JA, Crum BA. Intraoperative monitoring with free-running EMG. In: Handbook of clinical neurophysiology. Elsevier; 2008. p. 396–403. https://linkinghub.elsevier.com/retrieve/pii/S1567423107080276.
15. Tiel RL, Happel LT, Kline DG. Nerve action potential recording method and equipment. Neurosurgery. 1996;39(1):103–9.
16. Oberle JW, Antoniadis G, Rath SA, Richter HP. Value of nerve action potentials in the surgical management of traumatic nerve lesions. Neurosurgery. 1997;41(6):1337–43.
17. Nelson KR. Use of peripheral nerve action potentials for intraoperative monitoring. Neurol Clin. 1988 Nov;6(4):917–33.
18. Crum BA, Strommen JA. Intraoperative peripheral nerve stimulation and recording. In: Handbook of clinical neurophysiology. Elsevier; 2008. p. 364–70. https://linkinghub.elsevier.com/retrieve/pii/S1567423107080240.
19. Koht A, Sloan TB. Evoked response monitoring. In: Neuromonitoring techniques [Internet]. Elsevier; 2018. p. 147–77. https://linkinghub.elsevier.com/retrieve/pii/B9780128099155000061.
20. Robert EG, Happel LT, Kline DG. Intraoperative nerve action potential recordings: technical considerations, problems, and pitfalls. Neurosurgery. 2009;65(4):A97–104.
21. Zelenski NA, Oishi T, Shin AY. Indications and technique for the use of intraoperative Neuromonitoring in brachial plexus surgery. J Hand Surg Am. 2023;48:726.
22. Baker A, Widrich J. Somatosensory evoked potentials. In: StatPearls. Treasure Island (FL): StatPearls Publishing; 2023. http://www.ncbi.nlm.nih.gov/books/NBK544358/.
23. Sugioka H, Tsuyama N, Hara T, Nagano A, Tachibana S, Ochiai N. Investigation of brachial plexus injuries by intraoperative cortical somatosensory evoked potentials. Arch Orth Traum Surg. 1982;99(3):143–51.
24. Ying T, Wang X, Sun H, Tang Y, Yuan Y, Li S. Clinical usefulness of somatosensory evoked potentials for detection of peripheral nerve and brachial plexus injury secondary to Malpositioning in microvascular decompression. J Clin Neurophysiol. 2015;32(6):512–5.
25. Burkholder LM, Houlden DA, Midha R, Weiss E, Vennettilli M. Neurogenic motor evoked potentials: role in brachial plexus surgery: case report. J Neurosurg. 2003;98(3):607–10.
26. Turkof E, Millesi H, Turkof R, Pfundner P, Mayr N. Intraoperative electroneurodiagnostics (transcranial electrical motor evoked potentials) to evaluate the functional status of anterior spinal roots and spinal nerves during brachial plexus surgery. Plast Reconstr Surg. 1997;99(6):1632–41.
27. Kimura J. Electrodiagnosis in diseases of nerve and muscle: principles and practice. 4th ed. New York: Oxford University Press; 2013.

28. Gooch CL, Weimer LH. The Electrodiagnosis of neuropathy: basic principles and common pitfalls. Neurol Clin. 2007;25(1):1–28.
29. Schramm J, Møller AR. Intraoperative neurophysiologic monitoring in neurosurgery [Internet]. Berlin, Heidelberg: Springer; 2023. https://doi.org/10.1007/978-3-642-75750-1.
30. Galloway GM, Nuwer MR, Lopez JR, Zamel KM. Intraoperative neurophysiologic monitoring [internet]. 1st ed. Cambridge University Press; 2010. https://www.cambridge.org/core/product/identifier/9780511777950/type/book.
31. Crum BA, Strommen J. Intraoperative brachial plexus neurophysiological monitoring. In: Shin AY, Pulos N, editors. Operative brachial plexus surgery [internet]. Cham: Springer International Publishing; 2021. p. 111–9. Available from:. https://doi.org/10.1007/978-3-030-69517-0_9.
32. Wu G, Belzberg A, Nance J, Gutierrez-Hernandez S, Ritzl EK, Ringkamp M. Solutions to the technical challenges embedded in the current methods for intraoperative peripheral nerve action potential recordings. J Neurosurg. 2020 Sep;133(3):884–93.
33. Ashman BD, Tewari A, Castle J, Hasan SS, Bhatia S. Intraoperative Neuromonitoring for brachial plexus Neurolysis during delayed fixation of a clavicular fracture presenting as thoracic outlet syndrome: a case report. JBJS Case Connector. 2018;8(4):e85.

6 The Cutting Edge of Peripheral Nerve Surgery: A Look at Emerging Techniques

Debora Garozzo, Evelina Llorian, Vinícius M. Henriques, Gabriel Elias Sanches, Francisco José Lourenço Torrão-Junior, and Fernando Guedes

6.1 Introduction

Over the past few years, rapid advancements in peripheral nerve surgery have expanded the possibilities for repairing and restoring limb mobility, with significant improvements in surgical techniques such as nerve transfers, nerve grafts, tendon transfers, and tissue engineering. Additionally, the emergence of new technologies and devices like robotic and bionic devices has revolutionized peripheral nerve surgery, providing greater precision and accuracy during surgical procedures. These advancements offer hope to patients who were previously considered untreatable, enabling us to approach nerve injuries and disorders in a new way.

One such type of nerve injury occurs when the brachial plexus (BP) experiences injuries involving the avulsion of its nerve roots, leading to upper limb paralysis. These injuries are mainly caused by high-speed car accidents and typically affect young adults in their prime, with the most common mechanism of injury being high-energy traction on single nerve tracts. The consequences of global plexopathies can be severe, resulting in therapy-resistant pain, unemployment, decreased self-sufficiency, and negative socio-emotional impacts. Thus, immediate treatment for this intricate nerve injury must be initiated in addition to standard trauma management.

For patients with severe brachial plexus injuries causing complete loss of function, the primary objective is to restore shoulder function and stability, along with the biceps function, using various techniques such as nerve transfers, nerve grafts, and tendon transfers. However, these surgeries sometimes do not yield the expected improvement, while further therapeutic options are limited. Nonetheless, the combination of advanced surgical techniques and innovative technologies has led to exciting new developments in peripheral nerve surgery, paving the way for improved outcomes and greater hope for patients.

In the upcoming chapter, our focus will be on the latest technologies associated with peripheral nerve surgery. Specifically, we will discuss surgical advancements and alternative therapeutic options, particularly for cases where traditional treatment methods have proven ineffective in improving the affected limb, particularly with regard to the brachial plexus and upper limb.

D. Garozzo
Department of Neurosurgery, Mediclinic Parkview Hospital, Dubai, United Arab Emirates

E. Llorian (✉) · V. M. Henriques · G. E. Sanches · F. J. L. Torrão-Junior · F. Guedes
Department of Surgery, Division of Neurosurgery, Gaffrée and Guinle University Hospital, School of Medicine, Federal University of Rio de Janeiro State (UNIRIO), Rio de Janeiro, RJ, Brazil

F. Guedes et al. (eds.), *Nerve Transfers for Brachial Plexus Reconstruction after Trauma*,
https://doi.org/10.1007/978-3-031-92445-3_6

6.2 The Role of Amputation Surgery and Prosthetic Fitting in Enhancing Mobility

6.2.1 Overview

In certain circumstances, nerve repair or reconstructive surgery may not be the best solution for patients with severe brachial plexus injuries. This may be due to the seriousness of their condition, or these procedures may not result in a significant improvement in their situation. Consequently, these patients may be left with a limb that has little or no useful function. In these cases, rehabilitation options may be limited, including more conservative approaches such as hand control retraining or a functional arm orthosis, or more aggressive options like limb amputation and prosthetic restoration. It is worth noting that these types of procedures are more prevalent in North America than in Europe and Latin America.

For unstable limbs, orthopedic approaches may not be practical and offer limited functional benefits. In some cases, patients may choose to undergo amputation, either with or without prosthetic adjustment. However, since this is an irreversible procedure, the treatment team should only consider amputation after determining that there is no chance of further neurological recovery.

Patients with unstable limbs and little or no recovery are optimal candidates for this type of restoration. To allow some degree of function and prosthetic restoration, amputation is usually performed at the mid-transhumeral level, along with shoulder fusion. Shoulder fusion involves positioning the humerus between a maximum of 45° abduction and 45° flexion and a minimum of 30° abduction and 30° flexion [1]. Immobilizing the shoulder in this specific position enables a degree of simulated shoulder joint movement, achieved through the active contraction of the functioning scapular stabilizer muscles, the levator scapulae, and the trapezius muscles.

When considering amputation surgery as a treatment option for patients with brachial plexus injuries, the risk of significant neuropathic pain needs to be taken into account [2]. Despite the loss of the respective limb, pain may persist and can be localized to the affected limb. Some patients may assume that amputation will alleviate their pain, but studies have indicated that this is not the case. In fact, patients with neuropathic pain continue to experience it even after amputation surgery, and it is felt in the phantom limb. It is important to differentiate between neuropathic pain and mechanical shoulder pain, with the former generating a burning sensation in the affected limb, particularly in the forearm and hand, due to the deafferentation of sensory fibers. In contrast, mechanical shoulder pain is caused by joint subluxation, muscular atrophy, and a heavy, motionless limb.

It is worth noting that preoperative pain is a significant predictor of postoperative phantom limb pain in patients undergoing amputation. Therefore, it is vital that patients understand that amputation is not a solution for pain relief and other treatment options should be explored.

6.2.2 Indications

Amputation is generally considered a last resort for patients with traumatic brachial plexus injuries. However, under certain circumstances, it may be necessary to improve a patient's quality of life. In adult patients, some known criteria for amputation include (I) a limb that is heavy, stiff, and difficult to move, causing persistent mechanical pain in the shoulder that may be refractory to conservative treatment, (II) a claw hand that is painful and nonfunctional due to muscle atrophy, or (III) a patient with a strong motivation for the procedure [3]. A thorough evaluation of patients is essential to ensure that they fully understand the implications of the procedure and can manage the postoperative challenges.

Available options and the best prosthesis should also be contemplated to ensure that the patient's needs and preferences are considered and that the chosen prosthesis can provide adequate functionality and comfort. Evaluation of these options should be conducted before proceeding with the amputation to maximize the chances of a successful outcome.

In cases of pan-plexus injury, elective amputation may have a role to play when no recovery or only recovery of elbow flexion is observed after all other primary and rational secondary surgical procedures have been exhausted. To be considered for elective amputation, patients must meet certain criteria, including having complete information about the amputation process, understanding that amputation is not intended to relieve central neuropathic pain, and being aware that wearing a functional prosthesis requires scapulothoracic motor control, which is often absent in individuals with total brachial plexus root injury. This is necessary to ensure that the weight of the prosthesis can be supported by the upper limb. [4]

Patients must also understand that the aim of the procedure is to improve their ability to carry out everyday activities (Table 6.1). Discussions with the surgeon, rehabilitation staff, psychologists, the prosthetic team, and other amputees should be conducted to ensure that patients have a complete understanding of the procedure and post-amputation rehabilitation process.

6.2.3 Assessment Test for Prosthesis Candidates

Before considering the use of a bionic arm or prosthesis, a comprehensive evaluation of the upper extremity is essential. Objective assessments of hand function before and after bionic arm replacement can be conducted using the Action Research Arm Test (ARAT) and the Southampton Assessment Hand Procedure (SHAP) [5].

Table 6.1 Patient selection criteria for amputation surgery

Criteria for amputation surgery
• A heavy, stiff limb causing persistent shoulder pain refractory to conservative treatment
• A painful claw hand and nonfunctional due to muscle atrophy
• Patient with a strong motivation for the procedure
• Patients with scapulothoracic motor control
• Patients without neuropathic pain or patients understanding amputation do not relieve central neuropathic pain
• Patients that ensure they fully understand the implications of the procedure and can manage the postoperative challenges

The ARAT evaluates the patient's upper extremity mobility performance, with scores ranging from 0 to 57 points. A higher score of 57 indicates better performance. There are no specific cutoff scores for this assessment as it is a continuous measure based on observed mobility. The ARAT is particularly useful in predicting the functional recovery of the upper extremity in stroke rehabilitation. Scores below 10 points, between 10 and 56 points, and 57 points correspond to poor, moderate, and good recovery, respectively [6]

The Southampton Hand Assessment Procedure (SHAP) is a validated test used to assess hand function. Initially designed for evaluating the effectiveness of upper limb prostheses, it has been subsequently employed in the evaluation of musculoskeletal and neurological conditions. The SHAP involves 6 abstract objects and 14 Activities of Daily Living (ADL). Participants must complete timed tasks using these objects, minimizing any potential interference or reliance on the observer or clinician's reaction times. A score of 100 points on the SHAP indicates normal hand function.

Additionally, other evaluations such as the DASH questionnaire, visual analog scale (VAS) for pain assessment, and the SF-36 health survey should be administered to assess changes in quality of life.

6.2.4 Bionic Reconstruction

Bionic reconstruction procedures aim to expand the range of electromyography (EMG) signals available for prosthetic control. Individuals with global brachial plexus avulsion injuries often lose the ability to voluntarily activate muscles in their affected upper extremities. As part of targeted rehabilitation, these patients need to relearn how to selectively activate individual muscles. However, their weak muscle contractions do not result in actual movements because the brain no longer has a central representation of the disconnected limb [7].

While some patients can identify distinct surface EMG (sEMG) signals through intensive cognitive training and motor relearning with appropriate biofeedback, others may require additional muscles through free functional muscle transfer.

The primary objective when establishing surgical control signals for patients with global brachial plexus avulsion injuries is to create a limited number of stable myoelectric sites that enable simple and reliable cognitive control. Due to abnormal reinnervation and functional confusion in the reconstructed nerves, these patients often struggle with alternating (or antagonistic?) muscle contractions. Therefore, using a complex matrix of myosignals as a prosthetic control algorithm is likely to lead to frustration, malfunction, and abandonment of the prosthetic device. It is essential to employ cognitively "simple" control strategies specifically designed for this patient population [5].

Moreover, given the limited and confusing neurological input to the muscles in individuals with brachial plexus injuries, even basic two-signal prosthetic control requires extensive therapy, including sEMG biofeedback training, to establish reliable control.

In cases where there is a scarcity of EMG signals due to extensive muscle degeneration, targeted muscle reinnervation (TMR) can be performed, with implantation of a nerve or its fascicles into a viable muscle [8]. Another alternative is to use regenerative peripheral nerve interfaces (RPNI), which rely on free functional muscle transfers as targets for reinnervation, provided that viable motor axons are identified for nerve coaptation [9] (PP. Vu, 2020). Notably, the gracilis and adductor longus muscles have been frequently used in these bionic reconstruction procedures.

To ensure reliable signal control, voluntary muscle activation should consistently generate sEMG signals with amplitudes two to three times higher than those observed during relaxation. After nerve regeneration, the strength and activation patterns of the signals are regularly monitored during training using sEMG biofeedback, with the goal of achieving optimal functional outcomes during prosthetic fitting.

Along with myoelectric systems, nerve electrodes have also been used to interface with the peripheral nervous system (PNS), mainly for providing afferent sensory information for sensible control of prostheses. They may be classified according to their level of invasiveness as extraneural, interfascicular, or intrafascicular. Extraneural electrodes, such as the spiral cuff and the flat interface nerve electrode (FINE), have been shown to provide long-term selective and stable stimulation, as well as sensory information to the patient wearing a prosthesis [10–12].

Intrafascicular electrodes, which include the transverse intrafascicular multichannel electrode (TIME), have also been shown to successfully provide touch and proprioception sensory feedback to patients using prostheses with higher spatial resolution than their extraneural counterparts [13–17].

When initiating bionic reconstruction, it is crucial to consider and understand the patient's expectations. The extent of amputation, whether it is transhumeral or glenohumeral, must be thoroughly discussed with the patient, considering their neurobiological prerequisites (assessed through detailed myoactivity analysis before making any surgical decisions) and personal preferences.

Additionally, in cases of prolonged global avulsion injuries of the brachial plexus, there may be a subluxation of the glenohumeral joint caused by rotator cuff denervation. This highlights the importance of conducting a comprehensive assessment involving not only a neurosurgical team but also an orthopedist, physiotherapist, psychology team, and prosthetic team before subjecting the patient to such interventions. This approach ensures a holistic evaluation and supports an effective treatment plan.

6.3 Tissue Engineering

Peripheral nerve injuries have a profound impact on patients, resulting in functional loss and lifelong disabilities. Currently, autologous nerve grafting is the preferred surgical approach for repairing nerve gap injuries. However, this method has drawbacks, including the sacrifice of a healthy nerve and morbidity at the donor site [18].

To bridge nerve gaps when tension-free neurorrhaphy is not feasible, nerve guidance scaffolds are commonly employed. These scaffolds, typically made from biodegradable polymers or collagen-based hollow tubes, provide structural support to guide axonal regeneration and prevent neuroma formation and fibrous tissue invasion. Despite their potential, commercially available devices have not achieved the same regenerative outcomes as autologous nerve grafts and are limited in their effectiveness for short defects with poor functional recovery.

Recent advancements in tissue engineering have revolutionized neural scaffolds, transforming them from passive structures into active environments that promote neuronal growth and accelerate axonal regeneration. Surface modifications, such as grooves, electrospun fibers, gels, and films, have been explored to guide the growth and alignment of Schwann cells and neuronal cells [19]. Biomaterial chemistry has enabled the optimization of cellular behavior through the incorporation of short peptide sequences, enhancing cell adhesion and proliferation. Additionally, extracellular matrix molecules support cell attachment and stimulate the release of factors that promote neurite growth.

Currently, there are no clinically available pharmacological treatments for nerve injuries. However, peptides, hormones, and growth factors have shown promising results in reducing neuronal cell death and facilitating axonal regrowth. Neuroactive steroids like progesterone or allopregnanolone, as well as thyroid hormone and growth hormone, have demonstrated benefits in animal models of sciatic nerve injury. Neurotransmitters such as GABA, ATP, glutamate, and acetylcholine and their receptors have also been identified as potential targets for pharmacotherapies aimed at nerve repair.

While these treatment options are still under investigation and have limited availability, it is crucial to emphasize that autologous nerve grafts remain the preferred therapeutic choice due to their significantly superior benefits compared to other approaches.

The field of tissue engineering is making significant progress in developing new muscle tissue. In cases where the natural regenerative capacity of muscle is exhausted, the replacement of damaged tissue becomes necessary. An ideal tissue-engineered muscle construct should possess appropriate structural and mechanical properties to facilitate rapid muscle recovery.

A fundamental requirement for such a construct is a cell source that can be easily cultured, expanded, and differentiated into muscle lineage. While satellite cells and myoblasts are commonly considered, further research is needed to determine their optimal growth properties. Other cell types, including *ESC* (epithelial stem cell), *iPSC* (induced pluripotent stem cell), *pericytes*, and *MSC* (mesenchymal stem cell), have also undergone investigation [20].

Various scaffold types have been developed to mimic the natural extracellular matrix (ECM) of the muscle. These scaffolds, typically composed of resorbable materials, remodel as they degrade. Incorporating nano- and micro-scale topographic features into polymer scaffolds is essential for aligning myoblasts, promoting the assembly of myotubes, and organizing them into mature muscle fibers. Additionally, 3D gels like collagen and fibrin, as well as cell sheets, have demonstrated varying degrees of success. Gels offer the advantage of controlled release of growth factors such as IGF-1 and VEGF, which enhance myogenesis.

Adequate vascularization is crucial for cellular proliferation and differentiation within the constructs. While including endothelial cells is one approach, surgical anastomosis with existing vasculature is considered the optimal solution whenever feasible. Effective reinnervation support is also necessary, and new 3D models for neuromuscular junction connectivity are contributing to the design of these structures.

Recent advancements in progenitor/stem cell biology and scaffold technologies provide hope for the future development of clinically relevant tissue-engineered muscle constructs.

6.4 Artificial Nerve Conduits

When there is a gap of less than 1 cm between nerve injuries, direct end-to-end suturing without tension allows for proper regeneration. However, it is impossible to bring the nerve ends together without creating a substantial amount of tension for defects greater than 3 cm. To overcome this difficulty, nerve grafts can be used as a bridge. However, they come with disadvantages such as increased surgical complications, diameter mismatch between the nerve and graft, and immunological reactions. To address these limitations, nerve conduits have been proposed as an alternative strategy to bridge defective nerves and promote regeneration.

Nerve conduits are designed using nondegradable synthetic materials, providing a safer option compared to donor grafts without the need for immunosuppressant therapy. These conduits are designed to enhance peripheral nerve reconstruction and axon guidance while preventing the formation of fibrous scar tissues. Ideally, nerve conduits should have low immunogenicity, be bioabsorbable, and possess substantial mechanical properties to maintain alignment between proximal and distal nerve sites. There are two groups of biomaterials that can be used for this purpose: natural polymers and synthetic materials. However, most of these materials are controversial, and further studies are required [21].

Polyglycolic acid (PGA) is an FDA-approved synthetic polymer that is made from a more flexible and porous material, which enhances the nerve regeneration process. The use of PGA nerve conduits has shown better reconstruction outcomes for long nerve gaps compared to other synthetic polymer materials. In gaps less than 4 mm, PGA conduits have demonstrated a greater repair outcome compared to end-to-end regeneration. Polylactic acid (PLA), a biodegradable polyester, enhances neuron regeneration and supports neuron proliferation. It has also been shown to improve axon maturation. However, PLA generates lactic acid as a byproduct during degradation, which can result in neurotoxicity [21].

Poly(L-lactide-co-ε-caprolactone) (PLCL) theoretically produces less lactic acid during degradation, making it a more viable option due to its reduced toxicity. The efficacy of this conduit has been assessed with mixed outcomes [21].

In addition to synthetic nerve conduits, natural polymers have also been used to provide cell growth and support. Collagen and chitosan have been extensively employed in the manufacture of nerve conduits, and they exhibit minimal biodegradability and immunogenicity. Type I collagen has been widely used and constructs fibrils of the endoneurium in the basal lamina. Collagen conduits can bridge nerve gaps up to 20 mm and improve functional outcomes in nerve reconstruction. Studies have also shown reduced pain sensation. Chitosan, another natural polymer, has been researched for its ability to increase neurite growth and promote nerve cell adhesion [21].

6.5 Final Considerations

Revolutionizing peripheral nerve surgery through innovative techniques has opened new possibilities for patients with nerve injuries and disorders. The combination of advanced surgical techniques, such as nerve transfers, grafts, and tendon transfers, along with the integration of bionic and robotic technologies, has led to improved outcomes and increased hope for patients.

However, it is important to approach these advancements with caution and consider individual patient factors when determining the most appropriate treatment approach. While amputation and prosthetic fitting may enhance mobility for patients with severe brachial plexus injuries, it should be considered as a last resort after exhausting all other treatment options. Patients must be thoroughly evaluated and provided with comprehensive information about the procedure, its implications, and potential postoperative challenges.

In the field of tissue engineering, advancements in neural scaffolds and regenerative treatments show promise in promoting nerve regeneration and improving functional recovery. However, autologous nerve grafts remain the preferred choice due to their superior benefits. Ongoing research is focused on developing better biomaterials, growth factors, and pharmacological treatments to further enhance nerve repair.

In conclusion, the remarkable progress achieved in peripheral nerve surgery instills optimism and renewed hope for individuals grappling with nerve injuries and disorders. The integration of surgical techniques, bionic devices, tissue engineering, and artificial nerve conduit approaches has the potential to transform the field and improve the quality of life for individuals affected by peripheral nerve injuries. Continued research and advancements will further refine these techniques and expand their applicability, ultimately benefiting a larger population of patients in need.

References

1. Chung KC, Yang LJ-S, McGillicuddy JE. Rehabilitation concepts for adult brachial plexus injuries. In: Practical management of pediatric and adult brachial plexus palsies. Saunders/Elsevier; 2012.
2. Hruby LA, Sturma A, Mayer JA, Pittermann A, Salminger S, Aszmann OC. Algorithm for bionic hand reconstruction in patients with global brachial plexopathies. J Neurosurg. 2017;127(5):1163–71. https://doi.org/10.3171/2016.6.JNS16154.
3. Lombard A, Lavrard B, Pierrart J, Masmejean E. Indications for amputation after traumatic brachial plexus injury in adults: case report and review of new prosthetic technologies. Hand Surg Rehabil. 2022;41S:S71–5. https://doi.org/10.1016/j.hansur.2020.09.018.
4. Cantwell SR, Nelson AW, Sampson BP, et al. The role of amputation and myoelectric prosthetic fitting in patients with traumatic brachial plexus injuries. J Bone Joint Surg Am. 2022;104(16):1475–82. https://doi.org/10.2106/JBJS.21.01261.
5. Hruby LA, Gstoettner C, Sturma A, Salminger S, Mayer JA, Aszmann OC. Bionic Upper Limb Reconstruction: A Valuable Alternative in Global Brachial Plexus Avulsion Injuries-A Case Series. J Clin Med. 2019;9(1):23. Published 2019 Dec 20. https://doi.org/10.3390/jcm9010023.
6. Lyle RC. A performance test for assessment of upper limb function in physical rehabilitation treatment and research. Int J Rehabil Res. 1981;4(4):483–92. https://doi.org/10.1097/00004356-198112000-00001.
7. Socolovsky M, Malessy M, Lopez D, Guedes F, Flores L. Current concepts in plasticity and nerve transfers: relationship between surgical techniques and outcomes. Neurosurg Focus. 2017;42(3):E13. https://doi.org/10.3171/2016.12.FOCUS16431.
8. Cheesborough JE, Smith LH, Kuiken TA, Dumanian GA. Targeted muscle reinnervation and advanced prosthetic arms. Semin Plast Surg. 2015;29(1):62–72. https://doi.org/10.1055/s-0035-1544166.
9. Vu PP, Vaskov AK, Irwin ZT, et al. A regenerative peripheral nerve interface allows real-time control of an artificial hand in upper limb amputees. Sci Transl Med. 2020;12(533):eaay2857. https://doi.org/10.1126/scitranslmed.aay2857.
10. Polasek KH, Hoyen HA, Keith MW, Kirsch RF, Tyler DJ. Stimulation stability and selectivity of chronically implanted multicontact nerve cuff electrodes in the human upper extremity. IEEE Trans Neural Syst Rehabil Eng. 2009;17(5):428–37. https://doi.org/10.1109/TNSRE.2009.2032603.
11. Tan DW, Schiefer MA, Keith MW, Anderson JR, Tyler J, Tyler DJ. A neural interface provides long-term stable natural touch perception. Sci Transl Med. 2014;6(257):257ra138. https://doi.org/10.1126/scitranslmed.3008669.
12. Charkhkar H, Shell CE, Marasco PD, Pinault GJ, Tyler DJ, Triolo RJ. High-density peripheral nerve cuffs restore natural sensation to individuals with lower-limb amputations. J Neural Eng. 2018;15(5):056002. https://doi.org/10.1088/1741-2552/aac964.
13. Oddo CM, Raspopovic S, Artoni F, et al. Intraneural stimulation elicits discrimination of textural features by artificial fingertip in intact and amputee humans. elife. 2016;5:e09148. Published 2016 Mar 8. https://doi.org/10.7554/eLife.09148.
14. D'Anna E, Valle G, Mazzoni A, et al. A closed-loop hand prosthesis with simultaneous intraneural tactile and position feedback. Sci Robot. 2019;4(27):eaau8892. https://doi.org/10.1126/scirobotics.aau8892.
15. Petrini FM, Valle G, Bumbasirevic M, et al. Enhancing functional abilities and cognitive integration of the lower limb prosthesis. Sci Transl Med. 2019;11(512):eaav8939. https://doi.org/10.1126/scitranslmed.aav8939.
16. Petrini FM, Bumbasirevic M, Valle G, et al. Sensory feedback restoration in leg amputees improves walking speed, metabolic cost and phantom pain. Nat Med. 2019;25:1356–63. https://doi.org/10.1038/s41591-019-0567-3.
17. Petrini FM, Valle G, Strauss I, et al. Six-month assessment of a hand prosthesis with Intraneural tactile feedback. Ann Neurol. 2019;85(1):137–54. https://doi.org/10.1002/ana.25384.
18. Lischer M, di Summa PG, Petrou IG, et al. Mesenchymal stem cells in nerve tissue engineering:

bridging nerve gap injuries in large animals. Int J Mol Sci. 2023;24(9):7800. Published 2023 Apr 25. https://doi.org/10.3390/ijms24097800.
19. Faroni A, Mobasseri SA, Kingham PJ, Reid AJ. Peripheral nerve regeneration: experimental strategies and future perspectives. Adv Drug Deliv Rev. 2015;82–83:160–7. https://doi.org/10.1016/j.addr.2014.11.010.
20. Pereira C, Lazar SV, Wang A. Bioengineering approaches for nerve graft revascularization: current concepts and future directions [published online ahead of print, 2023 Apr 27]. WIREs Mech Dis. 2023;15:e1609. https://doi.org/10.1002/wsbm.1609.
21. Supra R, Agrawal DK. Peripheral nerve regeneration: opportunities and challenges. J Spine Res Surg. 2023;5(1):10–8. https://doi.org/10.26502/fjsrs0052.

7 Proximal Intra-and Extra-Plexal Nerve Transfers

Heather Rossong, Suganth Suppiah, and Rajiv Midha

The brachial plexus consists of five spinal nerve roots, C5, C6, C7, C8, and T1, and is divided proximally to distally into spinal nerve roots, trunks, divisions, cords, and terminal branches [1]. When evaluating patients for potential proximal brachial plexus transfers, it is important to clarify what function has been affected in brachial plexus injury, which therefore guides what target nerve will be used. A careful and systematic motor and sensory clinical examination is fundamental, and each muscle is graded using the British MRC system. The workup of these patients includes nerve conduction studies and electromyograms to not only understand the site of injury and muscles that are affected but also to understand which nerve are fully preserved and are viable candidates to be used as a donor. Imaging, using thin section myelography and CT scan previously, and more recently high-resolution MRI, to evaluate for nerve root avulsion(s), is important.

The physiological rationale for nerve transfers is relatively straightforward, with recovery of motor function being the main goal. Therefore, any potential donor nerve must have a reasonable amount of motor fibers that can be spared and the loss of innervation to the donor muscle must not lead to significant decline in function. The optimal nerve transfer options would be where the value of the recipient muscle being innervated greatly exceeds the utility or the function of the sacrificed one. Furthermore, an ideal compromise would be to use only a portion of the nerve as a donor, thereby retaining innervation of the donor muscle as well, as exemplified by taking a distal accessory nerve (sparing more proximal branches to trapezius) as a donor to suprascapular or other nerve recipients. Another principle of nerve transfers is to use synergistic muscles that behave similarly in complex movements, such as agnostic donors and recipients, which permits higher rates of cortical readaptation and thereby functional recovery. As a result, it is important that these patients are evaluated in multidisciplinary clinics involving neurologists, physiatrists, neurosurgeons, and plastic surgeons, along with physiotherapists, to determine the ideal candidates for surgery and optimal nerve transfer options. Follow-up and instruction by a dedicated

H. Rossong
Division of Neurosurgery, University of Calgary Cumming School of Medicine, Calgary, AB, Canada
e-mail: heather.rossong1@ucalgary.ca

S. Suppiah
Division of Neurosurgery, University Health Network, University of Toronto, Toronto, ON, Canada
e-mail: suganth.suppiah@uhnresearch.ca

R. Midha (✉)
Department of Clinical Neurosciences, Hotchkiss Brain Institute, Cumming School of Medicine, University of Calgary, Calgary, AB, Canada
e-mail: rajiv.midha@albertahealthservices.ca

F. Guedes et al. (eds.), *Nerve Transfers for Brachial Plexus Reconstruction after Trauma*,
https://doi.org/10.1007/978-3-031-92445-3_7

physiotherapist is essential to allow relearning and achieve optimal outcomes.

Proximal brachial plexus nerve transfers are often used for restoring shoulder function and/or elbow function [2]. When approaching proximal brachial plexus nerve transfers, localizing anatomy is critical to determine the best exposure. This knowledge allows for an appropriately planned incision and approach: supraclavicular for spinal roots/trunks, mixed supra-and infraclavicular for divisions or infraclavicular for cords/terminal branches. The different techniques can then be divided into whether the donor nerve is intra-plexal and extra-plexal [3]. Table 7.1 outlines the various approaches, divided into whether they are intra-or extra-plexal donors, what function is being restored, and what the donor and recipient nerves are. Other chapters in this textbook cover each transfer in great detail. Herein, we summarize the main transfer strategies described in the literature.

In intra-plexal nerve transfers, one functioning plexal nerve (or a portion of it at times) is transferred to an injured plexal nerve [4]. When targeting shoulder function (i.e., abduction), it is recommended to transfer to both the axillary and the suprascapular nerves. Donors that may be used to transfer to the axillary nerve within the brachial plexus include the C4 nerve root, median nerve, ulnar nerve, long thoracic nerve, thoracodorsal nerve, and the nerve to one of the heads of triceps. One of the intra-plexal donors to the suprascapular nerve within the brachial plexus is the dorsal scapular nerve [5]. For targeting elbow flexion, the primary target is the musculocutaneous nerve. The Oberlin nerve transfer was popularized in 1994 and includes using a fascicle of the ulnar nerve to a branch of the biceps. Oberlin and Mackinnon independently described the double fascicular nerve transfer using part of the median nerve (dominant for wrist flexion) to the brachialis nerve [6–8]. The double fascicular transfer had initially shown promising functional outcomes in elbow flexion [2, 9], but subsequent prospective analysis questions if the double transfer is superior to the Oberlin transfer alone

Table 7.1 Various intra-and extra-plexal nerve transfer techniques for brachial plexus injuries following trauma for shoulder function and elbow flexion

Intra-plexal			
Shoulder function		Elbow flexion	
Donor	Recipient	Donor	Recipient
C4 root	Axillary	Ulnar	Branch of biceps
Median	Axillary	Median	Musculocutaneous
Ulnar	Axillary	Double transfer (ulnar and median)	Musculocutaneous
Long thoracic	Axillary	Medial pectoral	Musculocutaneous
Nerve to long head of triceps	Axillary	Long thoracic	Musculocutaneous
Thoracodorsal	Axillary	Thoracodorsal	Musculocutaneous
Dorsal scapular	Suprascapular	Contralateral C7	Musculocutaneous, radial, triceps brachii, median
Contralateral C7	Shoulder abductors		
Extra-plexal			
Shoulder function		Elbow flexion	
Donor	Recipient	Donor	Recipient
Intercostal	Axillary	Intercostal	Musculocutaneous
Phrenic	Axillary	Phrenic	Musculocutaneous
Accessory	Axillary	Accessory	Musculocutaneous
Accessory	Suprascapular		
Phrenic	Suprascapular		

[10]. Other donors that may be used within the brachial plexus include the medial pectoral nerve [11] and rarely the long thoracic nerve and the thoracodorsal nerve [12].

In extra-plexal brachial plexus nerve transfers, the functioning donor nerve is outside of the brachial plexus and is transferred to an injured plexal nerve [3]. This is commonly employed when there are multiple brachial plexus spinal nerve root injuries, especially pan-plexus injuries, wherein intra-plexal transfers are not available. Once again, the axillary and suprascapular nerves are the recipients when targeting shoulder function. Extra-plexal nerves that have been commonly used include the intercostal nerve, phrenic nerve, or accessory nerve. Recently other nerves such as the one to levator scapulae have been utilized as donors [13]. The phrenic and accessory nerves have been used with either the axillary or suprascapular nerves as the recipient. The intercostal nerve is uncommonly used to transfer to the axillary nerve. For elbow function, the intercostal nerve, phrenic nerve, and the accessory nerve have been transferred to the musculocutaneous nerve [14–19]. For elbow extension, phrenic and intercostal nerves have been successfully transferred to triceps nerve in complete avulsion injuries [20, 21]. In rare cases of global avulsion injury that includes severe injury to the ipsilateral accessory nerve, Bhandari has proposed the use of the contralateral accessory nerve for neurotization of the suprascapular nerve [22]. In turn, transfers from redundant plexal elements can be utilized for reanimation of the trapezius muscle when the proximal accessory nerve stump is unavailable, for example, in the use of the lateral pectoral nerve for the distal accessory (Fig. 7.1).

It is important to elaborate further regarding the use of the contralateral C7 nerve root for both shoulder and elbow function restoration [23]. The contralateral C7 root has approximately 420,000 nerve fibers; therefore there is small risk to function (mostly sensory deficit and some patients with C7 neuropathic pain) associated with harvesting this nerve and studies have shown

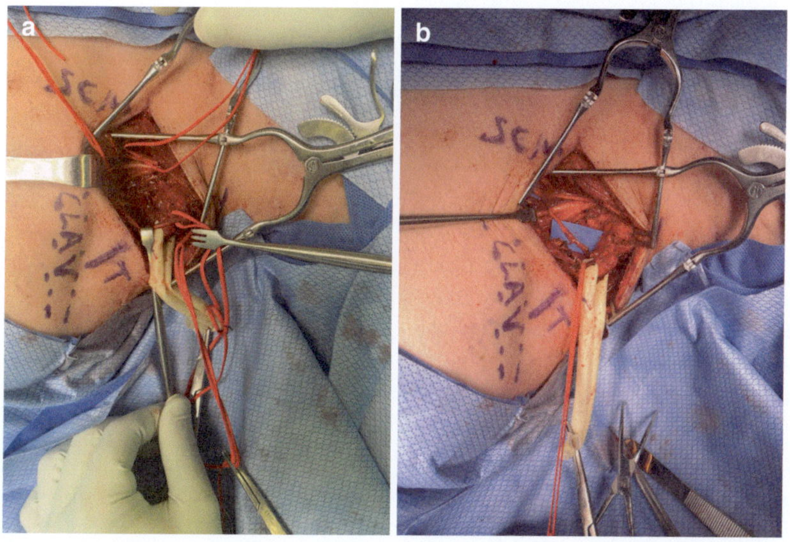

Fig. 7.1 This patient sustained a complex traumatic laceration of the proximal accessory nerve in the upper neck with complete loss of ipsilateral sternomastoid and trapezius muscle and presented 7 months after injury to our clinic. (**a**) The phrenic nerve (most medial vessel loop, near top of image), supraclavicular plexus, with its upper trunk and its anterior division exposed, with the lateral pectoral nerve identified (vessel loop just above clavicle and right angled retractor) and confirmed with stimulation. The accessory nerve was dissected away from scar and followed into the trapezius muscle (most lateral, lowest vessel loop). Surface representation markings on the skin: SCM, sternomastoid insertion; CLAV, clavicle; T, trapezius. (**b**) We used the lateral pectoral nerve as the donor with a direct end-end transfer to the distal accessory nerve

promising outcomes associated with the technique [24, 25]. This method is potentially indicated in global brachial plexus avulsion injuries that limits the amount of ipsilateral donor nerves that could be used. The contralateral C7 nerve may be transferred to the shoulder abductors and musculocutaneous, median, radial, and triceps brachii nerves [26, 27]. One of the main drawbacks is that independent arm function is rarely obtained so that the patient must initially consciously (and in time subconsciously) actively contract the donor limb muscles (triceps and pectoralis) to activate the reinnervated muscles in the recipient arm.

The use of intra-plexal transfers from C5 and/or C6 spinal nerve roots to the lower trunk to prioritize recovery of hand function in neonatal brachial plexus palsy has become well established. In adults, intra-plexal transfers have more recently been used in an attempt to reinnervate distal hand function (finger flexion), as with the innovative use of residual spinal nerve roots in near-complete avulsion injury by Wang and colleagues [28]. The same authors have performed "heroic" (extra-plexal) nerve transfer surgeries in complete avulsion injuries, with a paradigm combining contralateral C7 and ipsilateral phrenic and accessory nerve, along with deliberate limb shortening (to allow direct coaptation) in an attempt to reanimate the entire upper arm, with modest results reported [29–32].

The senior author's preferred approach for proximal plexus injuries is to explore the supraclavicular brachial plexus in all cases to assess for nerve continuity and testing for electrophysiological function. If the proximal spinal nerve roots are viable and surgery is within 6 months of injury, then intra-plexal nerve grafts are performed. If grafts are not performed or contraindicated and transfers are required, he prefers using distal accessory to suprascapular and a triceps fascicle to one of the divisions of the axillary nerve to reanimate the shoulder. A standard Oberlin transfer is done, with an ulnar nerve fascicle to biceps nerve branch to restore elbow function in all cases including ones where a proximal intra-plexal graft repair is done to maximize opportunity for elbow flexion recovery. For C5/6 and C5–7 palsies, the above triple transfer is standard. In complete loss of C7 function, we consider a double fascicular transfer for restoring elbow flexion. In pan-plexus injuries, we always carefully assess the C5 spinal root for viability and if viable lead grafts from it to upper trunk recipients. In addition, a distal accessory to suprascapular transfer is performed. For elbow flexion, three intercostal nerves are used to transfer to musculocutaneous nerve with direct coaptation and two intercostals to the long head of triceps. Sensory branches of intercostals are coapted to the lateral cord contribution to median nerve to bestow protective sensibility to the hand. We prefer not to use the phrenic nerve as a donor as our patients have high pulmonary morbidity from its use. We do not attempt contralateral C7 transfers in adult patients. In the rare adult patient with lower trunk palsies and avulsion of C8 and T1 spinal nerve roots, we perform distal transfers to regain finger extension (supinator to posterior interosseous nerve) and thumb index pinch (brachialis or more recently one branch of extensor carpi radialis brevis to anterior interosseous nerve) function.

References

1. Polcaro L, Charlick M, Daly DT. Anatomy, Head and Neck: Brachial Plexus. [Updated 2022 Aug 22]. In: StatPearls [Internet]. Treasure Island, FL: StatPearls Publishing; 2023. https://www.ncbi.nlm.nih.gov/books/NBK531473/.
2. Venkatramani H, Bhardwaj P, Faruquee SR, Sabapathy SR. Functional outcome of nerve transfer for restoration of shoulder and elbow function in upper brachial plexus injury. J Brachial Plex Peripher Nerve Inj. 2008;3:15. https://doi.org/10.1186/1749-7221-3-15. PMID: 18505571; PMCID: PMC2432056.
3. Addas BM, Midha R. Nerve transfers for severe nerve injury. Neurosurg Clin N Am. 2009;20:27–38.
4. Leechavengvongs S. Intraplexal nerve transfers. BMC Proc. 2015;9(Suppl 3):A27. https://doi.org/10.1186/1753-6561-9-S3-A27. PMCID: PMC4445334.
5. Augustine HFM, Coroneos CJ, Choi M, Bain JR. Adjunctive dorsal scapular nerve transfer to suprascapular nerve for brachial plexus birth injuries: case series. J Hand Surg Am. 2019;44(10):902.e1–9. https://doi.org/10.1016/j.jhsa.2018.12.008. Epub 2019 Feb 6.

6. Oberlin C, Béal D, Leechavengvongs S, Salon A, Dauge MC, Sarcy JJ. Nerve transfer to biceps muscle using a part of ulnar nerve for C5-C6 avulsion of the brachial plexus: anatomical study and report of four cases. J Hand Surg Am. 1994;19(2):232–7. https://doi.org/10.1016/0363-5023(94)90011-6.
7. Liverneaux PA, Diaz LC, Beaulieu JY, Durand S, Oberlin C. Preliminary results of double nerve transfer to restore elbow flexion in upper type brachial plexus palsies. Plast Reconstr Surg. 2006;117:915.
8. Mackinnon SE, Novak CB, Myckatyn TM, Tung TH. Results of reinnervation of the biceps and brachialis muscles with a double fascicular transfer for elbow flexion. J Hand Surg Am. 2005;30(5):978–85. https://doi.org/10.1016/j.jhsa.2005.05.014.
9. Goubier JN, Teboul F. Technique of the double nerve transfer to recover elbow flexion in C5, C6, or C5 to C7 brachial plexus palsy. Tech Hand Up Extrem Surg. 2007;11(1):15–7. https://doi.org/10.1097/01.bth.0000248360.14448.6b.
10. Martins RS, Siqueira MG, Heise CO, Foroni L, Teixeira MJ. A prospective study comparing single and double fascicular transfer to restore elbow flexion after brachial plexus injury. Neurosurgery. 2013;72(5):709–14. discussion 714-5; quiz 715. https://doi.org/10.1227/NEU.0b013e318285c3f6.
11. Brandt KE, Mackinnon SE. A technique for maximizing biceps recovery in brachial plexus reconstruction. J Hand Surg Am. 1993 Jul;18(4):726–33. https://doi.org/10.1016/0363-5023(93)90328-Z.
12. Midha R, Grochmal J. Surgery for nerve injury: current and future perspectives. J Neurosurg. 2019;130(3):675–85. https://doi.org/10.3171/2018.11.JNS181520.
13. Martins RS, Siqueira MG, Heise CO, Foroni L, Neto HS, Teixeira MJ. The nerve to the levator scapulae muscle as donor in brachial plexus surgery: an anatomical study and case series. J Neurosurg. 2021;135:1–8. https://doi.org/10.3171/2020.8.JNS201216.
14. Songcharoen P, Mahaisavariya B, Chotigavanich C. Spinal accessory neurotization for restoration of elbow flexion in avulsion injuries of the brachial plexus. J Hand Surg Am. 1996 May;21(3):387–90. https://doi.org/10.1016/S0363-5023(96)80349-2.
15. Nagano A, Yamamoto S, Mikami Y. Intercostal nerve transfer to restore upper extremity functions after brachial plexus injury. Ann Acad Med. 1995;24:42–5.
16. Ogino T, Naito T. Intercostal nerve crossing to restore elbow flexion and sensibility of the hand for a root avulsion type of brachial plexus injury. Microsurgery. 1995;16:571–7.
17. Gu YD, Wu MM, Zhen YL, Zhao JA, Zhang GM, Chen DS, Yan JQ, Cheng XM. Phrenic nerve transfer for treatment of root avulsion of the brachial plexus. Chin Med J. 1990;103(4):267–70.
18. Nagano A, Ochiai N, Okinaga S. Restoration of elbow flexion in root lesions of brachial plexus injuries. J Hand Surg Am. 1992;17(5):815–21. https://doi.org/10.1016/0363-5023(92)90450-4.
19. Pengked K, Laohaprasitiporn P, Monteerarat Y, Limthongthang R, Vathana T. Effect of shorter nerve graft and selective motor branch of recipient nerve on nerve transfer surgery for elbow flexion in patients with brachial plexus injury. J Neurosurg. 2023;139:1–7. https://doi.org/10.3171/2023.1.JNS222836. Epub ahead of print
20. Flores LP, Socolovsky M. Phrenic nerve transfer for reconstruction of elbow extension in severe brachial plexus injuries. J Reconstr Microsurg. 2016;32(7):546–50. https://doi.org/10.1055/s--0036-1583302. Epub 2016 May 4.
21. Goubier JN, Teboul F, Khalifa H. Reanimation of elbow extension with intercostal nerves transfers in total brachial plexus palsies. Microsurgery. 2011;31(1):7–11. https://doi.org/10.1002/micr.20822. Epub 2010 Nov 28.
22. Bhandari PS, Deb P. Use of contralateral spinal accessory nerve for ipsilateral suprascapular neurotization in global brachial plexus injury: a new technique. J Neurosurg Spine. 2016;24(1):186–8. https://doi.org/10.3171/2015.4.SPINE15108. Epub 2015 Sep 25.PMID: 26407088.
23. Gu YD, Zhang GM, Chen DS, Yan JG, Cheng XM, Chen L. Seventh cervical nerve root transfer from the contralateral healthy side for treatment of brachial plexus root avulsion. J Hand Surg Br. 1992;6(5):518–21. https://doi.org/10.1016/S0266-7681(05)80235-9.
24. Kim DH, Cho YJ, Tiel RL, Kline DG. Outcomes of surgery in 1019 brachial plexus lesions treated at Louisiana State University health sciences Center. J Neurosurg. 2003;98:1005–16.
25. Sun G, Wu Z, Wang X, Tan X, Gu Y. Nerve transfer helps repair brachial plexus injury by increasing cerebral cortical plasticity. Neural Regen Res. 2014;9(23):2111–4. https://doi.org/10.4103/1673-5374.147939. PMID: 25657729; PMCID: PMC4316477.
26. Xu WD, Gu YD. 30 years for contralateral C7 transfer (in Chinese). Chin J Hand Surg. 2016;32:247–9. https://doi.org/10.3760/cma.j.issn.1005-054X.2016.04.004.
27. Li WJ, He LY, Chen SL, Lyu YW, Wang SF, Yong Y, Tian W, Tian GL, Gu YD. Contralateral C7 nerve root transfer for function recovery in adults: a meta-analysis. Chin Med J. 2017;130(24):2960–8. https://doi.org/10.4103/0366-6999.220316. PMID: 29237929; PMCID: PMC5742924.
28. Wang SF, Li PC, Xue YH, Li F, Berger AJ, Bhatia A. Direct repair of the lower trunk to residual nerve roots for restoration of finger flexion after Total brachial plexus injury. J Hand Surg Am. 2021;46(5):423.e1–8. https://doi.org/10.1016/j.jhsa.2020.09.023. Epub 2020 Dec 14.
29. Wang SF, Xue YH. Contralateral C7 nerve transfer with direct Coaptation to restore lower trunk function after traumatic brachial plexus avulsion injuries: surgical technique. JBJS Essent Surg Tech. 2014;4(1):e5. https://doi.org/10.2106/JBJS.ST.M.00027. PMID: 30775112; PMCID: PMC6355036.

30. Wang SF, Li PC, Xue YH, Yiu HW, Li YC, Wang HH. Contralateral C7 nerve transfer with direct coaptation to restore lower trunk function after traumatic brachial plexus avulsion. J Bone Joint Surg Am. 2013;95(9):821–7, S1–2. https://doi.org/10.2106/JBJS.L.00039.
31. Wang SF, Li PC, Xue YH, Zou JY, Li WJ, Li Y. Direct Coaptation of the phrenic nerve with the posterior division of the lower trunk to restore finger and elbow extension function in patients with Total brachial plexus injuries. Neurosurgery. 2016;78(2):208–15. https://doi.org/10.1227/NEU.0000000000001008.
32. Li F, Wang SF, Li PC, Xue YH, Zou JY, Li WJ. Restoration of active pick-up function in patients with total brachial plexus avulsion injuries. J Hand Surg Eur. 2018;43(3):269–74. https://doi.org/10.1177/1753193417728405. Epub 2017 Sep 5.

Part II

Nerve Transfers for Restoration of Shoulder Function

Direct Nerve Transfer from the Upper Trunk to the Spinal Nerve

8

Belkheyar Zoubir, Cambon Adeline, and Oberlin Christophe

8.1 Principle of the Transfer

SAN lesions are mostly iatrogenic and consecutive to a lymph node biopsy in the posterior triangle of the neck [1]. The SAN transection leads to palsy of the sternocleidomastoid muscle and the trapezius muscle. Paralysis of the trapezius muscle alters scapula kinematics, with excessive lateral translation and various degrees of winging of the scapula [2]. In those patients, a sudden swing movement occurs when shoulder elevation reaches 90° [3]. Patients complain of shoulder pain and weak shoulder abduction. Diagnosis is frequently delayed because of late presentation of patients and insufficient awareness of this complication. In the complete loss of trapezius function for at least 2 months, with denervation on electromyography but remaining fibrillation potentials in the trapezius muscle at rest, exploration of the nerve is recommended [4]. A nerve graft is required when a direct suture is not possible. However, identification of the nerve in the scar tissue in the supraclavicular area is often difficult [4], time-consuming [5], and impossible in up to 25% of patients with a retracted proximal stump [6].

We proposed a direct transfer using a fascicle from the posterior division of the upper trunk to reinnervate the spinal accessory nerve [7] (Fig. 8.1). This technique has several advantages: dissection is conducted in healthy tissues and a tensionless suture is always possible. The donor fascicle is a pure motor nerve, with huge amount of axons, similar in diameter with the recipient nerve, and close to the effector end plates. Alternative donor nerves for transfer on the spinal accessory nerve were reported with grade 4 BMRC strength: a fascicule from the upper trunk related to the axillary nerve [8], or one fascicule of the C7 root dedicated to the pectoralis major muscle [9].

B. Zoubir · O. Christophe
Clinique du Mont Louis, Paris, France

C. Adeline (✉)
Orthopaedic and Traumatology Surgery Department, Sorbonne University, Saint-Antoine Hospital, Paris, France

F. Guedes et al. (eds.), *Nerve Transfers for Brachial Plexus Reconstruction after Trauma*,
https://doi.org/10.1007/978-3-031-92445-3_8

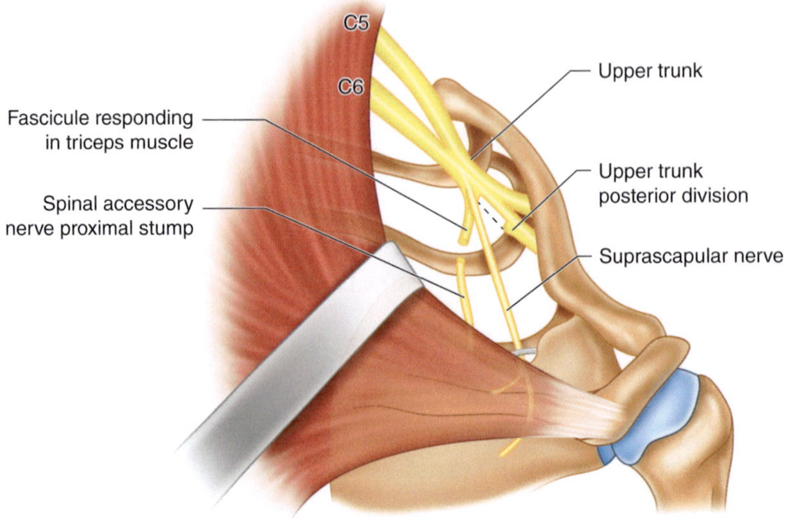

Fig. 8.1 Surgical technique of the transfer of a fascicule from the upper trunk posterior division to the spinal accessory nerve

8.2 Operative Technique

Surgery is performed under general anesthesia in the supine position, with the patient's head turned to the contralateral side. The SAN is identified through a V-shaped supraclavicular approach at the upper edge of the trapezius muscle, before its entry into the muscle belly. This area is usually free of scarring from previous surgery. Retrograde dissection is conducted to the distal stump. If the nerve is found in continuity, intraoperative electrostimulation is performed in search of trapezius muscle contraction. In its absence, the posterior division of the upper trunk is identified. Intraneural dissection is conducted under microscope magnification and using neurostimulation in order to select a fascicle dedicated to the triceps muscle or to the deltoid, with the same diameter as the spinal accessory nerve stump. A direct tensionless epiperineural suture is then performed with 10-0 nylon suture and fibrin glue. Postoperatively, the patient is immobilized for 3 weeks in an arm-to-body sling with the elbow in 90° of flexion, and then active and passive rehabilitation begins.

8.3 Expected Outcomes

In our experience, clinical signs of trapezius reinnervation may be visible on manual testing after a minimum of 9 months. In our published short series, active shoulder abduction improved significantly compared to preoperative values at final follow-up (Fig. 8.2). Active shoulder abduction reached 151° on average (90–180°) in the 11 patients, which represented 84% of the contralateral side, and trapezius muscle strength grade was M5 or M4 in ten cases, M3 in one case. Scapula was considered stable in seven cases. In patients with remaining unstable scapula, we observed that patients had recovered only the descending part of the trapezius muscle. We did not observe postoperative loss of strength in the deltoid or the triceps muscle, which is probably related to the fact that the donor nerve is not a terminal branch. Since then, this procedure is our favorite technique to deal with SAN lesions.

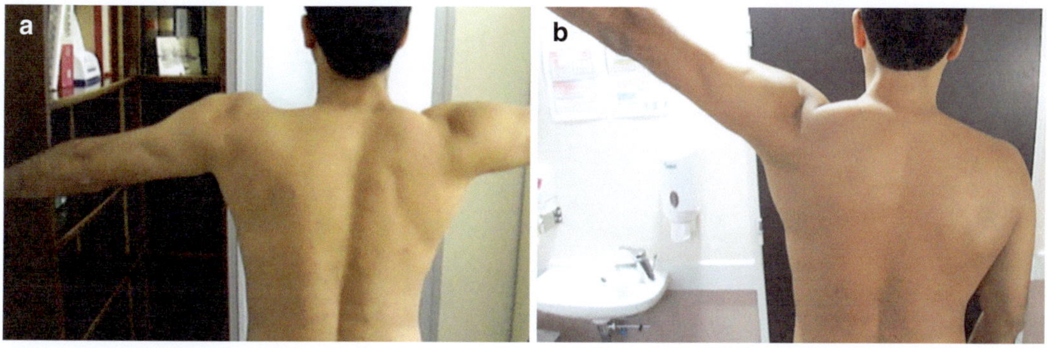

Fig. 8.2 Injury of the spinal accessory nerve after a cervical node biopsy in a 29-year-old man (**a**). On examination 53 months after the nerve transfer, shoulder abduction strength score was M4+, active shoulder abduction improved by 45°, and scapula was stable (**b**)

References

1. Boström D, Dahlin LB. Iatrogenic injury to the accessory nerve. Scand J Plast Reconstr Surg Hand Surg. 2007;41(2):82–7.
2. Bertelli JA, Ghizoni MF. Refinements in the technique for repair of the accessory nerve. J Hand Surg Am. 2006;31(8):1401–6.
3. Roren A, Fayad F, Poiraudeau S, Fermanian J, Revel M, Dumitrache A, Gautheron V, Roby-Brami A, Lefevre-Colau MM. Specific scapular kinematic patterns to differentiate two forms of dynamic scapular winging. Clin Biomech. 2013;28(8):941–7.
4. Kim DH, Cho YJ, Tiel RL, Kline DG. Surgical outcomes of 111 spinal accessory nerve injuries. Neurosurgery. 2003;53(5):1106–12.
5. Vastamäki M, Solonen KA. Accessory nerve injury. Acta Orthop Scand. 1984;55(3):296–9.
6. Alnot JY, Aboujaoude J, Oberlin C. Les lésions traumatiques du nerf spinal accessoire (n. accessorius). II: Etude clinique et résultats d'une série de 25 cas. Rev Chir Orthop Reparatrice Appar Mot. 1994;80:297–304.
7. Cambon-Binder A, Preure L, Dubert-Khalifa H, Marcheix PS, Belkheyar Z. Spinal accessory nerve repair using a direct nerve transfer from the upper trunk: results with 2 years follow-up. J Hand Surg Eur. 2018;43(6):589–95.
8. Mayer JA, Hruby LA, Salminger S, Bodner G, Aszmann OC. Reconstruction of the spinal accessory nerve with selective fascicular nerve transfer of the upper trunk. J Neurosurg Spine. 2019;31(1):133–8.
9. Goubier JN, Teboul F. Partial transfer from C7 root to external branch of accessory nerve for trapezius palsy. Hand Surg Rehabil. 2016;35(6):418–9.

Spinal Accessory to Axillary Nerve Transfer

9

Lukas Rasulic and Miroslav Samardžić

Abbreviations

AXN Axillary nerve
BP Brachial plexus
SAN Spinal accessory nerve

9.1 Introduction

In 1913, the American surgeon Tuttle introduced brachial plexus (BP) reinnervation with the spinal accessory nerve (SAN). In 1972, Kotani et al. used this nerve for the first time in the reinnervation of the upper trunk, the radial, or the musculocutaneous nerve, because of its close relation to the BP in its supraclavicular part. Imperfections and the unsatisfactory results of intercostobrachial anastomosis were the reasons for the introduction of SAN reinnervation in cases with upper and especially complete BP palsy following root avulsion. Direct anastomosis with the spinal nerves, C5 and C6 nerve roots, the upper trunk, and the suprascapular nerve, as well as indirect anastomosis with the radial nerve was later abandoned [1–3].

Restoration of shoulder function is somewhat controversial. Several authors recommended reinnervation of the suprascapular nerve since the supra-and infraspinatus muscles are important for the initiation of the arm abduction and some external rotation, and they reported good results for both functions [4–7]. On the contrary, other studies have demonstrated that paralyzed supraspinatus does not impede shoulder abduction. Accordingly, some others concluded that reinnervation of the shoulder function following the suprascapular nerve neurotization is not a promising option. In a significant number of our cases, we obtained good arm abduction and some external rotation reinnervating only the axillary nerve (AXN) [8–11]. This could be explained by reinnervation of the teres minor muscle and posterior part of the deltoid muscle that act as shoulder external rotators. Furthermore, the reinnervated biceps muscle contributes to shoulder stability through its long head and produces some external rotation. Probably, the best solution could be dual nerve transfer to both nerves although some research demonstrated similar strength of shoulder function after a single AXN transfer. However, the first muscle to be reinnervated attracts a majority of axons and in this case, the supraspinatus reduces the potential for reinnervation of the external rotator, the infraspinatus muscle [1, 10, 12, 13].

In some cases it is indicated to combine the donors, disregarding the opinion that if two

The original version of the chapter has been revised. A correction to this chapter can be found at https://doi.org/10.1007/978-3-031-92445-3_31

L. Rasulic (✉) · M. Samardžić
Faculty of Medicine, University of Belgrade, Belgrade, Serbia

Department of Peripheral Nerve Surgery, Functional Neurosurgery and Pain Management Surgery, Clinic for Neurosurgery, University Clinical Centre of Serbia, Belgrade, Serbia

F. Guedes et al. (eds.), *Nerve Transfers for Brachial Plexus Reconstruction after Trauma*,
https://doi.org/10.1007/978-3-031-92445-3_9

different nerves reinnervate the same muscle only one will ultimately function. The reason is anastomosis close to the end organs where the focalization of the nerve fibers for innervation of different muscles of their functional parts is located [3].

This chapter aims to present the author's experience concerning AN reinnervation using SAN as the donor, complemented by the literature review results. The surgical procedure, general considerations, and outcomes are discussed, as well as the advantages and disadvantages of the procedure.

9.2 General Considerations

The AXN contains between 4.967 and 8.437 myelinated fibers, with an average of 7.877, out of which 80% are motor. Number of the motor fibers in the anterior branch of the AXN ranges from 2.700 to 4.052 [14–19].

The SAN is a motor nerve with very few sensory fibers [1]. The number of motor fibers ranges from 1700 to 3000, with a mean value of about 2000 [3, 20]. The average diameter of the SAN is about 3 mm with an oligofascicular pattern, especially in its distal part.

9.2.1 Reasons for the Use of SAN as a Donor in BP Palsy Reinnervation

1. It originates from the C1 to C4 levels of the spinal cord.
2. There is a close relationship with BP.
3. Additional palsy of the trapezius muscle does not essentially alter the total functional deficit of the shoulder in a spinal root avulsion.
4. The function of the trapezius muscle, especially that of its distal part, which is important for the abduction of the shoulder blade and elevation of the arm over the horizontal plane, may be partially preserved, due to independent innervation from the C3 spinal nerve with an average of 740 motor fibers.
5. The SAN can be used without complete denervation of the trapezius muscle if it is transected distally to its branches. This is important in cases when the trapezius muscle does not receive independent innervation from the cervical plexus.
6. Trapezius muscle palsy may be sometimes compensated by the levator scapulae and the anterior serratus muscle. In cases of the trapezius and anterior serratus muscle palsy, the arm can be abducted 50″ to 70″ with considerable effort and winging of the scapula.
7. Finally, we must keep in mind that an active abduction of the arm is usually below the horizontal plane after reinnervation of the deltoid muscle [3, 16, 21, 22].

9.2.2 Advantages and Disadvantages of the Procedure

The advantages of this method compared to the other techniques of AXN reinnervation using extraplexal donors, such as the intercostal nerves, include a larger diameter of the nerve, three to four times greater number of motor fibers, and insignificant axonal mixing because the SAN is a motor nerve. A main disadvantage of this technique is the use of 7-to 20-cm-long cutaneous nerve grafts [3, 16].

9.3 Surgical Procedure

9.3.1 Approach to the SAN and Preparation of the Donor Branch

The SAN is approached in the lateral triangle of the neck, through a supraclavicular exploration of the BP (Figs. 9.1 and 9.2). The nerve enters this region at the posterior border of the sternocleidomastoid muscle, most often around 8 cm cranial to the clavicle, after which it takes a downward and backward course entering the

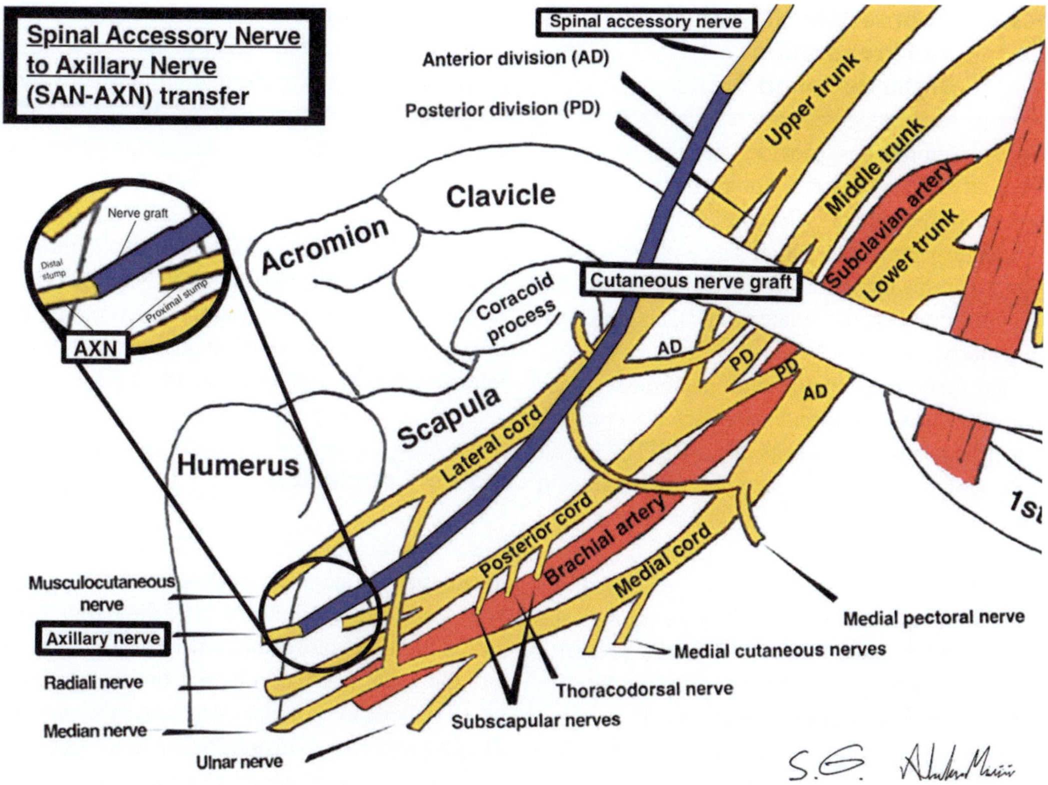

Fig. 9.1 Spinal accessory (SAN) to axillary (AXN) nerve transfer via the anterior approach (schematic illustration). With courtesy of Aleksa Mićić MD (University of Belgrade, Faculty of Medicine, Belgrade, Serbia) and Strahinja Gligorijević MSc (University of Belgrade, Faculty of Biology, Belgrade, Serbia)

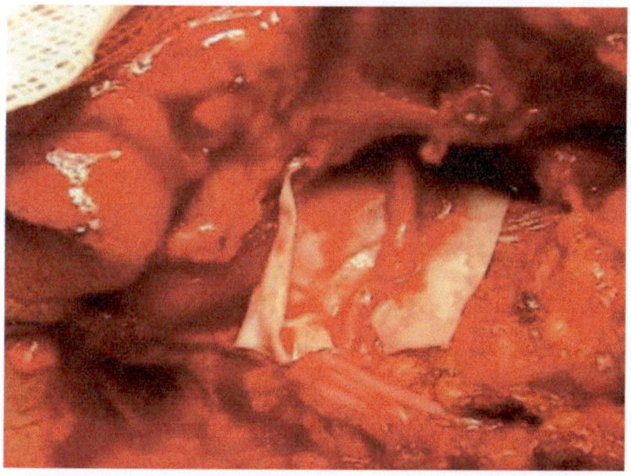

Fig. 9.2 Spinal accessory (SAN) to axillary (AXN) nerve transfer via the anterior approach (intraoperative photo)

trapezoid muscle at its deep surface, about 2 cm above the clavicle. The SAN gives two or three collateral branches before entering the muscle [19, 20].

During the procedure, a total palsy of the trapezius muscle must be avoided. In most cases, the SAN is sectioned distally with the preservation of its collateral branches. A distal section of the nerve gives only a part of the nerve fibers for reinnervation, but it partially spares the function of the trapezius muscle. The collateral branches can also be used for the reinnervation. The principle of distal exploration was also applied in cases of anastomosis with the AXN, with retrograde neurolysis [3, 23].

9.3.2 Approach to the AXN and Preparation of the Recipient Branch

Several approaches provide AXN exploration. The advantage of the anterior deltopectoral approach over others is the availability to explore proximal parts of the nerve. The anatomical key points for this approach are the cephalic vein, the clavipectoral fascia, the lateral cord, and the axillary artery.

The pectoralis major and pectoralis minor muscles must be cut and/or retracted to present the infraclavicular elements of the BP. The lateral cord and the axillary artery must be retracted medially to enable access to the posterior cord and AXN. The AXN exits the posterior cord at the level of the lower border of the pectoralis minor, curves backward, and passes through the quadrangular space together with the posterior circumflex humeral artery, where it divides into anterior and posterior branches [20–22].

9.3.3 Reinnervation of the AXN

The SAN to AXN transfer is performed indirectly, usually using 12–15-cm-long cutaneous nerve grafts. Depending on the diameters of the SAN and the nerve graft, up to two grafts are placed subcutaneously [3, 20, 24, 25]. A few epineurial sutures combined with a fibrin glue provide stability of the suture line without tension.

Due to the larger amount of motor fibers, and no sensitive fibers that could cause axonal mixing, the anterior branch of the AXN has a priority in reinnervation compared to the posterior [20, 26].

9.4 Outcomes

A useful motor recovery (MRC grade 3 or higher) was achieved in 60–70% of cases following SAN to AXN transfer. However, because of its importance for the scapular motions, it should not be considered particularly expendable [27, 28]. In many cases, a good arm abduction and some external rotation can be achieved, which could be explained by a reinnervation of the teres minor and posterior fibers of the deltoid muscle, which act as shoulder external rotators. In addition, the reinnervated biceps brachii muscle contributes to shoulder stability through its long head and produces some external rotation [12].

The best results are achieved with a combined use of donors, especially using the medial pectoral nerve. However, we cannot be sure whether this is the result of combined reinnervation or reinnervation by one nerve [3, 29].

9.5 Conclusion

The AXN reinnervation using SAN as a donor is a valuable technique in treatment of the patients with complete BP injuries following root avulsion. Due to its close anatomical origin with the BP, the SAN has the potential to address functional deficits in shoulder abduction even in cases of complete root avulsion, being more effective than the intercostal nerves and safer to use compared to the phrenic nerve.

Acknowledgments The first author would like to express his gratitude to his Ph.D. student, Aleksa Mićić, for his contribution to the preparation of this chapter.

References

1. Narakas AO. Thoughts on neurotization or nerve transfers in irreparable nerve lesions. Clin Plast Surg. 1984;11(1):153–9.
2. Kotani T. Trial surgical procedures of nerve transfer to avulsion injuries of plexus brachialis. Orthopaed Surg Traumatol. 1972;1972:348–50.
3. Samardzic M, Grujicic D, Antunovic V, Joksimovic M. Reinnervation of avulsed brachial plexus using the spinal accessory nerve. Surg Neurol. 1990;33(1):7–11.
4. Terzis JK, Kostas I. Suprascapular nerve reconstruction in 118 cases of adult posttraumatic brachial plexus. Plast Reconstr Surg. 2006;117(2):613–29.
5. Bertelli JA, Ghizoni MF. Transfer of the accessory nerve to the suprascapular nerve in brachial plexus reconstruction. J Hand Surg Am. 2007;32(7):989–98.
6. Suzuki K, Doi K, Hattori Y, Pagsaligan JM. Long-term results of spinal accessory nerve transfer to the suprascapular nerve in upper-type

paralysis of brachial plexus injury. J Reconstr Microsurg. 2007;23(06):295–9.
7. Malessy MJ, Thomeer RT, van Dijk JG. Changing central nervous system control following intercostal nerve transfer. J Neurosurg. 1998;89(4):568–74.
8. Howell SM, Imobersteg AM, Seger DH, Marone PJ. Clarification of the role of the supraspinatus muscle in shoulder function. J Bone Joint Surg Am. 1986;68(3):398–404.
9. Samardzic M, Grujicic D, Rasulic L, Bacetic D. Transfer of the medial pectoral nerve: myth or reality? Neurosurgery. 2002;50(6):1277–82.
10. Samardzic M, Rasulic LG, Grujicic DM, Bacetic DT, Milicic BR. Nerve transfers using collateral branches of the brachial plexus as donors in patients with upper palsy—thirty years' experience. Acta Neurochir. 2011;153:2009–19.
11. Samardzic MM, Grujicic DM, Rasulic LG, Milicic BR. The use of thoracodorsal nerve transfer in restoration of irreparable C5 and C6 spinal nerve lesions. Br J Plast Surg. 2005;58(4):541–6.
12. Narakas A, Hentz V. Neurotization in brachial plexus injuries: indication and results. Clin Orthop Relat Res. 1988;237:43–56.
13. Samardžić M, Rasulić L, Stanković L. Motor nerve transfers for restoration of upper arm function in adult brachial plexus injuries: basics, advantages, problems and strategies. Neurohirurgija Serbian J Neurosurg. 2022;1(1):9–16.
14. Bonnel F. Microscopic anatomy of the adult human brachial plexus: an anatomical and histological basis for microsurgery. Microsurgery. 1984;5(3):107–18.
15. Bonnel F, Rabischong P. Anatomie et systématisation du plexus brachial de l'adulte. Anat Clin. 1980;2(3):289–98.
16. Leechavengvongs S, Witoonchart K, Uerpairojkit C, Thuvasethakul P. Nerve transfer to deltoid muscle using the nerve to the long head of the triceps, part II: a report of 7 cases. J Hand Surg Am. 2003;28(4):633–8.
17. Samardzić M, Rasulić L, Grujicić D, Milicić B. Results of nerve transfers to the musculocutaneous and axillary nerves. Neurosurgery. 2000;46(1):93–101; discussion −3.
18. Mackinnon SE, Colbert SH. Nerve transfers in the hand and upper extremity surgery. Tech Hand Up Extrem Surg. 2008;12(1):20–33.
19. Nath RK, Mackinnon SE. Nerve transfers in the upper extremity. Hand Clin. 2000;16(1):131–9. ix
20. Samardzic M, Antunovic V, Joksimovic M, Bacetic D. Donor nerves in the reinnervation of brachial plexus. Neurol Res. 1986;8(2):117–22.
21. Brunelli G, Monini L. Neurotization of avulsed roots of brachial plexus by means of anterior nerves of cervical plexus. Clin Plast Surg. 1984;11(1):149–52.
22. Millesi H. Brachial plexus injuries. Management and results. Clin Plast Surg. 1984;11(1):115–20.
23. Millesi. Indications et traitement des lesions nerveuses. Rev Chir Orthop. 1977;63:82–7.
24. Narakas A. Surgical treatment of traction injuries of the brachial plexus. Clin Orthop Relat Res. 1978;133:71–90.
25. Samardžić M, , Rasulić L, , Stanković L,. Motor nerve transfers for restoration of upper arm function in adult brachial plexus injuries—basics, advantages, problems and strategies. Neurohirurgija Serbian J Neurosurg 2022 1:9–16.
26. Stecco C, Gagliano G, Lancerotto L, Tiengo C, Macchi V, Porzionato A, et al. Surgical anatomy of the axillary nerve and its implication in the transdeltoid approaches to the shoulder. J Shoulder Elb Surg. 2010;19(8):1166–74.
27. Tsuyama N. Reconstructive surgery for traumatic brachial plexus injuries. Clin Orthop. 1968;3:675–87.
28. Gu YD, Zhang GM, Chen DS, Yan JG, Cheng XM, Chen L. Seventh cervical nerve root transfer from the contralateral healthy side for treatment of brachial plexus root avulsion. J Hand Surg Br. 1992;17(5):518–21.
29. Leechavengvongs S, Witoonchart K, Uerpairojkit C, Thuvasethakul P, Malungpaishrope K. Combined nerve transfers for C5 and C6 brachial plexus avulsion injury. J Hand Surg Am. 2006;31(2):183–9.

Triceps Branch of the Radial Nerve to the Anterior Branch of the Axillary Nerve Transfer for Shoulder Abduction

10

Ellen Y. Lee and Alexander Y. Shin

10.1 Background

The radial to axillary nerve transfer dates to 1948 when Lurje described transferring two triceps radial nerve branches to the axillary nerve as part of his reconstruction for a 20-year-old female with an Erb's type palsy of 8-month duration [1]. He noted weakness of the triceps at 2 months after surgery, which improved with time. The patient recovered 35 degrees of shoulder abduction 14 months after surgery. Successful transfer of the superficial fascicular group supplying the triceps to the superolateral half of the axillary nerve was described in four patients by Nath and Mackinnon in 2000 [2]. In 2003, Leechavengvongs et al. published the long head of triceps branch of the radial nerve transfer to anterior branch of the axillary nerve [3, 4]. This transfer, with its modifications [5–7], has become an established method for reconstructing shoulder abduction in brachial plexus injuries (BPI). It is widely used to restore shoulder abduction in C5,6 or upper trunk injuries and isolated axillary nerve injuries.

E. Y. Lee (✉)
Department of Hand and Reconstructive Microsurgery, National University Health System, Singapore, Singapore

A. Y. Shin
Mayo Clinic Brachial Plexus Clinic, Departments of Orthopedics and Neurosurgery, Rochester, MN, USA
e-mail: shin.alexander@mayo.edu

The triceps is a multicompartment muscle with redundant motor nerve branches [8] and acts synergistically with the deltoid in extending the shoulder. Compared to other antagonistic donor nerves like medial pectoral or thoracodorsal nerves, the triceps' synergistic action facilitates postoperative rehabilitation. The nerve to the long head of the triceps is the first branch of the radial nerve and is the closest to the deltoid muscle [3]. It was the electromyographically least-involved muscle compartment in elbow extension [9], thus chosen over other triceps branches to limit donor morbidity. Transferring to the axillary nerve's anterior division directs the axons into the anterior and middle deltoid muscle and, in 57.5% of cases, the posterior deltoid muscle as well [10]. The anterior division as a target avoids regeneration into teres minor and superior lateral brachial cutaneous nerve.

10.2 Preoperative Assessments

Clinical examination of BPI patients should specifically test for triceps strength before performing this transfer. Patients should have at least British Medical Research Council (MRC) grade 4 elbow extension. This is tested by supporting their shoulder abducted more than 90 degrees and asking them to extend their elbow overhead against gravity. The active range of elbow extension motion should be the same as the passive

F. Guedes et al. (eds.), *Nerve Transfers for Brachial Plexus Reconstruction after Trauma*,
https://doi.org/10.1007/978-3-031-92445-3_10

range, and they should be able to hold their elbow extended against resistance without locking the joint in extension. In situations where patients have recovered triceps function, which was previously absent, preoperative electromyography (EMG) contributes to the decision to use as a donor. Improved shoulder abduction strength and motion were reported in patients with triceps EMG findings of full or decreased motor unit recruitment compared to donor muscles with discrete motor unit recruitment [11].

10.3 Surgical Technique

Our preferred technique is as originally described [4]. The surgery is performed under general anesthesia, without neuromuscular blockade, to allow intraoperative nerve stimulation. The patient is positioned supine with a sandbag under the affected shoulder and hip to facilitate rolling of the shoulder to the contralateral side. This allows for supraclavicular exploration and other nerve transfers necessary for C5,6 reconstruction to be performed in the same position without needing to re-prep and drape the patient. The shoulder is rolled anteriorly, resting the patient's forearm on the chest. A towel bump and assistant are necessary to hold the arm in place. A longitudinal incision is made over the quadrilateral space (Fig. 10.1a). Superficial dissection is through skin and subcutaneous tissue, and the posterior border of the deltoid is identified. The deltoid is denervated and slack so its posterior border can be retracted anteriorly without detaching it from the scapular spine. The sensory branch of the axillary nerve is identified. This sensory branch is traced toward the quadrilateral space where it will enter the posterior division of the axillary nerve. The quadrilateral space can also be identified by finding the long head of the triceps. The posterior division is traced anteriorly to identify the anterior division of the axillary nerve and a vessel loop is placed around the entire axillary nerve. The main axillary nerve is dissected as far anteriorly to maximize length. It is often quite scarred and ends in a rupture. The anterior division is neurolyzed from the posterior division and divided. The anterior division nerve is inspected for fascicular detail, serially trimmed back to good fascicles if necessary, and then delivered posteriorly into the wound.

The triangular interval is identified between the triceps' long and lateral heads. The radial nerve and its branches to the triceps are seen in this interval. The long head of triceps motor

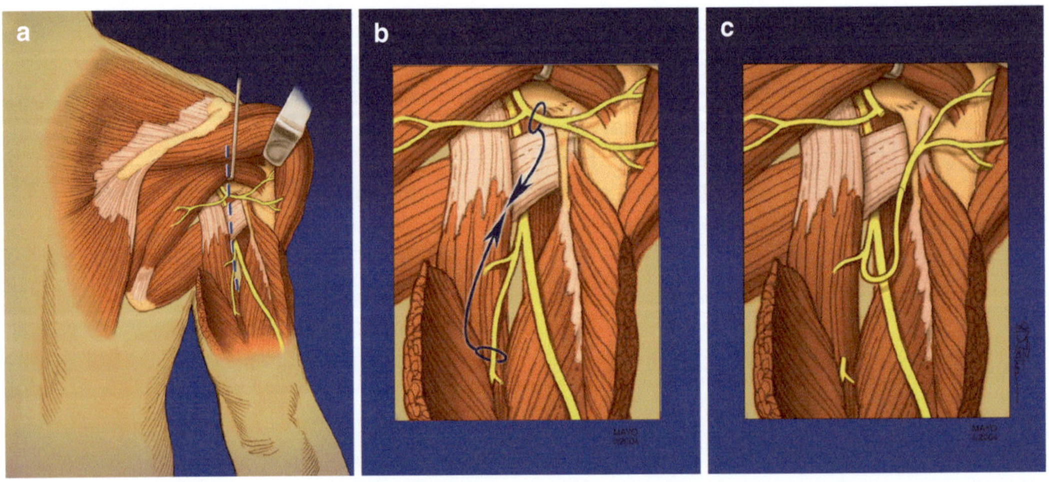

Fig. 10.1 Diagram of long head triceps motor branch transfer to the axillary nerve. (**a**) Incision over quadrilateral space. (**b**) Long head of the triceps motor branch in the triangular interval and anterior division of the axillary nerve in quadrilateral space. (**c**) Completed transfer. Used with permission of the Mayo Foundation for Medical Education and Research

branch is typically selected; however additional branches are identified as alternatives (Fig. 10.1b). This is especially important in patients who had triceps recovery after initial paralysis. The optimal nerve branch and its strength are tested with a nerve stimulator. The remaining branches of the triceps are stimulated to confirm adequate residual supply before harvesting. The chosen triceps branch is isolated distally before it branches into muscle fibers. The triceps branch is transected distally and turned proximally (Fig. 10.1c). If necessary, the teres major tendon can be partially incised to allow more proximal mobilization of the triceps motor branch for a tension-free direct repair. Partial release of the teres major also decreases the adduction force against the recovering deltoid. Nerve repair is performed under an operating microscope magnification using 9–0 nylon sutures. We verify the integrity of a tension-free repair by inspecting the repair after moving the shoulder. Patients are immobilized for 3 weeks in a sling to allow for soft tissue healing and maturation of the nerve coaptation.

We prefer the posterior approach because it provides direct access to the distal axillary and radial nerve branches in the quadrilateral space and triangular interval. This allows for a targeted distal transfer with a shorter regeneration time. Other approaches have since been described [12–14]. The deltopectoral approach and the anterior/modified axillary approach are applicable to brachial plexus reconstruction [13, 14]. The deltopectoral approach gives the surgeon access to other donor nerves, such as medial pectoral, thoracodorsal, median, or ulnar nerves [13]. However, this approach is more proximal. It exposes the first segment of the axillary nerve, where the lateral and medial fascicles are extensively intermingled [10]. Neurotization at this level has the disadvantage of losing axons to the teres minor and the superior lateral brachial cutaneous nerve, leading to suboptimal reinnervation of the deltoid. The anterior approach, modified from the axillary approach, offers easy positioning with the arm abducted and externally rotated. It has the advantage of gaining access to the second segment of the axillary nerve, where lateral and medial fascicular groups can already be identified [14]. Nerve transfer is performed to the lateral fascicular group because this forms the anterior branch at the quadrilateral space [10]. This approach has a higher risk of injury to the axillary vessels. This can be avoided by placing the patient in a slight reverse Trendelenburg position to prevent distention of the axillary vein, extending the transverse/axillary crease portion of the incision posteriorly for a wider field of view, and identifying and protecting the axillary artery first [14].

10.4 Outcomes

Restoration of shoulder function in C5,6 BPI is best achieved with the neurotization of both suprascapular and axillary nerves [6, 15–18]. Leechavenvong's original series of seven patients underwent both spinal accessory to suprascapular nerve and long head of triceps branch to anterior branch of axillary nerve transfers. All recovered MRC grade 4 deltoid power [4]. In a follow-up report of 15 patients, 13 patients recovered MRC grade 4 and 2 had MRC grade 3 deltoid recovery [17]. Bertelli and Ghizoni reported similarly good results in ten patients with shoulder abduction strength of MRC grade 4 in three patients and MRC grade 3 in seven patients after spinal accessory to suprascapular and long or lateral head triceps to axillary nerve transfers [6]. Both the supraspinatus and deltoid abduct the shoulder, so we cannot attribute shoulder abduction recovery to the radial to axillary nerve transfer alone.

In a systematic review of radial to axillary nerve transfers for isolated axillary nerve and brachial plexus injuries, 66 of 80 (82.5%) patients gained at least 40 degrees more of abduction. They recovered MRC grade 3 or more shoulder abduction strength [19]. A higher proportion of patients receiving multiple nerve transfers (95.6%) had clinically significant improvement compared to those with isolated radial to axillary transfers (65.7%) [19]. The overall shoulder abduction recovery is comparable to an earlier report of 22 of 27 (81.5%) similarly mixed patients recovering at least MRC grade 3 shoulder abduction strength after radial to axillary transfers [20]. This series could not assess the effect of concomitant transfers because of their small sample size [20]. Another series looked specifically at medial triceps motor nerve branch transfer to the axillary nerve. They reported 17 of 32 (53.1%) BPI patients recovering MRC grade 3 deltoid strength compared to 14 of 16 (87.5%) patients with isolated axillary nerve injuries [21].

In our cohort of 21 isolated axillary nerve injuries who underwent long head of triceps branch to anterior axillary nerve transfers alone, we find that 16 (76%) recovered deltoid strength of MRC grade 3 or stronger at an average of 6.7 months after surgery [22]. Greater deltoid strength recovery was associated with surgery performed less than 9 months from injury, age 39 years or younger, and lower body mass index [22]. However, in another cohort of 48 BPI patients who underwent triceps branch to anterior axillary nerve transfer, 12 (25%) recovered MRC grade 3 or stronger deltoid function [23]. Recovery of shoulder abduction in patients with isolated axillary nerve injuries was significantly better than in brachial plexus injury patients. Combining both cohorts, a weak (MRC grade 4 or below) triceps and the presence of triceps fibrillations in preoperative EMG were associated with less than MRC grade 3 deltoid recovery [23]. Similar findings were reported by Ferris et al. [24] Patients with MRC grade 5 triceps function before surgery recovered better shoulder abduction strength and range of motion after nerve transfer [24].

10.5 Conclusion

The long head of the triceps radial nerve branch transfer to anterior division of the axillary nerve is an established technique for reconstructing shoulder abduction in BPI. Transfer from a clinically normal (MRC grade 5) triceps is associated with improved recovery of deltoid strength and range of motion. This transfer is typically performed with neurotization for suprascapular nerve to achieve optimal shoulder function in BPI.

References

1. Lurje A. Concerning surgical treatment of traumatic injury to the upper division of the brachial plexus (Erb's type). Ann Surg. 1948;127(2):317–26.
2. Nath RK, Mackinnon SE. Nerve transfers in the upper extremity. Hand Clin. 2000;16(1):131–9.
3. Witoonchart K, Leechavengvongs S, Uerpairojkit C, Thuvasethakul P, Wongnopsuwan V. Nerve transfer to deltoid muscle using the nerve to the long head of the triceps, part I: an anatomic feasibility study. J Hand Surg. 2003;28(4):628–32.
4. Leechavengvongs S, Witoonchart K, Uerpairojkit C, Thuvasethakul P. Nerve transfer to deltoid muscle using the nerve to the long head of the triceps, part II: a report of 7 cases. J Hand Surg. 2003;28(4):633–8.
5. Kawai H, Akita S. Shoulder muscle reconstruction in the upper type of the brachial plexus injury by partial radial nerve transfer to the axillary nerve. Tech Hand Up Extrem Surg. 2004;8(1):51–5.
6. Bertelli JA, Ghizoni MF. Reconstruction of C5 and C6 brachial plexus avulsion injury by multiple nerve transfers: spinal accessory to suprascapular, ulnar fascicles to biceps branch, and triceps long or lateral head branch to axillary nerve. J Hand Surg. 2004;29(1):131–9.
7. Colbert SH, Mackinnon S. Posterior approach for double nerve transfer for restoration of shoulder function in upper brachial plexus palsy. Hand (N Y). 2006;1(2):71–7.
8. Lee EY, Sebastin SJ, Cheah A, Kumar VP, Lim AYT. Upper extremity innervation patterns and clinical implications for nerve and tendon transfer. Plast Reconstr Surg. 2017;140(6):1209–19.
9. Travill AA. Electromyographic study of the extensor apparatus of the forearm. Anat Rec. 1962;144(4):373–6.
10. Zhao X, Hung LK, Zhang GM, Lao J. Applied anatomy of the axillary nerve for selective neurotization of the deltoid muscle. Clin Orthop Relat Res. 2001;390(390):244–51.
11. Schreiber JJ, Feinberg JH, Byun DJ, Lee SK, Wolfe SW. Preoperative donor nerve electromyography as a predictor of nerve transfer outcomes. J Hand Surg Am. 2014;39(1):42–9.
12. Bertelli JA, Kechele PR, Santos MA, Duarte H, Ghizoni MF. Axillary nerve repair by triceps motor branch transfer through an axillary access: anatomical basis and clinical results. J Neurosurg. 2007;107(2):370–7.
13. Jerome JTJ. Long head of the triceps branch transfer to axillary nerve in C5, C6 brachial plexus injuries: anterior approach. Plast Reconstr Surg. 2011;128(3):740–1.
14. Bauer AS, Rabinovich RV, Waters PM. The anterior approach for transfer of radial nerve triceps fascicles to the axillary nerve. J Hand Surg Am. 2019;44(4):345.e1–6.

15. Chuang DC, Lee GW, Hashem F, Wei FC. Restoration of shoulder abduction by nerve transfer in avulsed brachial plexus injury: evaluation of 99 patients with various nerve transfers. Plast Reconstr Surg. 1995;96(1):122–8.
16. Merrell GA, Barrie KA, Katz DL, Wolfe SW. Results of nerve transfer techniques for restoration of shoulder and elbow function in the context of a meta-analysis of the English literature. J Hand Surg Am. 2001;26(2):303–14.
17. Leechavengvongs S, Witoonchart K, Uerpairojkit C, Thuvasethakul P, Malungpaishrope K. Combined nerve transfers for C5 and C6 brachial plexus avulsion injury. J Hand Surg Am. 2006;31(2):183–9.
18. Texakalidis P, Tora MS, Lamanna JJ, Wetzel J, Boulis NM. Combined radial to axillary and spinal accessory nerve (SAN) to suprascapular nerve (SSN) transfers may confer superior shoulder abduction compared with single SA to SSN transfer. World Neurosurg. 2019;126:e1251–6.
19. Wells ME, Gonzalez GA, Childs BR, Williams MR, Nesti LJ, Dunn JC. Radial to axillary nerve transfer outcomes in shoulder abduction: a systematic review. Plast Reconstr Surg Glob Open. 2020;8(9):e3096.
20. Desai MJ, Daly CA, Seiler JG, Wray WH, Ruch DS, Leversedge FJ. Radial to axillary nerve transfers: a combined case series. J Hand Surg Am. 2016;41(12):1128–34.
21. Krauss EM, Noland SS, Hill EJR, Jain NS, Kahn LC, Mackinnon SE. Outcome analysis of medial triceps motor nerve transfer to axillary nerve in isolated and brachial plexus-associated axillary nerve palsy. Plast Reconstr Surg. 2022;149(6):1380–90.
22. Lee JY, Kircher MF, Spinner RJ, Bishop AT, Shin AY. Factors affecting outcome of triceps motor branch transfer for isolated axillary nerve injury. J Hand Surg Am. 2012;37(11):2350–6.
23. Maldonado AA, Dittman LE, Loosbrock MF, Bishop AT, Spinner RJ, Shin AY. Factors associated with poorer outcomes from triceps motor branch to anterior axillary nerve transfer: a case-control study. World Neurosurg. 2022;167:e1115–21.
24. Ferris S, Withers A, Shukla L. Defining the reliability of deltoid reanimation by nerve transfer when using abnormal but variably recovered triceps donor nerves. Front Surg. 2021;8:8.

11 Long Thoracic to Axillary Nerve Transfer

Carlos Alberto Rodríguez-Aceves
and María Elena Córdoba-Mosqueda

Abbreviations

AN	Axillary nerve
BP	Brachial plexus
LTN	Long thoracic nerve
SAN	Spinal accessory nerve
SSN	Suprascapular nerve
TBPI	Total brachial plexus injury
TrBr	Triceps branch
UTBPI	Upper type brachial plexus injury

11.1 Introduction

Brachial plexus (BP) injury is a devastating condition that usually results from motor vehicle accidents, falls, gunshot wounds, and shoulder trauma, leading to several degrees of intraneural lesions because of stretching, laceration, or compression forces.

BP injuries are classified according to their extension in complete-, upper-, and lower-type injuries. The more severe the injury, the less chances for spontaneous recovery and the less workable donor elements to reconstruct [1–3].

Clinical and laboratory data concerning the feasibility of using the long thoracic nerve (LTN) as a donor in the reconstructive surgery of the BP regardless of the severity is scarce. However, a functional LTN may be considered a potential nerve donor when other nerves are not available during a primary reconstruction under certain conditions [4].

11.2 Anatomy

11.2.1 Axillary Nerve

The axillary nerve (AN) is a terminal branch of the BP formed by contributions from C5 and C6 roots. It arises from the posterior cord in the infraclavicular level at the axillary region, below the axillary artery.

Along with the circumflex humeral artery, the neurovascular bundle travels distal and lateral toward the quadrilateral space, which is limited proximally by the teres minor muscle, distally by the teres major muscle, medially by the long head of the triceps muscle, and laterally by the neck of the humerus. After exiting the quadrangular space, the nerve branches off into anterior and posterior divisions to innervate the anterolateral deltoid and posterior deltoid and teres minor muscles, respectively.

C. A. Rodríguez-Aceves (✉)
Peripheral Nerve Clinic, Neurological Center, The American British Cowdray Medical Center, Mexico City, Mexico

M. E. Córdoba-Mosqueda
Neurosurgery, Hospital Ángeles Pedregal, Mexico City, Mexico

F. Guedes et al. (eds.), *Nerve Transfers for Brachial Plexus Reconstruction after Trauma*,
https://doi.org/10.1007/978-3-031-92445-3_11

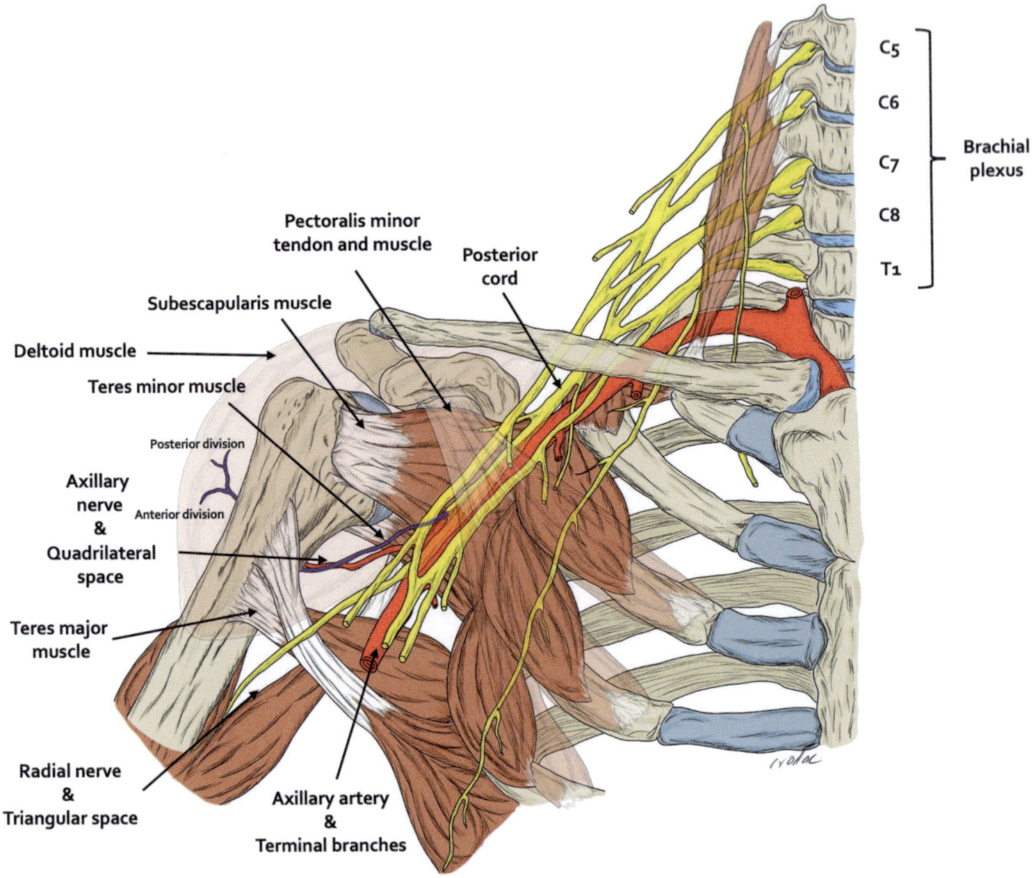

Fig. 11.1 Axillary nerve anatomy. Axillary nerve (blue) originating from posterior cord and behind the axillary artery, coursing through the quadrilateral space and branching off in the anterior and posterior divisions to innervate deltoid and teres minor muscles

The terminal segment of the posterior division forms the upper lateral brachial cutaneous nerve to provide sensory innervation to the lateral upper arm [5–8] (Fig. 11.1).

11.2.2 Long Thoracic Nerve

The LTN is a pre-truncal collateral pure motor branch of the BP, formed by contributions from C5, C6, and C7 roots at the foraminal level. After piercing the scalenus medius muscle, the C5 and C6 roots join the C7 root to form the main trunk of the LTN.

It descends dorsal to the proximal BP and ventral to the medius scalene muscle, the first rib, and the posterior angle of the second rib toward the upper lateral thoracic region at the level of the mid-axillary line, over the external surface of the serratus anterior muscle that innervates in its whole length.

Then the LTN divides into superior and inferior branches to innervate the upper serratus and the middle and lower serratus, respectively providing individual or segmental but complimentary innervation to each segment of the serratus anterior muscle [7–13] (Fig. 11.2).

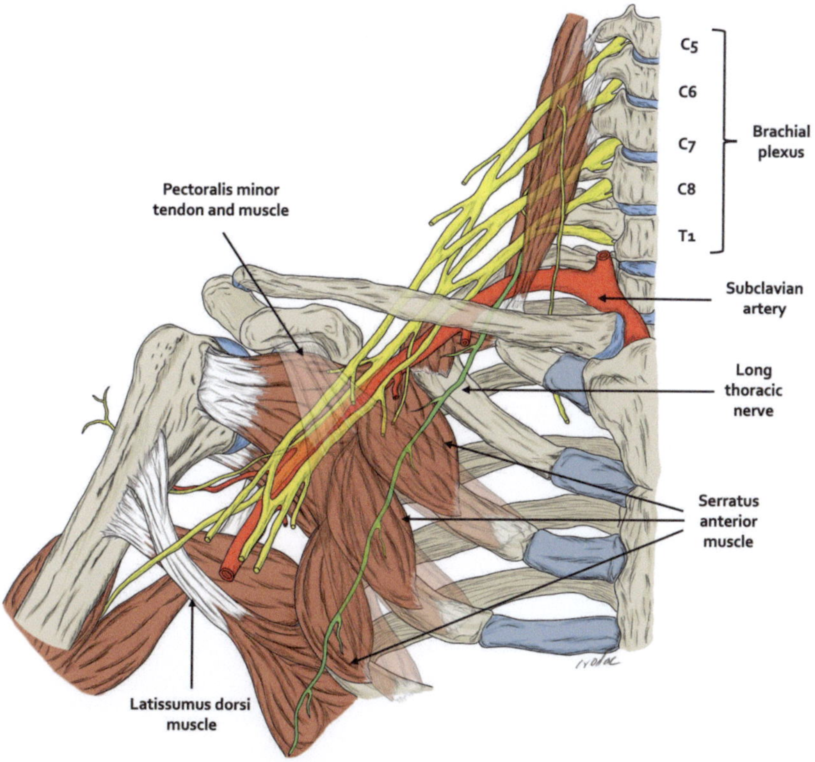

Fig. 11.2 Long thoracic nerve anatomy. Long thoracic nerve (green) originating from contributions by C5 to C7 roots behind the proximal brachial plexus, coursing distally to the lateral chest wall to innervate the serratus anterior muscle

11.3 Rationale and Indications

Upper-type (UTBPI), UTBPI *plus* C7, and total BP (TBPI) injuries lead to loss of shoulder function and stability because of the disconnection of the muscles innervated by both the suprascapular nerve (SSN) and AN [14].

In order to improve shoulder subluxation, abduction, and external rotation, the reinnervation of muscles supplied by these two nerves (SSN and AN) is one of the main priorities, preceded by elbow flexion restoration [15–17].

In supraclavicular BP injuries, identifying the pathological process (preganglionic or postganglionic) is paramount for the surgeon to determine the elements that remain intact and may serve as potential donors for reconstruction since BP reconstruction can be achieved through grafting or nerve transfers [1, 18, 19].

The main conditions for nerve transfers in BP reconstruction are the availability of functional, and expendable, neighboring synergistic healthy intraplexal or extraplexal nerve donors [20–22].

In such a way, for UTBPI pre- and postganglionic with intact C7 root, a dual nerve transfer including spinal accessory nerve (SAN) to SSN and radial triceps branch (TrBr) to AN yields the best outcomes in the present day [17, 23–27].

For UTBPI *plus* and TBPI, shoulder reinnervation may be achieved by grafting a remanent viable C5 or C6 root to the posterior division of the upper trunk, via the AN, and by transferring the SAN to the SSN in pre- and postganglionic injuries (when at least one root is available).

If the C7 root is damaged in an UTBPI *plus* with pre- or postganglionic pattern, then the TrBr cannot be used to reconstruct the AN and other nerve donors must be considered, such as intercostal, thoracodorsal, medial pectoral, phrenic, contralateral C7, partial median, partial ulnar, and LTN (if postganglionic) [17, 28–30].

Despite the extension of injury, in preganglionic injuries, the surgical treatment is challenging, because of a lack of available donors, and they should improve elbow flexion rather than AN function.

Although the LTN is not used routinely as a donor for primary reconstruction of the AN in BP injuries, or even in isolated injuries, the following features make its use workable as a donor: (1) is a neighboring pure motor nerve, (2) with enough length (23–30 cm) and diameter (2.5–3.5 mm), (3) containing 1135–1800 of myelinated axons, (4) easy to approach, and (5) with low risk of scapular winging because of the innervation pattern of the serratus anterior muscle [4, 9, 13, 31–34].

Therefore, the LTN could be used as an intraplexal donor to reconstruct the AN after BP injuries in extraforaminal postganglionic injuries distal to the origin of the contributions of the C5–C7 roots to this nerve, preganglionic UTBPI in where C7 root is preserved, and potentially in isolated AN injury, if no other donors are available, and the LTN preserves its function.

11.4 Surgical Technique

The patient is positioned supine, with the arm abducted at about 90°. The skin incision is outlined from along the deltopectoral sulcus, then is curved medially to the lateral thoracic wall, and longitudinally descends following the mid-axillary line as far as the sixth or seventh intercostal space. It can be traced continuously or leave a skin island at the mid-portion (axillary level) (Fig. 11.3).

For AN exposure, the deltopectoral sulcus is identified and opened, the pectoralis major muscle retracted medially, and the underlying pectoralis minor tendon is divided. After dissection of the underlying fat pad, the lateral cord and the axillary artery are visualized and retracted medially to expose the posterior cord and its division into the axillary and radial nerves, approximately at the distal border of the subscapularis muscle. AN is dissected and divided as proximal as possible [8, 35, 36] (Fig. 11.4).

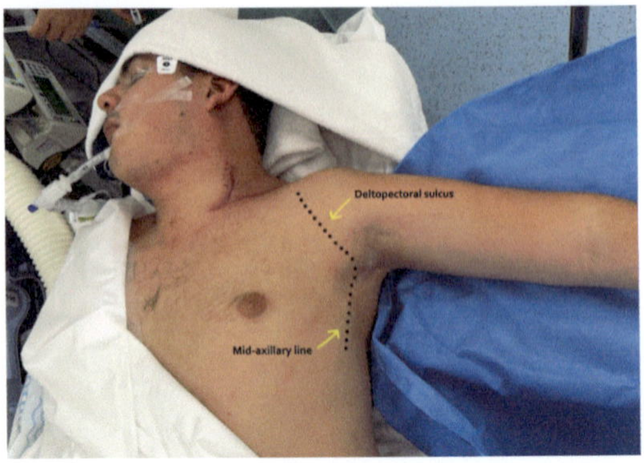

Fig. 11.3 Surgical positioning and incision. Outlined incision following the deltopectoral sulcus and the mid-axillary line to expose the axillary nerve and the long thoracic nerve, respectively

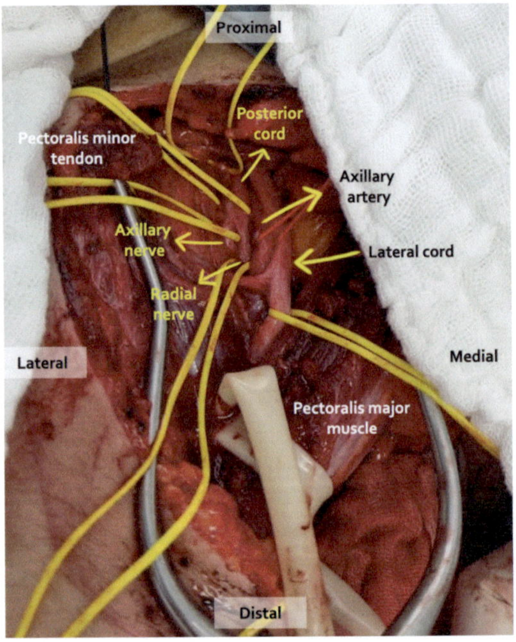

Fig. 11.4 Surgical exposure of the axillary nerve. Deep dissection after the retraction of the pectoralis major muscle and section of the pectoralis minor tendon. The axillary artery is visualized and retracted medially to expose the posterior cord and the origin of the axillary and radial nerves

For LTN distal exposure, after the skin incision at the mid-axillary line, the interval between the distal border of the pectoralis major and the anterior border of latissimus dorsi muscles over the serratus anterior muscle is signaled, and the fascia is opened.

The LTN is identified as descending in a longitudinal direction over the anterior surface of the serratus anterior muscle. Direct electrical stimulation confirms nerve identification and its functionality. Distal dissection is continued as far as the proximal border of the lower serratus anterior muscle, joining the thoracodorsal artery (Fig. 11.5).

The LTN is sectioned distally as necessary below the branches to the superior serratus anterior muscle. Then, the proximal stump is rerouted to the axillary region and coaptated (non-absorbable sutures and fibrin glue) without tension in an end-to-end fashion with the distal stump of the AN under a surgical microscope. The skin and subcutaneous tissue are closed by layers and immobilization for 3 weeks is required [4, 37–39] (Fig. 11.6). The use of surgical drain tubes is not necessary.

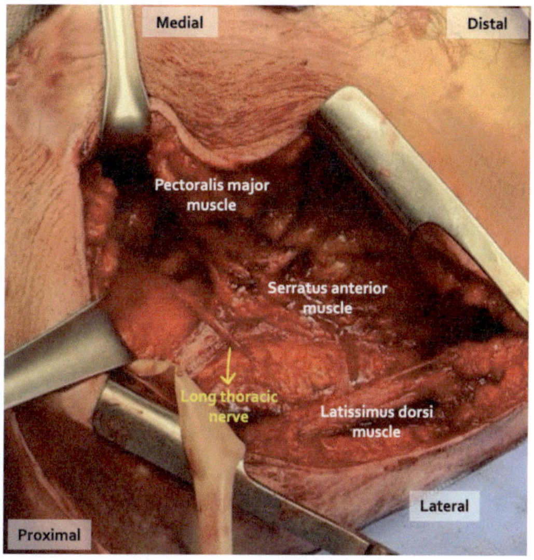

Fig. 11.5 Surgical exposure of the long thoracic nerve. The interval between the pectoralis major and latissimus dorsi muscles is opened. The long thoracic nerve is identified descending the lateral chest wall, lying over the serratus anterior muscle

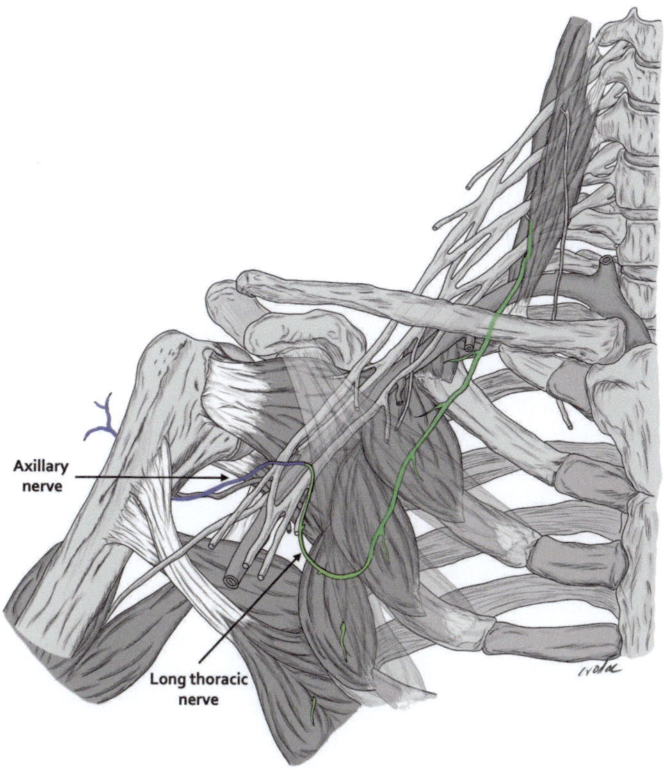

Fig. 11.6 Long thoracic to axillary nerve transfer. The functional proximal end of the long thoracic nerve (green) providing innervation to the distal serratus anterior muscle is sectioned and rerouted proximally for being anastomosed with the distal end of the axillary nerve (blue) in front of the axillary artery and terminal branches for a tensionless end to end coaptation

11.5 Complications

Since the upper segment of the serratus anterior muscle, together with the trapezius, serves as a primary stabilizer of the scapula, sectioning a functional LTN may result in varying degrees of scapular winging—typically characterized by medial displacement of the scapula—as well as shoulder weakness and limited range of motion, particularly during overhead activities. For that reason, a very proximal section of the donor nerve should be avoided. However, the denervation of the serratus anterior muscle may produce fewer functional consequences than those seen with the loss of shoulder abduction and elbow flexion. On the other hand, axonal dispersion during reinnervation may result in less strength of shoulder abduction, since the main trunk of the AN is neurotized, rather than only the anterior division, as in classical TrBr to AN transfer [32].

Other complications are related to unnoticed deepest dissection, such as pneumothorax and bleeding, and less frequent surgical wound dehiscence and infection, or rupture of the anastomosis if improper immobilization [39].

11.6 Results Based on Literature Review

Few studies report the use of the LTN as a donor for shoulder reinnervation in BP reconstructive surgery since was first described by Förster in 1929, alone or in combination with other nerve donors [4].

In 1992, Smardžić and colleagues reported functional recovery with the use of regional nerve transfers in 26/31 (83.3%) patients, from which 16 (84.2%) were treated using a single nerve donor, but they did not specify whether the LTN was used alone or combined with other donors and the selected target. Haninec and colleagues reported successful outcomes in 6/11 (55%) patients, similar to those reported by Kluemper and colleagues in 2/3 (66%) pediatric patients [4, 30, 40, 41].

11.7 Conclusion

Management of BP injuries has evolved in the last decades. Nerve transfers have changed the paradigm regarding the outcomes of this type of injury. Currently, many reports support the efficacy of dual reinnervation in improving shoulder function using the SAN and TrBr as donors targeted to the SSN and AN.

In UTBPI *plus* is not possible to reconstruct the AN with radial nerve branches, and other options have been described to substitute this strategy. Despite the scant experience using the LTN to reinnervate the AN, its inherent anatomical and physiological conditions may feasible the use of this nerve as a potential donor for primary surgery reconstruction if no other nerves are available, even when the LTN is initially involved in the injury, since there may be recovery over time as established by Kluemper.

Further clinical studies are necessary to demonstrate the efficacy of this technique when compared with other donors before the specific indications can be established.

References

1. Thatte M, Babhulkar S, Hiremath A. Brachial plexus injury in adults: diagnosis and surgical treatment strategies. Ann Indian Acad Neurol. 2013;16(1):26.
2. Siqueira MG, Martins RS. Surgical treatment of adult traumatic brachial plexus injuries: an overview. Arq Neuropsiquiatr. 2011;69(3):528–35.
3. Shin AY, Spinner RJ, Steinmann SP, Bishop AT. Adult traumatic brachial plexus injuries. J Am Acad Orthop Surg. 2005;13(6):382–96.
4. Kluemper C, Aversano M, Kozin S, Zlotolow DA. Long thoracic nerve transfer for children with brachial plexus injuries. J Pediatr Orthop. 2021;41(6):374–8.
5. Burkhead WZ, Scheinberg RR, Box G. Surgical anatomy of the axillary nerve. J Shoulder Elb Surg. 1992;1(1):31–6.

6. Leechavengvongs S, Teerawutthichaikit T, Witoonchart K, Uerpairojkit C, Malungpaishrope K, Suppauksorn S, et al. Surgical anatomy of the axillary nerve branches to the deltoid muscle: surgical anatomy of the axillary nerve branches to the deltoid muscle. Clin Anat. 2015;28(1):118–22.
7. Tubbs RS, Goodrich D, Watanabe K, Loukas M. Anatomic landmarks for selected nerves of the head, neck, and upper and lower limbs. In: Nerves and nerve injuries. Amsterdam: Elsevier; 2015. p. 575–88. https://linkinghub.elsevier.com/retrieve/pii/B9780124103900000457.
8. Maniker AH, editor. Operative exposures in peripheral nerve surgery. Stuttgart: Georg Thieme Verlag; 2005. http://www.thieme-connect.de/products/ebooks/book/10.1055/b-002-56118.
9. Tubbs RS, Salter EG, Custis JW, Wellons JC, Blount JP, Oakes WJ. Surgical anatomy of the cervical and infraclavicular parts of the long thoracic nerve. J Neurosurg. 2006;104(5):792–5.
10. Bertelli JA, Ghizoni MF. Long thoracic nerve: anatomy and functional assessment. J Bone Joint Surg Am. 2005;87(5):993–8.
11. Hamada J, Igarashi E, Akita K, Mochizuki T. A cadaveric study of the serratus anterior muscle and the long thoracic nerve. J Shoulder Elb Surg. 2008;17(5):790–4.
12. Smith R, Nyquist-Battie C, Clark M, Rains J. Anatomical characteristics of the upper serratus anterior: cadaver dissection. J Orthop Sports Phys Ther. 2003;33(8):449–54.
13. Ormsby NM, Hawkes DH, Ng CY. Variation of surgical anatomy of the thoracic portion of the long thoracic nerve. Clin Anat. 2022;35(4):442–6.
14. Moore A, Phillips B, Mackinnon SE. Nerve transfers to improve upper extremity function. In: Nerves and nerve injuries. San Diego: Elsevier; 2015. p. 275–306.
15. Brophy RH, Wolfe SW. Planning brachial plexus surgery: treatment options and priorities. Hand Clin. 2005;21(1):47–54.
16. Terzis JK, Papakonstantinou KC. The surgical treatment of brachial plexus injuries in adults. Plast Reconstr Surg. 2000;106(5):1097–124.
17. Sinha S, Khani M, Mansoori N, Midha R. Adult brachial plexus injuries: surgical strategies and approaches. Neurol India. 2016;64(2):289.
18. Garozzo D. Las lesiones de plexo braquial. Cómo diagnosticarlas y cuándo tratarlas. Ortho-tips. 2012;8(1):7–16.
19. Hems T. Nerve transfers for traumatic brachial plexus injury: advantages and problems. J Hand Microsurg. 2016;3(1):6–10.
20. Tung TH, Mackinnon SE. Nerve transfers: indications, techniques, and outcomes. J Hand Surg Am. 2010;35(2):332–41.
21. Robla-Costales J, Socolovsky M, Di Masi G, Domitrovic L, Campero A, Fernández-Fernández J, et al. Técnicas de reconstrucción nerviosa en cirugía del plexo braquial traumatizado Parte 1: Transferencias nerviosas extraplexuales. Neurocirugia. 2011;22(6):507–20.
22. Robla-Costales J, Socolovsky M, Di Masi G, Robla-Costales D, Domitrovic L, Campero A, et al. Técnicas de reconstrucción nerviosa en cirugía del plexo braquial traumatizado Parte 2: Transferencias nerviosas intraplexuales. Neurocirugia. 2011;22(6):521–34.
23. Texakalidis P, Tora MS, Lamanna JJ, Wetzel J, Boulis NM. Combined radial to axillary and spinal accessory nerve (SAN) to suprascapular nerve (SSN) transfers may confer superior shoulder abduction compared with single SA to SSN transfer. World Neurosurg. 2019;126:e1251–6.
24. Chuang DCC, Lee GW, Hashem F, Wei FC. Restoration of shoulder abduction by nerve transfer in avulsed brachial plexus injury: evaluation of 99 patients with various nerve transfers. Plast Reconstr Surg. 1995;96(1):122–8.
25. Terzis JK, Kostas I, Soucacos PN. Restoration of shoulder function with nerve transfers in traumatic brachial plexus palsy patients. Microsurgery. 2006;26(4):316–24.
26. Leechavengvongs S, Witoonchart K, Uerpairojkit C, Thuvasethakul P, Malungpaishrope K. Combined nerve transfers for C5 and C6 brachial plexus avulsion injury. J Hand Surg Am. 2006;31(2):183–9.
27. Leechavengvongs S, Malungpaishorpe K, Uerpairojkit C, Ng CY, Witoonchart K. Nerve transfers to restore shoulder function. Hand Clin. 2016;32(2):153–64.
28. Makeľ M, Sukop A, Kachlík D, Waldauf P, Whitley A, Kaiser R. Possible donor nerves for axillary nerve reconstruction in dual neurotization for restoring shoulder abduction in brachial plexus injuries: a systematic review and meta-analysis. Neurosurg Rev. 2022;45(2):1303–12.
29. Kang GHY, Yong FC. Shoulder abduction reconstruction for C5–7 avulsion brachial plexus injury by dual nerve transfers: spinal accessory to suprascapular nerve and partial median or ulnar to axillary nerve. J Plast Surg Hand Surg. 2022;56(2):87–92.
30. Samardzic M, Grujicic D, Antunovic V. Nerve transfer in brachial plexus traction injuries. J Neurosurg. 1992;76(2):191–7.
31. Raksakulkiat R, Leechavengvongs S, Malungpaishrope K, Uerpairojkit C, Witoonchart K, Chongthammakun S. Restoration of winged scapula in upper arm type brachial plexus injury: anatomic feasibility. J Med Assoc Thail. 2009;92(Suppl 6):S244–50.
32. Tubbs RS, Loukas M, Shoja MM, Shokouhi G, Wellons JC, Oakes WJ, et al. The contralateral long thoracic nerve as a donor for upper brachial plexus neurotization procedures: cadaveric feasibility study: laboratory investigation. J Neurosurg. 2009;110(4):749–53.

33. Tubbs RS, Shaffer WA, Loukas M, Shoja MM, Oakes WJ. The long thoracic nerve as a donor for facial nerve reanimation procedures: cadaveric feasibility study: laboratory investigation. J Neurosurg. 2008;108(6):1225–9.
34. Zhang D, Varadharajan V, Bhardwaj P, Venkatramani H, Sabapathy SR. Considerations in the selection of donor nerves for nerve transfer for reanimation of elbow and shoulder in traumatic brachial plexus injuries. J Hand Surg Asian Pac Vol. 2022;27(1):10–21.
35. Jerome JTJ, Rajmohan B. Axillary nerve neurotization with the anterior deltopectoral approach in brachial plexus injuries. Microsurgery. 2012;32(6):445–51.
36. Siqueira MG, Martins RS. Anatomia cirúrgica das vias de acesso aos nervos perifericos. São Paulo: Di Livros; 2006.
37. Noland SS, Krauss EM, Felder JM, Mackinnon SE. Surgical and clinical decision making in isolated long thoracic nerve palsy. Hand (N Y). 2018;13(6):689–94.
38. Hanna AS. Anatomy and exposures of spinal nerves. 1st ed. Cham: Springer International Publishing; 2015. Imprint: Springer; 2015. 1 p.
39. Laulan J, Lascar T, Saint-Cast Y, Chammas M, Le Nen D. Isolated paralysis of the serratus anterior muscle successfully treated by surgical release of the distal portion of the long thoracic nerve. Chir Main. 2011;30(2):90–6.
40. Haninec P, Šámal F, Tomáš R, Houstava L, Dubový P. Direct repair (nerve grafting), neurotization, and end-to-side neurorrhaphy in the treatment of brachial plexus injury. J Neurosurg. 2007;106(3):391–9.
41. Samardzic M, Rasulic LG, Grujicic DM, Bacetic DT, Milicic BR. Nerve transfers using collateral branches of the brachial plexus as donors in patients with upper palsy—thirty years' experience. Acta Neurochir. 2011;153(10):2009–19.

Median or Ulnar Nerve Fascicle to Axillary Nerve Transfer

12

Leandro Pretto Flores

12.1 Introduction

In approximately 15% of cases of traumatic brachial plexus injuries (BPI), deficits are limited to the C5 and C6 roots. Most commonly impaired functions include elbow flexion, shoulder flexion, abduction, and external rotation secondary to the palsy of the biceps, brachialis, brachioradialis, deltoid, teres minor, and *spinati* muscles [1]. In order to address shoulder deficits, two nerves need to be reinnervated, the suprascapular nerve (SSN) and the axillary nerve (AN).

In C5–6–7 brachial plexus avulsion injuries, shoulder abduction reconstruction by a spinal accessory nerve transfer to the suprascapular nerve usually demonstrate modest results [2]. In general, shoulder abduction at the glenohumeral joint is initiated by the supraspinatus muscle. Further abduction in the coronal plane to 90° requires external rotation of the humerus to clear the mechanical block of the acromial process. Full abduction typically requires a functioning deltoid muscle (nerve supply from the axillary nerve) [3].

Historically, interposition cabled sural nerve grafts were used from viable cervical root stump to the viable AN stump. In 2003, Leechavengvongs et al. described the transfer of the triceps long-head motor branch (TLHMB) of the radial nerve to the anterior division of the axillary nerve [4]. As this technique could be applied to both pre- and postganglionic lesions, it has gained popularity among surgeons as it has provided comparable functional outcomes to nerve grafting from the roots. However, in C5–6–7 brachial plexus avulsion injuries where the triceps is affected, the nerve to the triceps is not an ideal donor [1]. Alternative nerve transfer to the axillary nerve has been reported in these patients. These include a partial median nerve or partial ulnar nerves. Moreover, sural grafting and triceps transfer usually do not address the teres minor muscle and, if not reanimated, active shoulder external rotation mainly relies on the reinnervation of the infraspinatus muscle, which may lead to insufficient outcomes.

This chapter aims to report the results of studies that addressed the outcomes of nerve transfer of motor fascicles from the ulnar or the median nerve to reinnervate the axillary nerve or its branches innervating deltoid and teres minor muscles.

12.2 Results of the Reviewed Series

In 2012, Haninec and Kaiser [5] reported a first series of cases in which the axillary nerve was repaired by transfer of fascicle from the ulnar or

L. P. Flores (✉)
Department of Neurosurgery, Hospital das Forças Armadas, Brasília, Distrito Federal, Brazil

F. Guedes et al. (eds.), *Nerve Transfers for Brachial Plexus Reconstruction after Trauma*,
https://doi.org/10.1007/978-3-031-92445-3_12

median nerve, in upper brachial plexus palsy in adults. The study included 14 patients with C5–C6 and C5–C7 injuries where ulnar nerve fascicles were donor in 12. The infraclavicular approach was used in all patients, and all had concomitant spinal accessory nerve transfer to suprascapular nerve via the supraclavicular approach. The biceps was reinnervated by medial pectoral to musculocutaneous (MC) nerve transfer in all cases. Good recovery of deltoid muscle function—better than M3—was seen in seven cases (77.8%). Overall, the shoulder abduction ranged between 40° and 120°. The authors concluded that the results of ulnar motor fascicle transfer to the axillary nerve were very good and proposed an alternative approach for axillary nerve reinnervation in an upper brachial plexus palsy, especially in patients with concomitant radial nerve injury.

In 2021, Kang and Young [6] reported their outcomes with median or ulnar nerve fascicle transfer to axillary nerve for shoulder reinnervation in adult traumatic C5–C7 root avulsion. They reported nine patients with triceps motor power less than M4. The transfer was accomplished by an anterior axillary approach and all had spinal accessory to the suprascapular nerve transfers. The MC nerve was approached by the same incision and reinnervated with motor fascicles from the ulnar or the median nerve (i.e., one to the biceps and the other one to the axillary nerve). According to the authors, all patients achieved shoulder abduction better than M3, which was graded as M4 in six. The mean abduction range was 114.4° (range 90°–180°). Outcomes for external rotation were available in only four cases, reported as 136.3° (range 135°–140°). Authors concluded that partial median or ulnar to axillary nerve was a good option for shoulder abduction reconstruction in C5–6 ± C7 brachial plexus avulsion injuries where the tríceps is impaired.

Lafosse et al., in 2020 [7], published their results of double-nerve transfer to the axillary nerve in traumatic upper trunk brachial plexus injuries. The authors performed an anatomical and clinical analysis of transferring a triceps motor branch (from the radial nerve) to the anterior division of the axillary nerve and one motor fascicle from the ulnar nerve to the teres minor motor branch (off the posterior division of the axillary nerve). Their technique aimed to improve shoulder external rotation. The study included six cases sustaining C5–C6 injuries, and surgery was performed via an anterior axillary approach. Reinnervation of the suprascapular nerve was performed by a motor fascicle transfer from ipsilateral C7 in all cases. The axillary nerve was dissected to identify its terminal division, giving an anterior division (i.e., anterior division of the axillary nerve (ADAN)) and a posterior division (posterior division of the axillary nerve (PDAN)). Further dissection of the posterior division allowed identifying a subsequent branching, giving two branches as well, including one motor, posterior (i.e., branch to the teres minor (TMB)), and one sensory. The radial nerve and the nerve to the long head of the triceps (LHTB) were isolated. The LHTB was transferred to the ADAN; a proximal motor branch from the ulnar nerve was transferred to the MC nerve; and a second distal motor branch from the same ulnar nerve was transferred to the TMB. The authors reported no permanent motor deficits in the harvested nerve's territory; M3 strength or above was observed in all patients, both in the deltoid and teres minor muscles. Subsequently, all patients achieved at least 90° (128° ± 34°) of active shoulder flexion and 89° ± 67° of active shoulder external rotation. The study concluded that a double-nerve transfer to the anterior and posterior motor branches of the axillary nerve is anatomically feasible and appears to provide satisfactory clinical outcomes in terms of shoulder external rotation without increasing the morbidity of the reconstruction.

12.3 Surgical Technique

The distal nerve transfer from either a partial median or ulnar nerve to the axillary nerve is frequently reported in association with an anterior axillary approach. The axillary nerve must be identified anteriorly, at the inferior border of the subscapularis muscle, before it enters the quadrangular space. Zhao et al. [8] reported that although the nerve has not yet divided into its divisions at this level, two fascicular groups can be identified: one lateral and one medial. They are enclosed within an outer epineurial layer. The lateral fascicular group continues as the anterior division of the axillary nerve, while the medial fascicular group continues as the posterior division. A vessel loop is placed around the nerve for later identification after the prepared donor nerve is ready for cooptation to the axillary nerve.

The donor median or ulnar nerve is identified via the same anterior axillary incision, extended distally. A partial longitudinal epineurotomy is made on the donor nerve for intraoperative nerve stimulation to identify suitable donor fascicles. For the median nerve, suitable donors include the fascicles to wrist or finger flexors (*flexor carpi radialis* (FCR) *or flexor digitorum superficialis* (FDS)), or forearm pronator (*pronator teres* (PT)). The suitable donor fascicles from the ulnar nerve include those to *the flexor carpis ulnaris* (FCU) muscle. (Please detail further how the authors select the donor fasciles and how many—often there are multiple muscles contracting not just the FCU or FCR.)

The selected donor nerve fascicles are mobilized to the level of the recipient nerve stump distally. The donor fascicles must be transected distally and brought proximally, to be coopted to the recipient nerve stump without tension. End-to-end nerve cooptation is performed under operative microscope magnification using 10–0 nylon sutures and the repair site is reinforced with biological adhesive.

12.4 Conclusions

There are very few published series of cases addressing the transfer of ulnar or median nerve motor fascicles for reinnervation the axillary nerve. Existing series include only a few cases. Hence, it is difficult to make definitive conclusions regarding the outcomes.

However, it should be considered as an option for cases sustaining upper root avulsions of the brachial plexus, especially those cases with C5 to C7 nerve injury in which reconstruction of the axillary nerve with nerve transfers from triceps motor branches is not feasible. Alternatively, these techniques may be useful in cases sustaining C5–C6 or C5–C7 where the biceps has been reinnervated via a different donor than the ulnar/median nerve and in cases where the biceps is considered normal and the axillary nerve is the main goal of the surgery.

The anterior axillary approach is the best choice for performing these nerve transfers. It offers the opportunity to explore all of the donors and recipient nerves, by using one single incision and avoiding spending time with intraoperative positional changes. Moreover, tension-free sutures between donors (ulnar or median nerve) and recipients (axillary nerve or its branches) can be performed.

The reported studies also provided valuable learning in the sense that surgeons should pay more attention to the teres minor branch of the axillary nerve in brachial plexus surgery. The teres minor muscle is of key importance regarding shoulder function. Ackland et al. [9] reported on the primary role that both the teres minor and the infraspinatus muscle played regarding posterior glenohumeral stabilization in the transverse plane, balancing the action of the internal rotators. Such biomechanical data appear to be of crucial importance when considering glenohumeral function and have already been confirmed clinically. Despite these biomechanical and clinical findings, teres minor reinnervation is not commonly performed in upper brachial plexus injuries; therefore, active shoulder external rotation will mainly rely on the reinnervation of the infraspinatus. However, Terzis and Kostas [10] showed that, following suprascapular nerve reconstruction, infraspinatus activity was significantly lower than supraspinatus activity, justifying the need to increase the attention for reinnervation of the teres minor in such cases.

In summary, all of the few case series that evaluated the outcomes of shoulder abduction and external rotation associated with reinnervating the axillary nerve by motor fascicles from the median or the ulnar nerve reported some satisfactory outcomes. However, such results must be carefully considered, given the low number of enrolled cases and the lack, to date, of comparative or controlled studies.

References

1. Tung TH, Moore AM. Brachial plexus injuries. In: Mackinnon SE, editor. Nerve surgery. 5th ed. New York: Thieme Medical Publishers; 2015. p. 391–467.
2. Malessy MJA, De Ruiter GCW, De Boer KS, et al. Evaluation of suprascapular nerve neurotization after nerve graft of transfer in the treatment of brachial plexus traction lesions. J Neurosurg. 2004;101(3):377–89.
3. Saha AK. Biomechanics of shoulder movements: functional classification of muscles elevating the shoulder. In: Surgery of the paralysed and flail shoulder. Acta Orthopaedica Scandinavica, Supplement No. 97. Copenhagen: Munksgaard; 1967. p. 14–32.
4. Leechavengvongs S, Witoonchart K, Uerpairojkit C, Thuvasethakul P. Nerve transfer to deltoid muscle using the nerve to the long head of the triceps, part II: a report of 7 cases. J Hand Surg Am. 2003;28(4):633–8.
5. Haninec P, Kaiser R. Axillary nerve repair by fascicle transfer from the ulnar or median nerve in upper brachial plexus palsy. J Neurosurg. 2012;117(3):610–4.
6. Kang GH, Young FC. Shoulder abduction reconstruction for C5–7vavulsion brachial plexus injury by dual nerve transfers: spinal accessory to suprascapular nerve and partial median or ulnar to axillary nerve. J Plast Surg Hand Surg. 2022;56(2):87–92.
7. Lafosse T, Gerosa T, Serane J, Bouyer M, et al. Double-nerve transfer to the axillary nerve in traumatic upper trunk brachial plexus injuries using an axillary approach: anatomical description and preliminary case series. Oper Neurosurg (Hagerstown). 2020;19(2):E131–9.
8. Zhao X, Hung LK, Zhang GM, et al. Applied anatomy of the axillary nerve for selective neurotization of the deltoid muscle. Clin Orthop Relat Res. 2001;390:244–51.
9. Ackland DC, Pandy MG. Lines of action and stabilizing potential of the shoulder musculature. J Anat. 2009;215(2):184–97.
10. Terzis JK, Kostas I. Suprascapular nerve reconstruction in 118 cases of adult posttraumatic brachial plexus. Plast Reconstr Surg. 2006;117(2):613–29.

13 Restoring Suprascapular Nerve Function in Brachial Plexus Injuries: Spinal Accessory Nerve to Suprascapular Nerve Transfer

Fernando Guedes, Evelina Llorian, Vinícius M. Henriques, Gabriel Elias Sanches, and Francisco José Lourenço Torrão-Junior

13.1 Introduction

Shoulder injuries can be debilitating, especially when involving the upper brachial plexus. Such injuries can significantly impact the quality of life, making restoring shoulder function a crucial objective. The primary goal of treatment of brachial plexus injuries is to restore elbow flexion and then to stabilize the glenohumeral joint and restore shoulder function, in particular external rotation and abduction [1].

These injuries are particularly prevalent in the young, socioeconomically active population, underscoring the importance of successful treatment and rehabilitation to minimize their impact on individuals, families, and society.

There are methods for reconstructing the injured brachial plexus and restoring shoulder function in patients. A common technique involves the transfer of the spinal accessory nerve to the suprascapular nerve. In this chapter, we will delve into the latest advancements in this nerve transfer and its potential in restoring shoulder function.

F. Guedes · E. Llorian (✉) · V. M. Henriques · G. E. Sanches · F. J. L. Torrão-Junior
Division of Neurosurgery, Department of Surgery, Gaffrée and Guinle University Hospital, School of Medicine, Federal University of Rio de Janeiro State (UNIRIO), Rio de Janeiro, RJ, Brazil
e-mail: evelinallorian@gmail.com

13.2 Incidence

Brachial plexus injuries represent approximately one-third of peripheral nerve injuries [2]. They occur in slightly more than 1% of trauma patients. More than 60% of these injuries occur in the supraclavicular plexus and are more severe than infraclavicular, leading to a greater need for surgical intervention (52% of cases) compared to infraclavicular injuries (which require surgical intervention in 17% of cases).

Shoulder dysfunction can occur when the C5 and C6 root of the brachial plexus is injured. The mechanisms of injury vary, but typically are high energy injuries with car accidents/motorcycle crashes being the most frequent mechanism. Obstetric injuries during childbirth, tumors, and inflammatory disorders may also contribute to brachial plexus injury. The extent of the injury can range from a minor stretch of the nerve to a complete avulsion of the nerve root from the spinal cord [3].

One of the most significant problems associated with superior brachial plexus palsy is the loss of shoulder abduction. To address this issue, it is necessary to target the suprascapular and axillary nerves.

Nerve transfer surgery is an effective and reliable method for reconstructing the brachial plexus and restoring shoulder function in patients who have available donor nerves. A common technique used in brachial plexus reconstruction

F. Guedes et al. (eds.), *Nerve Transfers for Brachial Plexus Reconstruction after Trauma*,
https://doi.org/10.1007/978-3-031-92445-3_13

is the transfer of the spinal accessory nerve to the suprascapular nerve, using the proximal portion of this nerve for the transfer. The spinal accessory nerve (SAN), which innervates the sternocleidomastoid and trapezius muscles, is transferred to the suprascapular nerve. To minimize denervation of the trapezius muscle's upper portion, the spinal accessory nerve should be divided distal to its first or second branches. The goal is to achieve a tension-free direct end-to-end transfer of the spinal accessory nerve to the suprascapular nerve.

13.3 Anatomy

Understanding the anatomy of the suprascapular nerve (SSN) and the spinal accessory nerve (SAN) is important for successful surgical interventions. The SSN originates from the upper trunk of the brachial plexus, receiving nerve fibers primarily from C5 and C6 spinal nerves. Anatomically, the SSN is the only branch that originates directly from a trunk of the brachial plexus. The SSN provides sensory and motor innervation to the supraspinatus and infraspinatus muscles and the glenohumeral joint. The nerve exits the brachial plexus in the posterior triangle of the neck, passes laterally and downward across the triangle, and goes through the suprascapular notch beneath the transverse scapular ligament, deep to the supraspinatus and infraspinatus muscles.

The supraspinatus and infraspinatus muscles play an important role in shoulder movement, with the supraspinatus initiating abduction and the infraspinatus initiating external rotation. If SSN function is not properly restored or fully recovered, it can result in motion difficulties and positioning the hand and elbow in front of the body [4, 5].

The SAN exits the skull through the jugular foramen and runs between the heads of the sternocleidomastoid muscle before appearing at the posterior border of the muscle. It is covered only by skin and fascia as it travels through the posterior triangle toward the trapezius muscle. When the neck is viewed from the side, a line drawn from the atlas' transverse process to the posterior lateral point of the acromion indicates the path of the SAN.

The nerve passes between the heads of the sternocleidomastoid muscle and appears to penetrate its upper anterior border. The nerve supplies the sternocleidomastoid muscle before it reaches the posterior border of the muscle, which is located two-thirds of the distance between the muscle's lower and upper attachments. The nerve then branches into multiple short branches, which innervate the trapezius muscle directly [4, 5].

Understanding the precise anatomy of both nerves, the location, pathway, and relationship of the nerves to surrounding structures, is essential for successful surgical interventions and can impact the patient's overall recovery and functional outcome. During the anterior approach, the insertion point of the inferior belly of the omohyoid muscle can serve as a reliable marker to locate the suprascapular notch. Conversely, when adopting a posterior approach, a line drawn from the transverse process of the atlas to the posterior lateral point of the acromion can be utilized as a guide to delineate the pathway of the accessory nerve that pertains to the shoulder.

13.4 Diagnosis

In order to achieve an accurate diagnosis of brachial plexus injuries that may require a nerve transfer from the SAN to the SSN, a comprehensive approach is necessary, as the identification of viable roots if available. It should include a thorough physical examination, imaging studies (preferably MRI), and electro-neurophysiological tests to determine the extent and severity of the injury and guide the selection of an appropriate surgical procedure at a later stage. Additionally, it is essential to evaluate the main nerves that can be used as donor's nerves during nerve transfer surgery. By carefully considering all these factors, a customized treatment plan can be developed that effectively addresses the unique requirements of each individual patient.

13.4.1 Clinical Evaluation

A comprehensive evaluation is crucial for identifying the specific elements of a plexus injury. This evaluation should include a detailed medical history, physical examination, and the use of electrodiagnostic and imaging tests. Several factors are associated with a poorer prognosis, such as the time to surgery, presence of root avulsions, and body mass index [6]. The MRC scale is the recognized system for quantifying the extent of injury, providing a standardized assessment of muscle strength and function on a scale from 0 to 5 (Table 13.1). This scale enables better communication and consistent reporting of the severity of injury among medical professionals and institutions. Evaluating the presence of Tinel's sign is also important.

Additionally, valuable information that can help predict the outcome includes the time of injury when the patient seeks consultation. It is known that patients who present within 6 months of the trauma have a better surgical outcome compared to those with a longer duration of symptoms. However, patients with more than 6 months to a year after the trauma should still be considered as candidates for surgery, depending on their clinical, imaging, and electrophysiologic status [7].

The evaluation of shoulder function involves examining both passive and active ranges of motion, specifically the ability to perform abduction and external rotation in various positions [8, 9]. The examiner should identify any contractures present during the passive range of motion assessment for abduction, external rotation in adduction, and external rotation in maximal abduction. Also, glenohumeral total active and passive forward flexion and abduction should be recorded. To evaluate the patient's strength, they should be asked to tilt their spine to the opposite side while holding their arm in maximum abduction; meanwhile some authors test external rotation with 90° of abduction, determining if they are able to perform glenohumeral abduction against gravity at MRC Grade 3. It's important that the patient remains standing during the evaluation to eliminate any interference from spinal movements or pectoralis major activity.

Table 13.1 The British Medical Research Council scale

MRC scale for muscle strength	
0	No contraction
1	Flicker or trace of contraction
2	Full range of active movement, with gravity eliminated
3	Active movement against gravity
4	Active movement against gravity and resistance
5	Normal power

13.4.2 Imaging Studies and Electrophysiologic Exams

Imaging studies and electrophysiologic exams play a crucial role in evaluating and planning SAN transfer for SSN surgery. These diagnostic tools provide valuable information about nerve integrity, anatomical variations, and the feasibility of successful nerve transfer.

Magnetic resonance imaging (MRI) is a tool that can be used to assess the preoperative condition of the brachial plexus, specifically focusing on the spinal accessory and suprascapular nerve, often utilizing MR neurography (MRN). High-resolution MRIs are valuable in pinpointing the precise location and extent of nerve injuries and any accompanying soft tissue abnormalities. When conducting imaging, it is recommended to utilize the coronal and sagittal planes. The sagittal plane is particularly effective in assessing compartments such as the interscalene, costoclavicular, and pectoralis minor regions, which are located above and below the clavicle, thus aiding in surgical treatment planning [10].

MRN employs high-resolution, fat-suppressed, T2-weighted STIR sequences aligned with peripheral nerves. Its primary objective is to obtain selective images of nervous tissue, enabling the identification and evaluation of various morphological characteristics of the nerves. This technique allows for the observation of internal fascicular patterns, longitudinal variations in signal intensity and size, as well as connections and relationships with other nerves or plexuses. Additionally, it aids in distinguishing the signal intensity between intact nerves and muscles, with injured nerves typically exhibiting a higher signal intensity. In cases of moderate-to-severe stretch injuries, the brachial plexus can exhibit edema and fibrosis, causing the injured nerves to swell and appear twisted, resulting in diffuse increases in signal intensity over significant lengths in MR neurograms.

Electromyography (EMG) and nerve conduction studies (NCS) are electrophysiologic tests used to assess the electrical activity and conduction abilities of nerves and muscles in patients with brachial plexus injuries. These tests offer valuable information that allows for an assessment of the extent of brachial plexus damage, the degree of denervation, and the potential for functional recovery. EMG helps locate the site of injury and determine the severity of nerve damage, while NCS measures the speed and amplitude of nerve signals. These tests aid in patient selection, surgical planning, and monitoring of postoperative nerve regeneration [11].

Given the importance of these studies, it is imperative to assess the condition of the trapezius, supraspinatus, and infraspinatus muscles before proceeding with any surgical intervention. This evaluation should be conducted alongside their prior clinical assessment to ascertain the status of the SAN and SSN [12]. Intraoperative electrophysiologic monitoring plays a crucial role in spinal accessory nerve transfer surgery. This involves using EMG and nerve stimulation techniques to assess nerve function. Intraoperative EMG ensures precise placement and tensioning of the transferred nerve by providing real-time feedback on muscle activation. Nerve stimulation is employed to confirm the integrity and excitability of the transferred nerve, ensuring its potential for functional recovery.

During the surgical procedure, the nerve stimulus intensity gradually increases, typically ranging from 3 to 15 V for healthy nerves, while damaged nerves may require higher levels (usually below 100 V). The stimulus duration is set between 0.05 and 0.1 ms, with a frequency of 2–3 Hz. Amplification settings are adjusted incrementally, starting from 50 μV/division and increasing to 5 mv/division, with the time base usually set at 0.5 ms per division. A positive response, indicated by a visible regenerative NAP (negative action potential), confirms the presence of at least 4000 partially myelinated axons with a diameter greater than 5 μ between the stimulating and recording electrodes. The repetitive summation can further enhance small responses.

Abnormal EMG results, indicating muscle abnormalities or dysfunctions, and intraoperative testing revealing compromised nerve conduction can raise concerns about the success of the transfer procedure. The surgeon must carefully evaluate these findings to determine their potential impact on the procedure's success and expected functional outcomes.

The timing and decision to proceed or cancel the transfer procedure depend on various factors. If the EMG and intraoperative testing indicate normal nerve function and no significant abnormalities, the transfer can proceed as planned. However, if the results suggest compromised nerve function or abnormalities, the surgeon may need to reconsider the timing or cancel the transfer altogether. This decision will be based on a thorough evaluation of the patient's condition, the extent of nerve dysfunction, and the likelihood of achieving successful outcomes.

In conclusion, including EMG and NCS in the preoperative evaluation process for SAN transfer to SSN surgery is essential, aiding in surgical decision-making and forecast. However, if abnormal findings are revealed during the EMG and intraoperative testing, the timing of the transfer procedure may need to be adjusted or canceled, depending on the individual case and the likelihood of achieving favorable outcomes.

13.5 Surgical Technique

When performing a nerve transfer from the spinal accessory nerve to the suprascapular nerve, there are generally two approaches to consider: the anterior and the posterior route. It is important to evaluate each approach carefully to determine which is most suitable for the situation [2, 4, 5, 13–17].

For patients with blunt and stretch injuries of the brachial plexus, it is recommended to undergo surgery within 6 months of the injury [18]. However, waiting up to 9 months is also acceptable, especially for mild-to-moderate injuries that are typically associated with C5 and C6 root lesions. These types of injuries have a higher chance of spontaneous recovery, while injuries associated with C7 lesions or complete plexus lesions have a lower percentage of spontaneous recovery [19]. Nevertheless, early surgery is generally considered to be more beneficial for recovery, regardless of the level of injury. It is important, however, to always consider the potential for spontaneous recovery.

13.5.1 Anterior Approach

To perform the anterior approach, the patient is positioned supine with folded sheets under the shoulder, head, and neck to raise the shoulder area off the operating table [14]. The head is turned away from the surgical site. General anesthesia is used, avoiding the use of neuromuscular blocker.

A transverse incision of approximately 10 cm in length is made above the clavicle, parallel to it, and extending laterally from the posterior border of the sternocleidomastoid muscle to the acromioclavicular joint (Fig. 13.1). The skin, subcutaneous tissue, and platysma muscle are separated. The SSN can be located through a supraclavicular exposure by following the upper trunk to its divisions or by using the omohyoid and transverse cervical vessels if the upper trunk has been displaced distally by an injury [2].

The deep cervical fascia is detached from the trapezius muscle a few centimeters above the clavicle to identify and preserve the SAN. If necessary, the trapezius muscle's insertion in the clavicle is retracted posteriorly, detached, and reinserted later to aid in dissection [3].

A nerve stimulator is used to confirm the nerve's functionality and the proximal branches to the upper part of the trapezius are preserved

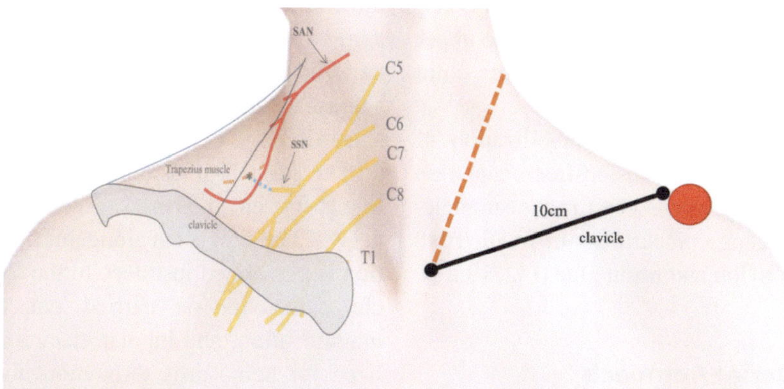

Fig. 13.1 Anatomic diagram of the anterior approach for SAN to SSN nerve transfer. Acromioclavicular joint (*red dot*); posterior border of the sternocleidomastoid muscle (*orange dashed line*); incision for supraclavicular approach (*black line*), 10 cm approximately. The spinal accessory nerve (SAN) typically emerges from the sternocleidomastoid muscle (SCM) at a location approximately two-thirds of the distance between its insertion on the clavicle and its origin on the mastoid process. It is important to consider that the specific branch intended for the transfer is one of the branches responsible for innervating the trapezius muscle. The suprascapular nerve (SSN) can be located through supraclavicular exposure by tracing the upper trunk to its divisions or by using the omohyoid and transverse cervical vessels as landmarks if the upper trunk has been displaced distally due to injury

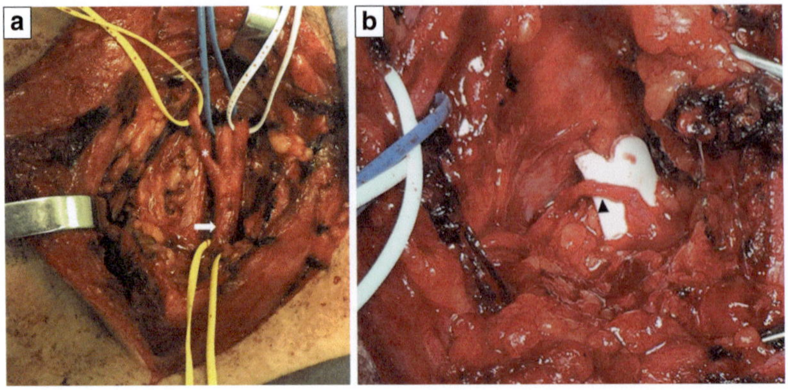

Fig. 13.2 Surgical image illustration of the anterior approach of the SAN to SSN transfers. (**a**) The suprascapular nerve is precisely located through a supraclavicular exposure, tracing its path from the upper trunk (*white arrow*) to its divisions. Suprascapular nerve (*asterisk*); posterior division of the upper trunk (*blue band*); anterior division of the upper trunk (*white band*). (**b**) The nerve transfer is executed (blackhead arrow) using the anterior approach after confirming the functionality of the SAN with a nerve stimulator, ensuring a tension-free coaptation of the SAN with the SSN during the surgical procedure

upper trapezius function. The terminal branch of the nerve is dissected and divided close to the muscle's entrance after the origin of one or two branches for the lower part of the muscle. The inferior belly of the omohyoid muscle is identified and retracted, and the SSN is exposed by dissecting the supraclavicular fat in the distal part of the posterior triangle of the neck. The SSN is isolated and dissected proximally toward the upper trunk and transected at the closest healthy point to its division from the upper trunk.

Finally, the dissection and mobilization of both nerves allow for a tension-free coaptation under the operating microscope in the supraclavicular fossa, using epineural sutures with 10–0 monofilament nylon and fibrin glue (Fig. 13.2).

13.5.2 Posterior Approach

It is crucial to mark the relevant landmarks before surgery to facilitate the identification of the distal accessory and suprascapular nerves. The dorsal midline and acromion are marked to locate the distal accessory nerve. Additionally, a point located 40% of the distance from the dorsal midline to the acromion along the superior border of the scapula is marked to approximate the location of the distal accessory nerve [14, 15]. To identify the SSN, the superior angle of the scapula and acromion are marked, and a point midway between these two points identifies the area of the suprascapular notch that transmits the nerve (Fig. 13.3).

The surgical incision is planned in a straight line between the marks identifying the two nerves. The skin is cut along this line, and dissection is performed just deep to the trapezius muscle. Dissection is carried out under loupe magnification, and bipolar electrocautery is utilized for hemostasis throughout the procedure. The superior border of the scapula is palpated, and dissection is carried out deep through or above the supraspinatus muscle toward the notch,

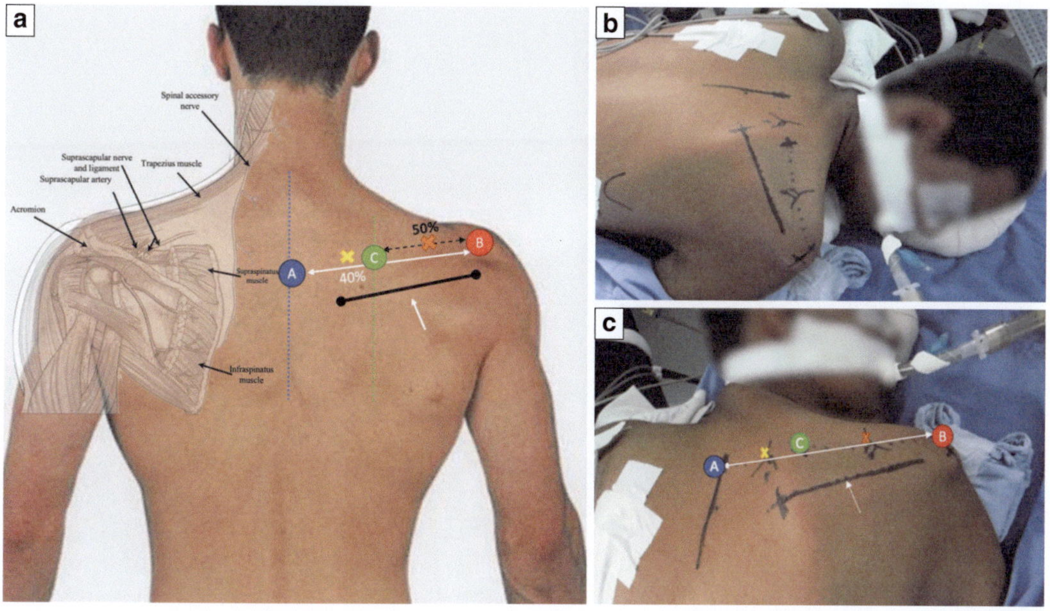

Fig. 13.3 (**a**) Anatomical diagram of the posterior approach for nerve transfer from the spinal accessory nerve to the suprascapular nerve. A. *Blue line and dot*: Dorsal midline. B. *Red dot*: Acromion. *Green line*: Medial border of the scapula C. *Green dot*: Superior angle of the scapula. Segment A–B (*white line*): Distance between the spinous processes and the acromion. The spinal accessory nerve (*yellow cross*) is located at 40% of the segment A–B, starting from A. Segment B–C (*black dash line*): Distance between the superior angle of the scapula and the acromion. The suprascapular nerve (*orange cross*) is located halfway (50%) of segment B–C. (**b**, **c**) Posterior surgical approach. (**b**) Patient in prone position, with arms adducted to both sides of the body. (**c**) Surgical application of anatomical diagram and approach detailed in (**a**); the incision is planned transversally to expose both nerves (*white arrow*)

with careful attention paid to identifying the suprascapular artery. The suprascapular notch is located by palpating the superior transverse scapular ligament with the index finger, and the hollow of the foramen is felt below the ligament. The ligament is palpated as a sharp band and is exposed bluntly with a "peanut" sponge or Kittner gauze. The ligament is then divided sharply under direct vision. In most cases, the nerve is not identified until the ligament has been divided. The nerve is exposed as it passes through the suprascapular notch and distally. The nerve stimulator is used to verify that the nerve is not active.

Once the SSN is isolated, the trapezius muscle is separated medially toward the location of the spinal accessory nerve. The presence of the nerve is typically indicated by adipose tissue, and its course is observed to be running in a superolateral-to-inferomedial direction as it enters the deep surface of the trapezius muscle. A nerve stimulator is used to aid in identification. The SAN is divided distally as necessary to allow for transfer without tension. After preparing the nerve ends, the proximal segment of the SAN is transferred and sutured to the distal segment of the SSN using interrupted 9–0 nylon under an operating microscope (Fig. 13.4).

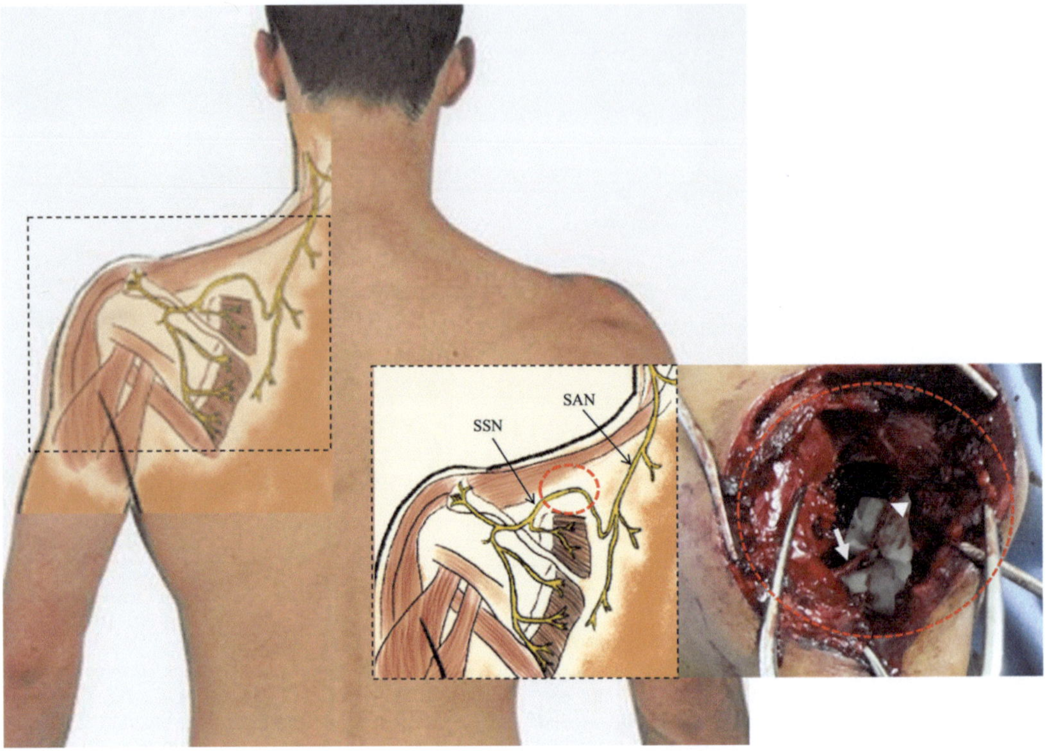

Fig. 13.4 Anatomical diagram illustrating nerve coaptation between the spinal accessory nerve (SAN) and the suprascapular nerve (SSN). Nerve transfer is executed using a posterior approach, ensuring tension-free coaptation of the SAN (*head arrow*) with the SSN (arrow) during the surgical procedure

13.6 Rehabilitation

Rehabilitation is a crucial component of recovery for patients who have undergone spinal accessory nerve to suprascapular nerve transfer for brachial plexus injuries. The primary objective of rehabilitation is to help patients regain strength, mobility, and range of motion in the affected shoulder. The transfer of the SAN to the SSN has the potential to restore external rotation and abduction by reinnervating the infraspinatus and supraspinatus muscles, respectively, and has shown better results than other nerve transfers with an index equal to or greater than M3, when performed at the appropriate time post-injury.

Physical therapy typically begins a few weeks after surgery and includes a combination of exercises, stretching, and massage to alleviate pain, stiffness, and muscle atrophy. The exercises focus on flexion, extension, abduction, and rotation of the shoulder to improve strength and mobility. The intensity of the exercises can be gradually increased over time using resistance bands, free weights, or other equipment to facilitate progress.

The rehabilitation process can be prolonged, and ongoing therapy is necessary to achieve optimal outcomes. However, with proper care and dedication, many patients can achieve significant improvement in shoulder function and return to their daily activities with greater ease and comfort. This underscores the importance of an individualized and comprehensive rehabilitation program to maximize the benefits of SAN transfer for the treatment of brachial plexus injuries.

13.7 Pearls and Pitfalls

When considering the two approaches, anterior and posterior, for performing a nerve transfer from the SAN to the SSN in brachial plexus injuries, there are advantages and disadvantages to each method [15, 17, 20–22].

The anterior approach has the benefit of allowing exploration of the supraclavicular brachial plexus, along with positioning, repair, and reconstruction in the same procedure. Additionally, there is a greater proportion of axons from the SAN available for transfer. However, this approach also has its drawbacks. One is the scarred supraclavicular region resulting from prior surgery or injury that can potentially cause denervation of a part of the trapezius muscle, which is crucial in maintaining shoulder stability and function that we aim to restore or improve with this approach.

The posterior approach offers notable advantages, including the preservation of upper trapezius functions and the possibility of near-nerve transfer to the target muscle, making it particularly valuable in cases where there are suspected SSN lesions at multiple levels. However, it is important to acknowledge several disadvantages associated with this approach. These include the need for specific surgical adjustments, such as transitioning from a supine to a prone position, during a brachial plexus reconstruction. Furthermore, substantial incisions in the back are required, involving the detachment of the trapezius muscle from its attachment to the scapular spine. It is also worth noting that the reduced axonal counts in the distal part of the SAN can be considered a disadvantage as well (Table 13.2).

Table 13.2 Advantages and disadvantages of anterior and posterior approach for the spinal accessory nerve (SAN) to suprascapular nerve (SSN)

Approach	Advantages	Disadvantages
Anterior	Allows exploration of the supraclavicular brachial plexus	Scarred supraclavicular region from prior surgery or injury can cause denervation of a part of the trapezius muscle, which is crucial in maintaining shoulder stability and function
	Allows for positioning, repair, and reconstruction in one procedure	Greater proportion of axons from the spinal accessory nerve available for transfer
Posterior	Preserves the functions of the upper part of the trapezius	Need to change position from supine to prone
	Near-nerve transfer to the target muscle	Large incisions in the back involve detaching the trapezius muscle from its attachment to the scapular spine
	Useful in cases of suspicion of SSN lesions at multiple levels	Reduced axonal counts in the distal part of SAN

13.8 Conclusions

Nerve repair techniques, particularly nerve transfer surgery involving the spinal accessory nerve (SAN) and the suprascapular nerve (SSN), play a vital role in restoring functionality to individuals with brachial plexus injuries. Accurate diagnosis and surgical planning are essential for achieving successful outcomes, highlighting their importance.

Two commonly employed surgical methods, the anterior and posterior approaches, are used for performing nerve transfers from the SAN to the SSN. Although the anterior approach is typically the preferred option, the posterior route may be utilized as a secondary method in cases where the anterior approach presents greater challenges or limitations.

References

1. Bhandari PS, Deb P. Dorsal approach in transfer of the distal spinal accessory nerve into the suprascapular nerve: histomorphometric analysis and clinical results in 14 cases of upper brachial plexus injuries. J Hand Surg Am. 2011;36(7):1182–90. https://doi.org/10.1016/j.jhsa.2011.02.025.
2. Wilson T, Yang LJS. Peripheral nerve neurosurgery. Oxford: Oxford University Press; 2018. https://play.google.com/store/books/details?id=kzdtDwAAQBAJ.
3. Emamhadi M, Alijani B, Andalib S. Long-term clinical outcomes of spinal accessory nerve transfer to the suprascapular nerve in patients with brachial plexus palsy. Acta Neurochir. 2016;158(9):1801–6. https://doi.org/10.1007/s00701-016-2886-1.
4. Mackinnon SE. Nerve surgery. New York: Thieme; 2015. https://play.google.com/store/books/details?id=Ozu9YgEACAAJ.
5. Rigoard P. Atlas of anatomy of the peripheral nerves: the nerves of the limbs—student edition. Cham: Springer International Publishing; 2017. https://play.google.com/store/books/details?id=7ucGDQEACAAJ.
6. Socolovsky M, Di Masi G, Bonilla G, Malessy M. Spinal to accessory nerve transfer in traumatic brachial plexus palsy: is body mass index a predictor of outcome? Acta Neurochir. 2014;156(1):159–63. https://doi.org/10.1007/s00701-013-1896-5.
7. Chung KC, Yang LJ-S, McGillicuddy JE. Chapter15—Nerve repair/nerve transfer strategies for adult brachial plexus palsies. In: Practical management of pediatric and adult brachial plexus palsies. London: Saunders/Elsevier; 2012.
8. Malessy MJA, de Ruiter GCW, de Boer KS, Thomeer RTWM. Evaluation of suprascapular nerve neurotization after nerve graft or transfer in the treatment of brachial plexus traction lesions. J Neurosurg. 2004;101(3):377–89. https://doi.org/10.3171/jns.2004.101.3.0377.
9. Guarantors of the Brain. Aids to the examination of the peripheral nervous system. London: Saunders; 2010. https://play.google.com/store/books/details?id=69xYpwAACAAJ.
10. Chung KC, Yang LJ-S, McGillicuddy JE. Chapter 18, Radiographic assessment of adult brachial plexus injuries. In: Practical management of pediatric and adult brachial plexus palsies. London: Saunders/Elsevier; 2012.
11. Kline DG, Hackett ER, May PR. Evaluation of nerve injuries by evoked potentials and electromyography. J Neurosurg. 1969;31(2):128–36. https://doi.org/10.3171/jns.1969.31.2.0128.
12. Suzuki K, Doi K, Hattori Y, Pagsaligan JM. Long-term results of spinal accessory nerve transfer to the suprascapular nerve in upper-type paralysis of brachial plexus injury. J Reconstr Microsurg. 2007;23:295.
13. Socolovsky M, Martins RS, Di Masi G, Bonilla G, Siqueira MG. Influence of body mass index on the outcome of brachial plexus surgery: are there any differences between elbow and shoulder results? Acta Neurochir. 2014;156(12):2337–44. https://doi.org/10.1007/s00701-014-2256-9.
14. Kim D, Hudson AR, Kline DG. Atlas of peripheral nerve surgery: expert consult—online and print. Amsterdam: Elsevier Health Sciences; 2012. https://play.google.com/store/books/details?id=NgtuvTBx-1QC.
15. Colbert SH, Mackinnon S. Posterior approach for double nerve transfer for restoration of shoulder function in upper brachial plexus palsy. Hand (N Y). 2006;1(2):71–7. https://doi.org/10.1007/s11552-006-9004-4.
16. Bertelli JA, Ghizoni MF. Transfer of the accessory nerve to the suprascapular nerve in brachial plexus reconstruction. J Hand Surg Am. 2007;32(7):989–98. https://doi.org/10.1016/j.jhsa.2007.05.016.
17. Makel M, Sukop A, Kachlík D, Waldauf P, Whitley A, Kaiser R. Is there any difference between anterior and posterior approach for the spinal accessory to suprascapular nerve transfer? A systematic review and meta-analysis. Neurol Res. 2023;45(5):489–96. https://doi.org/10.1080/01616412.2022.2156721.
18. Martin E, Senders JT, DiRisio AC, Smith TR, Broekman MLD. Timing of surgery in traumatic brachial plexus injury: a systematic review. J Neurosurg. 2018;130(4):1333–45. https://doi.org/10.3171/2018.1.JNS172068.

19. Kline DG. Timing for brachial plexus injury: a personal experience. Neurosurg Clin N Am. 2009;20(1):24–6. https://doi.org/10.1016/j.nec.2008.07.030, v.
20. Maurya S, Renganathan G, Venkatnarayanan R, Bharti R. Outcomes of shoulder functions in spinal accessory to suprascapular nerve transfer in brachial plexus injury: a comparison between anterior and posterior approach. Indian J Plast Surg. 2021;54(2):152–6. https://doi.org/10.1055/s-0041-1731255.
21. Chuang DC, Lee GW, Hashem F, Wei FC. Restoration of shoulder abduction by nerve transfer in avulsed brachial plexus injury: evaluation of 99 patients with various nerve transfers. Plast Reconstr Surg. 1995;96(1):122–8. https://doi.org/10.1097/00006534-199507000-00019.
22. Bhatnagar A. Spinal accessory nerve transfer to the suprascapular nerve to restore shoulder function in brachial plexus injury: management nuances. Neurol India. 2019;67(Suppl):S29–31. https://doi.org/10.4103/0028-3886.250725.

14 Transfer of a C7 Fascicule for the Pectoralis Major to the Suprascapular Nerve

Belkheyar Zoubir, Cambon Adeline, and Oberlin Christophe

14.1 Principle of the Transfer

In C5–C6 plexus brachial roots injuries, targeted nerves to restore shoulder function include the SSN and the axillary nerve. When root grafting is not possible between C5 root and SSN, SAN transfer is the main donor nerve used for reanimation of the SSN. Despite the satisfactory results reported by various team [1, 2], this transfer has one disadvantage, the weakening of an essential scapula stabilizer: the trapezius muscle. This periscapular muscle is the main scapula retropulsor. As a consequence, its paralysis causes scapular dyskinesia [3]. Moreover, in patients with insufficient external shoulder rotation following nerve surgery, previous harvesting of SAN could jeopardize results of palliative surgical options such as lower trapezius transfer and scapulohumeral arthrodesis [4, 5]. Since 2015, in the goal of sparing the SAN, we transfer one fascicule from C7 root for the PM to the SSN when graft between the roots and distal nerve targets is not feasible (Fig. 14.1).

This transfer has several advantages. The donor fascicule is a pure motor nerve, not a terminal branch, and close to the recipient nerve, so a direct, tensionless suture is always possible. In our experience, shoulder external rotation is clinically noticeable 6 months earlier than after a SAN transfer to the SSN. Finally, we observed superior outcomes after this transfer than in our previous published series of SAN to SSN transfer, in terms of range of motion and strength: half of the 19 patients had recovered external rotation strength inferior to M4 [6].

B. Zoubir · O. Christophe
Clinique du Mont Louis, Paris, France

C. Adeline (✉)
Orthopaedic and Traumatology Surgery Department,
Sorbonne University, Saint-Antoine Hospital,
Paris, France

F. Guedes et al. (eds.), *Nerve Transfers for Brachial Plexus Reconstruction after Trauma*,
https://doi.org/10.1007/978-3-031-92445-3_14

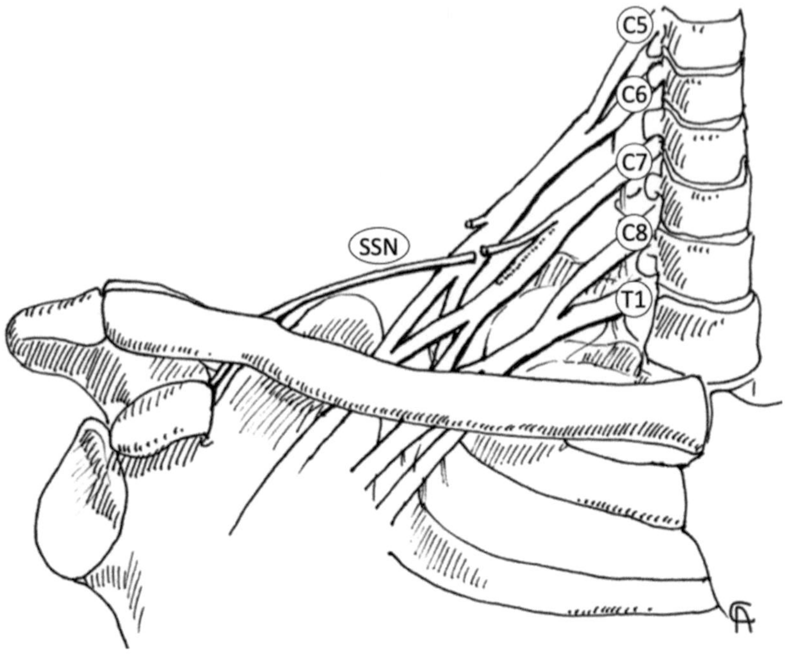

Fig. 14.1 Transfer of a fascicule from C7 root to the suprascapular nerve

14.2 Surgical Technique

Under general anesthesia, the patient is placed on supine position. A V-shaped cervical incision is done along the posterior border of sternocleidomastoid muscle and upper border of the clavicle. First, the upper primary trunk, the C5 and C6 roots, and the distal SSN are identified. Electrostimulation of the SSN is done to confirm its paralysis. Next, intraneural dissection of the C7 root is performed under microscope magnification with the help of electrostimulation in order to select a fascicule from its supero-anterior part, responding in the PM on, but not in the triceps muscle. The fascicule is cut proximal to the division of the middle trunk and dissected proximally over 3 cm. The SSN is then cut in a healthy area as proximal as possible. A tensionless suture is done between the two nerve ends by using simple epiperineural stitches with fibrin-based biological glue.

The patient's shoulder is splinted in abduction for 3 weeks. Rehabilitation is then initiated.

14.3 Expected Outcomes

In patients of our published series, first contractions were observed at a mean postoperative delay of 6 months [7]. Nine of the ten patients reached M4 shoulder external rotation strength. Patients recovered 58 degrees of external rotation in average (Fig. 14.2).

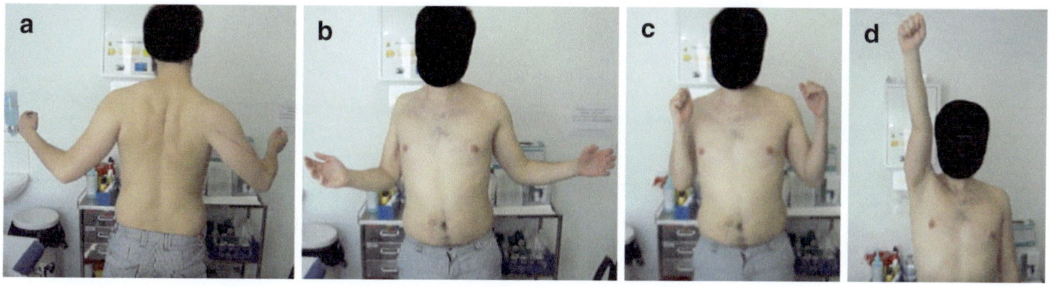

Fig. 14.2 Postoperative result in a 17-year-old man with a C5–C6 brachial plexus palsy. Nerve surgery 4 months after the trauma included the transfer of one C7 fascicule to the SSN, transfers from fascicules of the ulnar and median nerves, respectively, to the biceps motor branch and brachialis motor branch of the musculocutaneous nerve, and of the branch of the lateral head of the triceps to the anterior branch of the axillary nerve. On examination 41 months later, the patient had recovered 35° of active external shoulder rotation (**a**, **b**), 140° of elbow flexion (**b**), complete elbow flexion (**c**) and complete shoulder elevation (**d**). Pectoralis major muscle strength and triceps muscle strength were graded as M4+, with 28% loss of strength compared to the contralateral triceps

References

1. Bertelli JA, Ghizoni MF. Transfer of the accessory nerve to the suprascapular nerve in brachial plexus reconstruction. J Hand Surg Am. 2007;32:989–98.
2. Merrell GA, Barrie KA, Katz DL, Wolfe SW. Results of nerve transfer techniques for restoration of shoulder and elbow function in the context of a meta-analysis of the English literature. J Hand Surg Am. 2001;26:303–14.
3. Oberlin C, Durand S, Belkheyar Z, Shafi M, David E, Asfazadourian H. Nerve transfers in brachial plexus palsies. Chir Main. 2009;28:1–9.
4. Elhassan B. Lower trapezius transfer for shoulder external rotation in patients with paralytic shoulder. J Hand Surg Am. 2014;39:556–62.
5. Atlan F, Durand S, Fox M, Levy P, Belkheyar Z, Oberlin C. Functional outcome of glenohumeral fusion in brachial plexus palsy: a report of 54 cases. J Hand Surg Am. 2012;37:683–8.
6. Pages L, Le Hanneur M, Cambon-Binder A, Belkheyar Z. C5/C6 brachial plexus palsy reconstruction using nerve surgery: long-term functional outcomes. Orthop Traumatol Surg Res. 2020;106(6):1095–100. S1877-0568(20)30196-1.
7. Cambon-Binder A, Belkheyar Z. Transfer of a C7 fascicle for the pectoralis major to the suprascapular nerve: a 3-year follow-up patient series. Plast Reconstr Surg. 2022;149(3):672–5.

15 Phrenic Nerve for Shoulder Reinnervation

Luccie M. Wo and Johnny Chuieng-Yi Lu

Abbreviations

Ph	Phrenic nerve
SAN	Spinal accessory nerve
SSN	Suprascapular nerve

15.1 Introduction

The restoration of shoulder function is a significant goal in brachial plexus reconstruction. The glenohumeral joint is a ball-in-socket joint that allows for a wide range of motion in multiple planes, including shoulder abduction, adduction, flexion, extension, and external and internal rotation [1]. However, restoring shoulder abduction and external rotation allows the patient to reach for objects and move the upper extremity away from the thorax. This enables a better appreciation of restored elbow flexion [2]. The main targets for shoulder reinnervation include the (1) suprascapular nerve (SSN), which controls the supraspinatus and infraspinatus muscle, and (2) axillary nerve, which controls the deltoid and teres minor muscles. Achieving a full range of motion requires reinnervation of the muscles above. However, using one donor nerve for shoulder function may be the only option in extended brachial plexus injuries such as C5–8 avulsions (or total root avulsions) with a lack of donor nerves. As such, SSN becomes the primary target for restoration because it is responsible for initiating shoulder abduction from 0° to 60° while also providing external rotation to provide room for elbow flexion [1].

The choice of donor's nerve for reinnervating the SSN has long-term sequelae in the primary and secondary reconstruction strategies for brachial plexus injuries. The more severe the injury, the more functions that require reinnervation; consequently, the demand for reinnervation exceeds the availability of donor nerves. Donor nerve selection for shoulder abduction depends on the patient's condition and the surgeon's expertise. According to current literature, the spinal accessory nerve (SAN) is the preferred choice for nerve transfer to restore shoulder abduction. Alternative options include nerve grafting from ruptured spinal roots, phrenic nerve (Ph), deep cervical motor branches, hypoglossal nerve, and

L. M. Wo
Division of Reconstructive Microsurgery, Department of Plastic Surgery, Chang Gung Memorial Hospital, Chang Gung Medical University, Linkou, Taiwan

Division of Plastic and Reconstructive Surgery, Department of Surgery, Yale School of Medicine, New Haven, CT, USA
e-mail: luccie.wo@yale.edu

J. C.-Y. Lu (✉)
Division of Reconstructive Microsurgery, Department of Plastic Surgery, Chang Gung Memorial Hospital, Chang Gung Medical University, Linkou, Taiwan

F. Guedes et al. (eds.), *Nerve Transfers for Brachial Plexus Reconstruction after Trauma*,
https://doi.org/10.1007/978-3-031-92445-3_15

Table 15.1 Comparison of the phrenic nerve and spinal accessory nerve

	Phrenic nerve	Spinal accessory nerve
Axon count	~2600	~2100
Surgical approach	Anterior: concurrent brachial plexus exploration	Anterior: concurrent brachial plexus exploration Posterior: outside zone of injury from brachial plexus injury
Advantages	• Proximity to suprascapular nerve • Stimulation of target muscle is constant and spontaneous	• Proximity to suprascapular nerve • Induction of movement synergistic with shoulder
Disadvantage	• Permanent ipsilateral diaphragm paralysis • Transient decrease in pulmonary function	• Middle and lower trapezius paralysis and atrophy • Possible transient shoulder pain • Decreased scapular stability
Contraindications	• C2–C4 injury • Infantile obstetric brachial plexus injury • Chronic lung disease (relative) • BMI >35 (relative) • Heavy smoker (relative)	• Spinal accessory nerve injury • Denervated scapulothoracic muscles

contralateral C7. The Ph is the first choice at our institute as a donor nerve to the SSN.

The technique of using the Ph as a donor's nerve was first conceptualized by Lurje in 1948 [3] and popularized by Gu for clinical application in the 1990s [4]. The Ph is primarily comprised of motor axons [5]. At rest or during quiet respiration, the diaphragm is controlled by autonomic input from the Ph. The Ph can also initiate powerful and voluntary diaphragm contractions during deep inspiration [5, 6]. Thus, following nerve transfer with Ph, patient rehabilitation involves aerobic exercises such as running and stair climbing to practice Ph induction for purposeful movements.

We select the ipsilateral Ph as our first choice for several reasons. First, the Ph is already exposed during the exploration of the supraclavicular brachial plexus. Second, it lies close to the SSN, often allowing for a direct coaptation without using a nerve graft. Furthermore, patients report easy adaption following Ph transfer, demonstrating good brain plasticity for regaining volition control of the targeting function [7]. Additionally, rehabilitation for Ph transfers involves aerobic exercises that encourage mobility and promote early rehabilitation. Finally, using the Ph spares the SAN. For instance, the SAN is a commonly used nerve for free-functioning muscle transplantation, which is indicated for elbow flexion following failed nerve reconstruction or for pan-brachial plexus injuries [8]. Recent literature has advocated for preserving SAN to maintain shoulder stability better. The distal trapezius muscle tendon can be used for tendon transfer to restore external rotation at the shoulder [9, 10]. In patients with failed nerve reconstruction that require subsequent shoulder arthrodesis, preserving the trapezius is critical to maintaining scapulothoracic stability [11]. Table 15.1 compares the use of Ph and SAN for the restoration of the shoulder function.

The Ph is efficacious in restoring elbow flexion and shoulder abduction [4, 5, 12, 13]. Our preference is to transfer Ph to the SSN for a better match in axon count: the Ph axon count is approximately 2600+ motor fibers, and the SSN is approximately 3500+ fibers, which matches the 70% target of donor-to-recipient axon count ratio [14–16]. While Ph can also be transferred to C5 to reach more muscle targets (such as supraspinatus, deltoid, and triceps), the axon count mismatch leads to unpredictable results unless Ph is combined with other donor nerves [17].

15.2 Applied Anatomy and Preoperative Assessment

The Ph is a motor nerve that innervates the diaphragm to initiate inspiration for pulmonary expansion. The Ph arises from the C4 root with variable contributions from C3 to C5 [18]. The anterior rami of the C3, C4, and C5 rootlets join from the Ph along the upper-lateral border of the anterior scalene muscle [19]. Ph travels medially and caudally along the anterior scalene muscle's anterior surface parallel to the internal jugular vein [19]. The Ph most commonly travels deep to the transverse cervical artery at the inferomedial border of the anterior scalene muscle before it enters the thorax between the subclavian artery and subclavian vein [19]. Variations in Ph occur at the rootlets, with some cadaveric studies demonstrating isolated contributions only from C4 or contributions only from C4 to C5 [18, 20]. Variations along its cervical course are rare, with some reports of the Ph being anterior to the subclavian vein, emitting a communicating branch to the root of C5 of the brachial plexus, or occasionally bifurcating into two branches along the anterior scalene muscle [20]. The most described variation is an accessory phrenic nerve incidence, which can occur in as many as 60% of cases [20]. The accessory phrenic nerve usually originates from the subclavian nerve and joins the Ph in the thorax [20]. The Ph can reliably be identified during a supraclavicular brachial plexus exploration and conveniently used as a donor nerve, thus preserving the XI nerve for other purposes in brachial plexus reconstruction.

Contraindications for Ph transfer are concurrent C2–C4 level root injuries, infantile obstetric brachial plexus injury, chronic lung disease, morbid obesity (BMI >35 kg/m^2), heavy smoking (relative contraindication), and noncompliant or poorly motivated patients (relative contraindication) [17]. Furthermore, preoperative assessment should include inspiratory and expiratory chest X-rays, ultrasound study of diaphragmatic movement, and pulmonary function testing for greater accuracy. These tests not only establish a baseline preoperative lung function but can diagnose any occult Ph injury. Concurrent Ph dysfunction-associated brachial plexus trauma occurs in 10–20% of injuries. Preoperative chest X-ray has a sensitivity of 56% and specificity of 93% for identifying phrenic nerve palsy [21].

15.3 Surgical Technique

An extensive supraclavicular brachial plexus exploration is required to expose the Ph and target nerves fully. The patient is supine with the injured arm extended and the head turned toward the uninjured side. A C-curve incision is designed on the lateral neck starting from the mastoid, extending medially to the jugular notch and laterally along the clavicle shaft. A platysma musculocutaneous flap is elevated, and dissection is carried down to the sternocleidomastoid muscle, which is then retracted medially. The omohyoid muscle is identified and retracted medially. There is a variable amount of adipofascial tissue lying above the plexus that requires retraction, and thus, a c-shaped adipofascial flap is elevated laterally by separating the connections between the internal jugular vein and the adipofascial tissue before the anterior scalene muscle is exposed. Care should be taken to preserve the transverse cervical artery and vein deep to the adipofascial flap because the vessels intersect with the nerve at the anteromedial margin of the anterior scalene muscle. When the anterior scalene muscle is exposed along with the plexus, it is highly recommended to use a nerve stimulator to identify the Ph and elicit intraoperative diaphragmatic movement. It is essential to examine the health of the Ph for any signs of scarring or ruptures along its entire length in the neck to the clavicle; Fig. 15.1 demonstrates Ph's relation to the brachial plexus. It is better to start dissection of the Ph more dis-

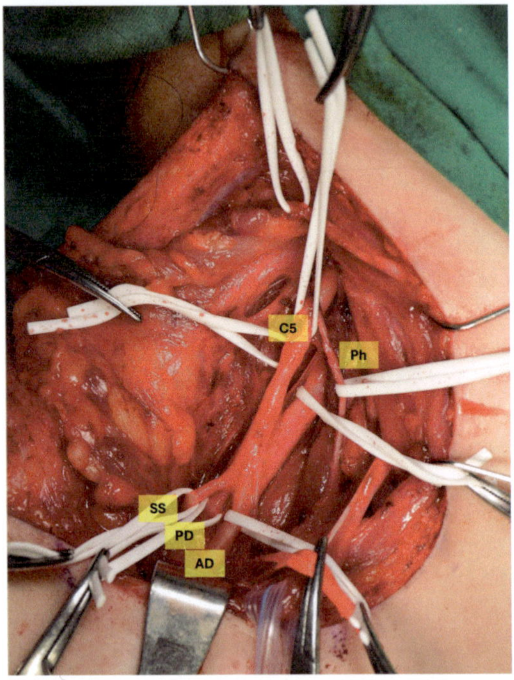

Fig. 15.1 Phrenic exposure. The phrenic nerve is exposed during brachial plexus exploration and dissected from distal to proximal in preparation for nerve transfer. C5: cervical spinal nerve 5, Ph: phrenic nerve, SS: suprascapular nerve, PD: posterior division of the brachial plexus, AD; anterior division of the brachial plexus

tally as it reaches the thorax rather than proximally as it connects with the C5 spinal nerve or the upper trunk. If C5 root avulsion was impressed before surgery, be wary of concurrent C4 injury, which may render the Ph unhealthy. If the Ph is unusable, alternatives include the SAN, the cervical motor branch, the hypoglossal nerve, or the levator scapulae branch. In the left neck, accidental ligation of the thoracic duct should be prevented to avoid chylous leakage after surgery.

The SSN is the upper trunk's first branch, usually found beneath the transverse cervical artery. It exits the upper trunk and travels posteriorly towards the scapula notch. The division medial to the SSN is the posterior division of the upper trunk, which travels in the posterior plane. The Ph can be transferred to the SSN for reinnervation of supraspinatus (abduction) and infraspinatus (external rotation) muscles or to the posterior division of the upper trunk for deltoid (abduction) and teres minor (external rotation) muscles. In pure level I injuries, Ph can reach SSN by direct coaptation; however, if the injury extends to level II or retroclavicular regions, the SSN may be tractioned distally and have larger zones of trauma that may extend to the scapular notch. A nerve graft may be required if a tension-free coaptation cannot be achieved. If there is a high suspicion of SSN injury near the scapular notch, a posterior approach to examine SSN may be needed, followed by SAN as the intended donor nerve.

15.4 The Results of Phrenic Nerve Transfer for Shoulder Abduction

Lu et al. demonstrated that the Ph nerve can achieve equivalent results in restoring shoulder abduction compared to the SAN [17]. A retrospective review of 132 cases revealed that patients gained an average of 61.9 + 38.7° of shoulder abduction with Ph to SSN and 51.1 + 37.3° with SAN to SSN, with a minimum follow-up of 2 years [17]. Dual transfer of Ph and SAN can achieve even better results [22–24]. Nevertheless, the lack of donor nerves in panplexus injuries precludes the reconstruction of one function with two donors.

15.5 Respiratory Function Following Phrenic Nerve Transfer

The primary concern regarding the Ph as a donor nerve is the effects of ipsilateral diaphragm paralysis on pulmonary function. Past reports by groups commonly using the Ph as a donor demonstrated that decreased pulmonary function did not permanently affect daily function. Gu et al. series of 180 patients only had 1 report of clinically significant but transient respiratory problems in a 5-year-old patient who had concurrent neurotization using the Ph and three intercostal nerves [4]. Subclinically, patients may have elevated ipsilateral diaphragm elevation on imaging and decreased pulmonary capacity, but this resolves in most patients after 1 year of follow-up [4, 25, 26]. In a study of pulmonary function in 19 brachial plexus injuries with received Ph and multiple intercostal nerve transfers, the postoperative patients had, on average, an 8% decrease in inspiratory capacity, forced vital capacity (FVC), and total lung capacity but an 11% increase in diffusing capacity at 3 years follow-up [26]. Even so, patients reported recovery from respiratory symptoms starting at 6 months following surgery. Nevertheless, using the Ph as a donor is not recommended in infants with obstetric brachial plexus injury and adults with BMI >35, chronic lung disease, or contralateral Ph injury [24].

15.6 Alternative Nerves for Shoulder Abduction

Suppose the Ph is injured and SAN is not available. In that case, other donor nerves for shoulder reinnervation include the hypoglossal nerve, deep cervical motor branches of the cervical plexus, contralateral C7, levator scapula motor nerve, and nerve grafting from ruptured spinal roots [27–29]. Cambon-Binder et al. demonstrated that a nerve transfer between the pectoralis major branch of ipsilateral C7 to SSN restored shoulder abduction to an average of 99° at a 3-year follow-up in ten patients [28]. Goubier et al. used the rhomboid for SSN transfer to restore shoulder rotation and elevation in eight patients [30]. Cadaveric studies have also demonstrated the feasibility of using the levator scapular motor nerve for nerve transfer to the SSN [29]. Ultimately, the choice of nerve transfer for restoration of shoulder abduction depends mainly on the patient's anatomy and injury presentation, as well as the surgeon's preference. In addition to nerve transfers, patients can receive tendon transfers or shoulder arthrodesis to improve shoulder function and stability [9, 10]. These techniques can be used as alternatives to nerve transfer or in conjunction with nerve transfers in a staged fashion.

15.7 Summary

The Ph is a reliable donor nerve for the reinnervation of shoulder function. Using the Ph conveys several advantages: convenience to target nerves when exploring the plexus in the supraclavicular region provides constant and spontaneous motor stimulation to target nerves and offers an alternative to SAN, which can free up options for other aspects of brachial plexus reconstruction. The decision to sacrifice the phrenic nerve due to the fear of permanent pulmonary dysfunction, although rare, ultimately depends on the surgeon's judgment and the specific patient population.

References

1. Chang LR, Anand P, Varacallo M. Anatomy, shoulder and upper limb, glenohumeral joint. In: StatPearls. Treasure Island, FL: StatPearls Publishing; 2024. http://www.ncbi.nlm.nih.gov/books/NBK537018/.
2. Yang LJS, Chang KWC, Chung KC. A systematic review of nerve transfer and nerve repair for the treatment of adult upper brachial plexus injury. Neurosurgery. 2012;71(2):417–29.
3. Lurje A. Concerning surgical treatment of traumatic injury to the upper division of the brachial plexus (Erb's type). Ann Surg. 1948;127(2):317–26.
4. Gu YD, Ma MK. Use of the phrenic nerve for brachial plexus reconstruction. Clin Orthop Relat Res. 1996;323:119–21.
5. Luedemann W, Hamm M, Blömer U, Samii M, Tatagiba M. Brachial plexus neurotization with donor phrenic nerves and its effect on pulmonary function. J Neurosurg. 2002;96(3):523–6.
6. Adrian ED, Bronk DW. The discharge of impulses in motor nerve fibres. J Physiol. 1928;66(1):81–101.
7. Socolovsky M, Barillaro K, Bonilla G, Masi GD, Malessy M. Nerve transfers for brachial plexus injuries: grading of volitional control. J Neurosurg. 2022;138(5):1419–25.
8. Doi K, Muramatsu K, Hattori Y, Otsuka K, Tan SH, Nanda V, et al. Restoration of prehension with the double free muscle technique following complete avulsion of the brachial plexus: indications and long-term results. J Bone Joint Surg Am. 2000;82(5):652.
9. Elhassan B. Lower trapezius transfer for shoulder external rotation in patients with paralytic shoulder. J Hand Surg Am. 2014;39(3):556–62.
10. Elhassan B, Bishop AT, Hartzler RU, Shin AY, Spinner RJ. Tendon transfer options about the shoulder in patients with brachial plexus injury. J Bone Joint Surg. 2012;94(15):1391–8.

11. Atlan F, Durand S, Fox M, Levy P, Belkheyar Z, Oberlin C. Functional outcome of glenohumeral fusion in brachial plexus palsy: a report of 54 cases. J Hand Surg Am. 2012;37(4):683–8.
12. Siqueira MG, Martins RS. Phrenic nerve transfer in the restoration of elbow flexion in brachial plexus avulsion injuries: how effective and safe is it? Neurosurgery. 2009;65(4):A125–31.
13. Xu WD, Gu YD, Xu JG, Tan LJ. Full-length phrenic nerve transfer by means of video-assisted thoracic surgery in treating brachial plexus avulsion injury. Plast Reconstr Surg. 2002;110(1):104.
14. Ma JJ, Zhang GM, Xu JG, Gu YO. Histochemical study on the donor nerves for nerve transfer in treatment of the brachial plexus injuries. Chin J Hand Surg. 1997;13:235–7.
15. Lee D, Neviaser RJ. Operative techniques: shoulder and elbow surgery. Amsterdam: Elsevier Health Sciences; 2018. 747 p.
16. Schreiber JJ, Byun DJ, Khair MM, Rosenblatt L, Lee SK, Wolfe SW. Optimal axon counts for brachial plexus nerve transfers to restore elbow flexion. Plast Reconstr Surg. 2015;135(1):135e–41e.
17. Lu JCY, Lin JAJ, Lee CH, Chang TNJ, Chuang DCC. Phrenic nerve as an alternative donor for nerve transfer to restore shoulder abduction in severe multiple root injuries of the adult brachial plexus. J Hand Surg Am. 2023;48(9):954.e1–954.e10.
18. Mendelsohn AH, DeConde A, Lambert HW, Dodson SC, Daney BT, Stark ME, et al. Cervical variations of the phrenic nerve. Laryngoscope. 2011;121(9):1920–3.
19. Canella C, Demondion X, Delebarre A, Moraux A, Cotten H, Cotten A. Anatomical study of phrenic nerve using ultrasound. Eur Radiol. 2010;20(3):659–65.
20. Prates Júnior A, Vasques L, Bordoni L. Anatomical variations of the phrenic nerve: an actualized review. J Morphol Sci. 2015;32(01):53–6.
21. Crowe CS, Pulos N, Spinner RJ, Bishop AT, Wigle DA, Shin AY. The diagnostic utility of inspiratory-expiratory radiography for the assessment of phrenic nerve palsy associated with brachial plexus injury. Acta Neurochir. 2023;165(9):2589–96.
22. Cardenas-Camarena L, Dorado C, Guerrero MT, Nava R. Surgical masculinization of the breast: clinical classification and surgical procedures. Aesth Plast Surg. 2017;41(3):507–16.
23. Chuang DCC, Lee GW, Hashem F, Wei FC. Restoration of shoulder abduction by nerve transfer in avulsed brachial plexus injury: evaluation of 99 patients with various nerve transfers. Plast Reconstr Surg. 1995;96(1):122.
24. Boyd KU, Nimigan AS, Mackinnon SE. Nerve reconstruction in the hand and upper extremity. Clin Plast Surg. 2011;38(4):643–60.
25. Chalidapong P, Sananpanich K, Kraisarin J, Bumroongkit C. Pulmonary and biceps function after intercostal and phrenic nerve transfer for brachial plexus injuries. J Hand Surg. 2004;29(1):8–11.
26. Chuang ML, Chuang DCC, Lin IF, Vintch JRE, Ker JJW, Tsao TCY. Ventilation and exercise performance after phrenic nerve and multiple intercostal nerve transfers for avulsed brachial plexus injury. Chest. 2005;128(5):3434–9.
27. Chuang DC. Brachial plexus injuries: adult and pediatric. Plast Surg. 2013;6:789–816.
28. Cambon-Binder A, Belkheyar Z. Transfer of a C7 fascicle for the pectoralis major to the suprascapular nerve: a 3-year follow-up patient series. Plast Reconstr Surg. 2022;149(3):672–5.
29. Saltzman EB, Krishnan K, Winston MJ, Das De S, Lee SK, Wolfe SW. A cadaveric study on the utility of the levator scapulae motor nerve as a donor for brachial plexus reconstruction. J Hand Surg Am. 2021;46(9):812.e1–5.
30. Goubier JN, Echalier C, Dubois E, Teboul F. Transfer of the rhomboid nerve for restoration of shoulder external rotation in partial brachial plexus palsy. Injury. 2020;51:S84–7.

16 Thoracodorsal Nerve to Long Thoracic Nerve Transfer

Juan Pablo Martinez and Mariano Socolovsky

Abbreviations

BP	Brachial plexus
LTN	Long thoracic nerve
TDN	Thoracodorsal nerve

16.1 Introduction

The lesion or paralysis of the LTN produces dysfunction of the serratus anterior target muscle, which originates in the ribs and ends its insertion in the scapula. On physical examination, the first evident thing is a scapular asymmetry—winged scapula—first described in 1723 by Winslow [1, 2]. Subsequently, Sir Charles Bell detailed this nerve in its anatomy and function in 1821 in a communication to the Royal Society, thus bearing his name—Bell's long thoracic nerve or external respiratory nerve [3, 4]. Since then, at the beginning of the twentieth century, different treatments have been reported to correct this dysfunction. Regarding the surgical approach, the first proposed treatments were mainly related to traumatological and orthopedic techniques, which were to be modified over time and enter the modern era, where we find the first reports of this type of transfer.

This chapter will analyze this technique, briefly reviewing the nerve anatomy, the main etiologies, its clinical presentation, and treatment. We will describe the current literature, and finally, we will present a patient successfully treated by our team, reported in the Surgical Neurology International.

16.2 Applied Anatomy

Previous chapters exposed the topographic and organizational anatomy of BP, but this chapter will describe some considerations regarding the anatomy of the long thoracic nerve and thoracodorsal nerve.

The long thoracic nerve is formed immediately from the spinal roots—anterior branches C5, C6, and frequently C7—directly related to the BP [4, 5]. In a few cases, C8 fibers might contribute [6]. Horwitz and Tocantins performed nerve dissection in 100 cadavers, identifying the previously mentioned roots. After the nerve is formed, it generally descends between the middle and anterior scalene muscles, and then through the second rib, to end in the different digitations of the serratus anterior muscle, reaching a length

J. P. Martinez
Department of Neurosurgery, Hospital Universitario Fundación Favaloro, Buenos Aires, Argentina

M. Socolovsky (✉)
Division of Neurosurgery, Hospital de Clínicas, University of Buenos Aires School of Medicine, Buenos Aires, Argentina

F. Guedes et al. (eds.), *Nerve Transfers for Brachial Plexus Reconstruction after Trauma*,
https://doi.org/10.1007/978-3-031-92445-3_16

of approximately 25–30 cm in its entire course, being located in the lateral and superficial part of the thorax, being more vulnerable to traumatic injuries at this level [4, 6].

The thoracodorsal nerve, in turn, originates in the roots of C5, C6, and C7 mainly in the last one, emerging as a branch of the posterior cord of the BP [7]. It continues its course, inferiorly and laterally, to form part of the pedicle of the latissimus dorsi, positioning itself superficial to the thoracodorsal artery and vein, finally entering the muscle on its medial tendinous surface to extend to its inferior border [8]. In axillary procedures, the nerve may be located 2 cm from the confluence of the lateral thoracic vein and the axillary vein [8–10]. In anatomical and histological studies of the C7 root—the main component of the thoracodorsal nerve—it was proved in successive sections under microscopic vision and staining with acetylcholinesterase, the conformation mainly of motor axons, in addition to sympathetic and sensory fibers, showing most of the motor axons located in the posterior region, which will give origin to the thoracodorsal nerve. In this way, its usefulness and good results were reported in nerve repairs of the BP and transfer to the long thoracic nerve [7, 11–16].

16.3 Biomechanics

The serratus anterior muscle is a broad and flat muscle extending at the midaxillary line level. Far from being a single structure, it comprises multiple digitations extending from the superior aspect of the first 8–9 ribs to insert into the ventral scapular portion [17].

It is a muscle that presents three different belly components directly related to its scapular insertion: a superior component, which attaches to the superior and medial border of the scapula, which has the function of anchoring the upper limb during its rotation above the head; a middle muscular component, which connects the third, fourth and fifth ribs, with the vertebral border of the scapula, stabilizing the scapula on the thorax and elevating the ribs, when a patient holds an object or exerts pressure with his upper limbs on a surface—respiratory function. Finally, the inferior component is composed of the last ribs that converge at the inferior angle of the scapula to rotate it upward and laterally [18]. In summary, the serratus anterior muscle contributes to the dynamic abduction and elevation of the shoulder on the horizontal plane, stabilizing the scapula on the thorax [19].

16.4 Etiology

The etiology of long thoracic nerve injury can be classified into nontraumatic and traumatic. In the first group, there are reports of infectious, inflammatory, anatomical, postradiation, familial, radiculopathy, and myelopathic causes [20–27].

The second group is the most frequent, reaching more than 50% in some cases series [27]. The typical pattern is a sudden jerk of the arm, forward or backward, and strenuous manual activities related to carpenters of large structures and builders, among other activities. Another important group is sportspeople and athletes, represented by ballet dancers to tennis, golf, and basketball players, among other activities, where the mechanism of injury is stretching the long thoracic nerve, producing different levels of disability [27]. Then there is a particular group—iatrogenic injuries—which represent about 11%, including procedures in regions related to the nerve pathway through the neck, axilla, and chest wall [27–31]. The bibliographic reports detail as the leading cause, resections of the first rib through the axillary approach, a vulnerable region of the nerve pathway due to its superficiality as described above, followed by surgical procedures related to breast and lymph node pathology, neck pathology treated through the supraclavicular approach, and anesthetic blocks of the brachial plexus, among others [29].

16.5 Initial Approach and Results of the Thoracodorsal Nerve Transfer in Long Thoracic Nerve Injury

The nerve injury produces paralysis of the serratus muscle, expressed clinically by a winged scapula, omalgia, and altered mobility of the homolateral shoulder [4, 21, 23, 27, 28, 32, 33].

Patients with mild to moderate partial injuries would benefit from initially conservative treatment, including clinical observation and an established routine physiotherapy program [13, 21, 23, 34–38]. Patients with more severe injuries, such as iatrogenic traumatic injuries, will require surgical intervention by primary nerve reconstruction, nerve transfer, or trauma-orthopedic surgery [28, 30, 33, 36, 39–43].

In experimental and clinical models of peripheral nerve injury, recovery is directly related to the location, severity, and mechanism of injury [5, 44], with the outcome being more favorable in idiopathic inflammatory cases and worse in traumatic cases [5, 39, 44]. It is recommended to perform a nerve transfer approach within 1 year of the onset of symptoms [32, 36, 39, 43, 45].

Surgical options are extensive, although recently, according to literature reports, both nerve transfer and modified pectoralis major muscle-tendon transfer have gained prominence [11–13, 19, 30, 36, 41, 46, 47].

Only three papers (two case reports and one case series) describe thoracodorsal to long thoracic nerve transfer. These are summarized in Table 16.1. The first record of this technique was published by Christine B. Novak in 2002. It is about a 17-year-old male patient, right-handed, with a history of physical exercise with weights, who the next day after training developed pain in the right shoulder and subsequently intense pain and restriction of unilateral movement in a transient manner, with no other remarkable history. Physical examination revealed a right-winged scapula with shoulder flexion and a less pronounced winged scapula with shoulder abduction. Active shoulder abduction and flexion range of motion were 90°, and passive range of motion was complete. Electromyography 6 weeks after the onset of weakness revealed fibrillations and positive sharp waves in the right serratus anterior muscle. All other muscles revealed no abnormal muscle activity, including the right deltoid, biceps brachii, triceps, trapezius, infraspinatus, and latissimus dorsi. Subsequently, electromyographic studies were repeated and revealed decreased muscle activity (positive sharp waves and fibrillations) without evidence of muscle reinnervation. After 3.5 months with no recovery and weakness of the serratus anterior muscle, it was decided to perform the exploration and transfer of the thoracodorsal nerve to the long thoracic nerve. A bandage was applied, and the patient was immobilized in internal rotation and shoulder adduction for 2 weeks. As the patient lived a long way from the hospital, he was unable to attend checkups, where he presented after 6.5 years, with total resolution of the winged scapula and total functional recovery [12].

Then, in 2011, Ray et al. described a case report of a 46-year-old man with a history of a fall on a mountain bike with a fracture of the left distal radius that required a traumatological procedure. He presented a good recovery, and in the first month, he added severe right shoulder pain, which only prompted him to attend a neurological evaluation 3 months after the onset of symptoms. Physical examination showed a right-winged scapula without involvement of other muscles. The electromyogram showed positive fibrillation potentials and no motor unit potentials, which is compatible with the absence of motor reinnervation. He was first treated by physiotherapy with periodic controls. After 7 months of clinical and electromyographic controls with no evidence of improvement, nerve transfer was performed at two levels, one superior, which included an end-to-end neurorrhaphy of fascicles of the pectoral nerve and the proximal segment of the long thoracic nerve and a simple inferior transfer, from the thoracodorsal

Table 16.1 Summary of studies. Literature reports of nerve transfer from thoracodorsal nerve to long thoracic nerve

Author	Country	Study design	Total (analyzed population)	Key findings	Electromyographic studies	Outcomes
Christine B. Novak, 2002	United States	Case report	1	• First report of thoracodorsal nerve to long thoracic nerve transfer technique • 17-year-old male patient, right-handed • History of excessive physical exercise • Reason for consultation: right shoulder weakness, winged scapula, and omalgia	• Presence of sharp waves and fibrillations in the right serratus anterior muscle	• Transfer of thoracodorsal nerve to long thoracic nerve was performed • Patient returned for follow-up 6.5 years later, with full shoulder flexion without scapular winging. She reported no functional limitation in her shoulder or at the donor site
Wilson Z. Ray, 2011	United States	Case report	1	• Second case report of the technique • 46-year-old male patient • History of a mountain bike accident, with fracture of the left distal radius that required surgical treatment • At 30 days, he develops omalgia and right-winged scapula	• Positive fibrillation potentials, without motor units in the right serratus anterior muscle	• A double nerve transfer was performed: an inferior thoracodorsal to long thoracic nerve and an upper one via a pectoral fascicle from the middle trunk to long thoracic nerve • 7 months, right shoulder range of motion recovery • 11 months, full recovery of shoulder strength and mobility
Shelley S. Noland, 2017	United States	Serie de casos	19	• Mean age 32 years • Nerve injury was present in 58% • Parsonage-Turner syndrome 32% • Shoulder surgery 10% • All patients had scapular winging, and 16 patients had a limitation to shoulder flexion to 90°	• Eight patients had evidence of denervation as determined by the presence of fibrillations and positive sharp waves • In 13 patients, active motor unit potentials were detected in the serratus anterior muscle • Five patients had no evidence of motor unit	• All patients underwent nerve decompression • Only three patients underwent nerve transfer (two patients with traumatic etiology and one with inflammatory etiology). Two patients underwent thoracodorsal nerve to long thoracic nerve transfer, and one patient underwent double transfer

nerve to the long thoracic nerve. Subsequently, the patient was immobilized, and motor physical therapy sessions were initiated, focusing primarily on patient education and passive range of motion and promoting greater patient compression and participation. After 11 months, the patient almost recovered full strength in anterior and lateral shoulder abduction, with nearly total resolution of scapular movement [13].

Several years later, Shelley S. Noland published a case series of 19 patients with isolated paralysis of the long thoracic nerve of different etiologies. All patients were preoperatively studied with electromyography and compared with the intraoperative findings to design a study protocol for this lesion. Only three patients were treated by nerve transfer; one received a double transfer, as explained before, and two others were treated by single nerve transfer, from thoracodorsal nerve to long thoracic nerve [11].

In our limited experience, we treated a single case of a 32-year-old male patient, a right-handed athlete, who presented for 12 months with bilateral (predominantly right) abduction paresis with changes in the coloring and paresthesia in the upper limbs. As relevant history, he had a resection of the right first rib in another institution after being diagnosed with thoracic vascular operculum syndrome. After surgery, the previous symptoms persisted, adding loss of strength and decreased right shoulder flexion. On physical examination, there was a significant right-winged scapula and decreased flexion extension of the homolateral shoulder, with no other muscle involvement (Fig. 16.1). A magnetic resonance imaging of that region was performed, where no structural lesions were evidenced, neither muscular-tendinous nor of the rotator cuff. Due to his history, our first diagnostic presumption was traumatic nerve injury, which was confirmed by electromyographic studies. The patient underwent physiotherapy for 6 months without improvement. Due to the absence of response, it was decided to perform a nerve transfer from the thoracodorsal to the long thoracic nerve at 8 months. This indication was due to the absence of improvement in the paralysis observed up to that moment. The patient was positioned in dorsal decubitus, with the right upper limb in 90° abduction. A 15-cm skin incision was made on the right mid-axillary line, following the free border of the latissimus dorsi muscle (Fig. 16.2). Dissection of the subcutaneous cellular tissue and aponeurosis of the latissimus dorsi muscle was continued until the right thoracodorsal nerve was identified by dissection and neurostimulation (Fig. 16.3). Subsequently, the aponeurosis of the serratus anterior muscle was opened, which allowed the identification of the right long thoracic nerve, which had not responded to intraoperative motor stimulation (Fig. 16.4). A donor branch of the right thoracodorsal nerve of similar size to that of the recipient was repaired to perform a nerve transfer in which the former would function as the axon donor and the latter as the recipient. End-to-end neurorrhaphy was performed under

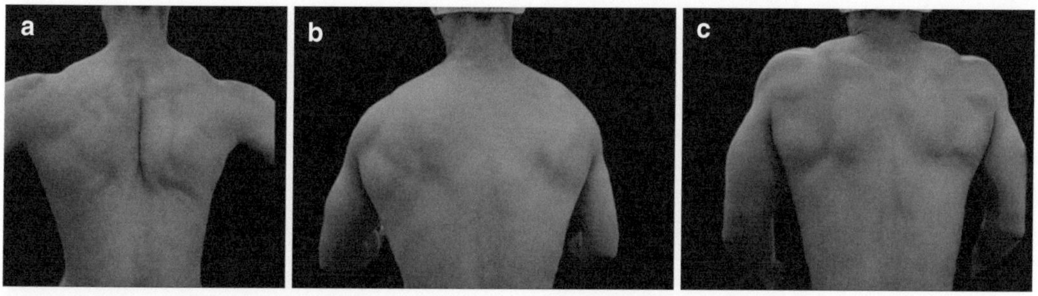

Fig. 16.1 Preoperative examination. (**a**, **b**) Shoulder flexion at 90° and (**c**) shoulder extension. The important right-winged scapula is observed. (Extracted from: Martinez J, Lovaglio A, Di Masi G, Mandolesi J, Zancolli P, Socolovsky M. Thoracodorsal to long thoracic nerve transfer in a patient with traumatic injury: A case report. Surgical Neurology International. 2024 May)

microscopic magnification using a 9–0 nylon microsuture. Fibrin glue was used to coat the repair. The patient was monitored 6 months after surgery, with partial improvement of the winged scapula and good recovery of flexion and function of the right shoulder. At 12 months, the winged scapula was resolved, with full functional recovery and muscle strength of both the latissimus dorsi and pectoralis muscles. The patient reported that he could complete all his routine activities normally and showed a decrease in preoperative pain measured with the Visual Analog Scale, 5/10–2/10 (Fig. 16.5) [48].

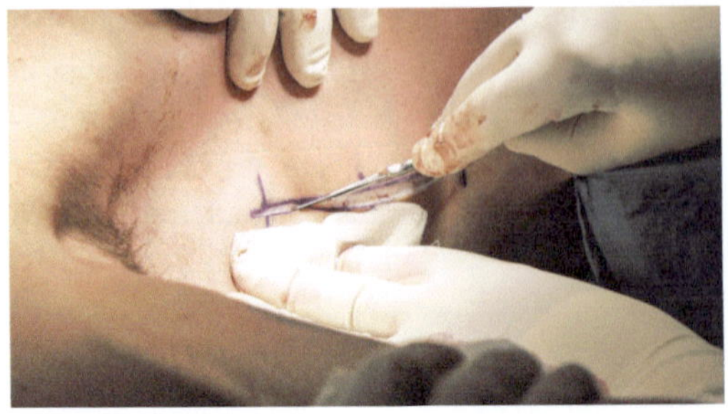

Fig. 16.3 Intraoperative picture. A dissection of the latissimus dorsi. (Extracted from: Martinez J, Lovaglio A, Di Masi G, Mandolesi J, Zancolli P, Socolovsky M. Thoracodorsal to long thoracic nerve transfer in a patient with traumatic injury: A case report. Surgical Neurology International. 2024 May)

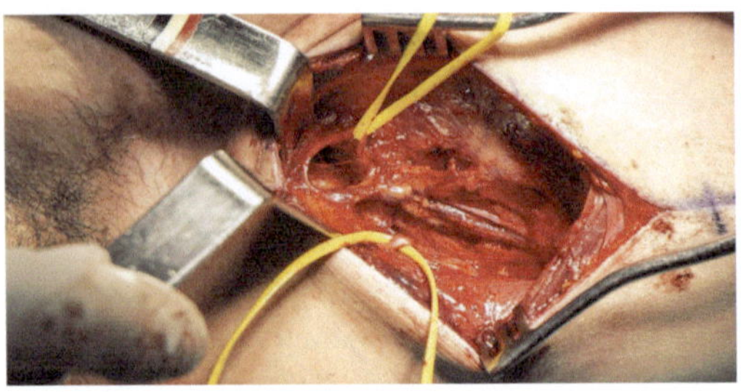

Fig. 16.2 Intraoperative picture. The skin incision over the midaxillary line and following the lateral border of the thoracodorsal muscle. (Extracted from: Martinez J, Lovaglio A, Di Masi G, Mandolesi J, Zancolli P, Socolovsky M. Thoracodorsal to long thoracic nerve transfer in a patient with traumatic injury: A case report. Surgical Neurology International. 2024 May)

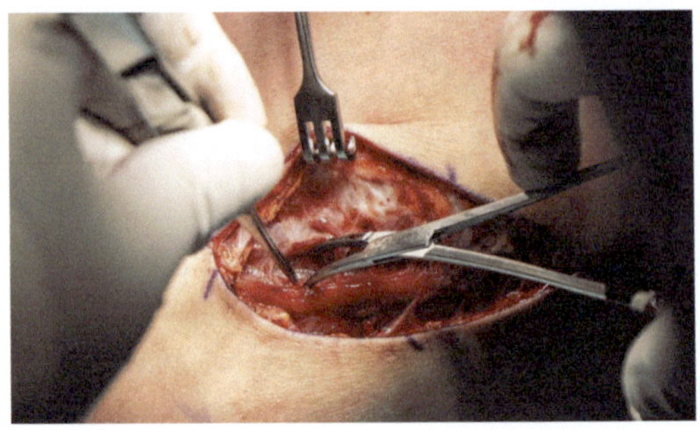

Fig. 16.4 Intraoperative picture. A separate thoracodorsal nerve on the inferior and the long thoracic nerve on the superior side. (Extracted from: Martinez J, Lovaglio A, Di Masi G, Mandolesi J, Zancolli P, Socolovsky M. Thoracodorsal to long thoracic nerve transfer in a patient with traumatic injury: A case report. Surgical Neurology International. 2024 May)

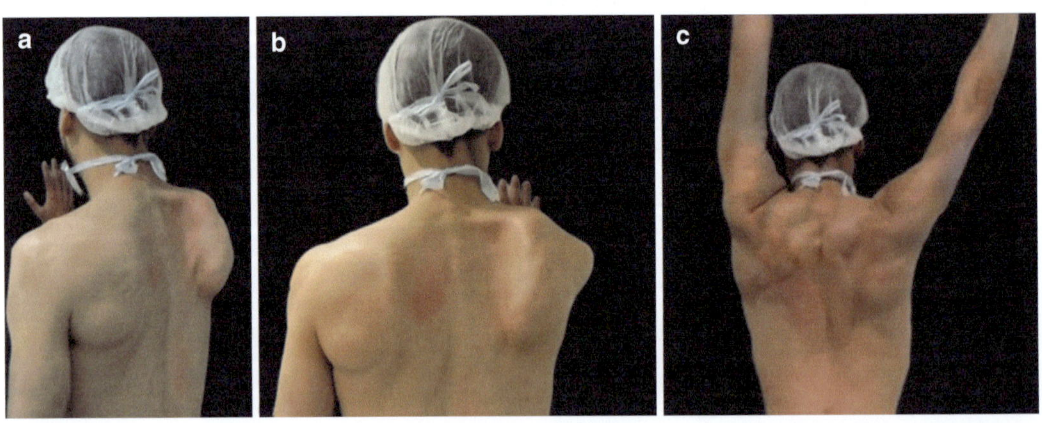

Fig. 16.5 Postoperative examination at 12 months: (**a**) Total resolution of the winged scapula, functional recovery, and muscle strength; (**b**) total resolution of the winged scapula, functional recovery, and muscle strength; and (**c**) total resolution of the winged scapula, functional recovery, and muscle strength. (Extracted from: Martinez J, Lovaglio A, Di Masi G, Mandolesi J, Zancolli P, Socolovsky M. Thoracodorsal to long thoracic nerve transfer in a patient with traumatic injury: A case report. Surgical Neurology International. 2024 May)

16.6 Summary

The thoracodorsal nerve has proven to be a valuable donor for injuries of different etiologies of the long thoracic nerve, reporting good reinnervation of the serratus anterior muscle, expressed clinically with improvement of the winged scapula and excellent functional recovery of the affected shoulder. Although very scarce, published reports of the success of this technique should bring it into the surgical armamentarium of nerve transfers. To optimize the results, it is necessary to correctly select the patient and establish a physiotherapy regimen before and after the transfer. We recommend indicating this transfer within 12 months of the onset of symptoms, under compatible electromyography and lack of response to medical treatment.

References

1. Post MP. Pectoralis major transfer for winging of the scapula. J Shoulder Elb Surg. 1995;4:1–9.
2. Winslow M. Sur quelques mouvements extraordinaires des omoplates et des bras, et sur une nouvelle espece de muscles. Chez, Panckouke; 1723
3. Grzybowski A, Kaufman MH. Sir Charles Bell (1774-1842): contributions to neuro-ophthalmology. Acta Ophthalmol Scand. 2007;85:897–901.
4. Martin RM, Fish DE. Scapular winging: anatomical review, diagnosis, and treatments. Curr Rev Musculoskelet Med. 2008;1:1–11.
5. Sunderland S. The anatomy and physiology of nerve injury. Muscle Nerve. 1990;13:771–84.
6. Horwitz MT, Tocantins LM. An anatomic study of the role of the long thoracic nerve and the related scapular bursae in the pathogenesis of local paralysis of the serratus anterior muscle. Anat Rec. 1938;71:375–85.
7. Lu W, Xu JG, Wang DP, Gu YD. Microanatomical study on the functional origin and direction of the thoracodorsal nerve from the trunks of brachial plexus. Clin Anat. 2008;21(6):509–13.
8. Takahashi N, Watanabe K, Koga N, Rikimaru H, Kiyokawa K, Saga T, Nakamura M, Tabira Y, Yamaki K. Anatomical research of the three-dimensional route of the thoracodorsal nerve, artery, and veins in latissimus dorsi muscle. Plast Reconstr Surg Glob Open. 2013;1(2):1–7.
9. Zin T, Maw M, Oo S, Pai D, Paijan R, Kyi M. How I do it: simple and effortless approach to identify thoracodorsal nerve on axillary clearance procedure. Ecancermedicalscience. 2012;6:255.
10. Anthony DJ, Basnayake BMOD, Ganga NMG, Mathangasinghe Y, Malalasekera AP. An improved technical trick for identification of the thoracodorsal nerve during axillary clearance surgery: a cadaveric dissection study. Patient Saf Surg. 2018;12:18.
11. Noland SS, Krauss EM, Felder JM, Mackinnon SE. Surgical and clinical decision making in isolated long thoracic nerve palsy. Hand (N Y). 2018;13:689–94.
12. Novak CB, Mackinnon SE. Surgical treatment of a long thoracic nerve palsy. Ann Thorac Surg. 2002;73:1643–5.
13. Ray WZ, Pet MA, Nicoson MC, Yee A, Kahn LC, Mackinnon SE. Two-level motor nerve transfer for the treatment of long thoracic nerve palsy. J Neurosurg. 2011;115:858–64.
14. Xu JG, Hu SN, Wang H, Gu YD. Histochemical study on C7 roots and its clinical significance. Chin J Clin Anat. 1996;14:243.
15. Soldado F, Ghizoni MF, Bertelli J. Thoracodorsal nerve transfer for triceps reinnervation in partial brachial plexus injuries. Microsurgery. 2016;36(3):191–7.
16. Soldado F, Ghizoni MF, Bertelli J. Thoracodorsal nerve transfer for elbow flexion reconstruction in infraclavicular brachial plexus injuries. J Hand Surg Am. 2014;39(9):1766–70.
17. Martin JT. Postoperative isolated dysfunction of the long thoracic nerve: a rare entity of uncertain etiology. Anesth Analg. 1989;69(5):614–9.
18. Gregg JR, Labosky D, Harty M, et al. Serratus anterior paralysis in the young athlete. J Bone Joint Surg. 1979;61:825–32.
19. Segonds JM, Alnot JY, Asfazadourian H. Paralysie isolée du muscle serratus antérieur d'origine traumatique [Isolated traumatic serratus anterior muscle palsy]. Rev Chir Orthop Reparatrice Appar Mot. 2002;88:751–9.
20. Del Sasso L, Mondini A, Brambilla S. A case of isolated paralysis of serratus anterior. Ital J Orthop Traumatol. 1988;14:533–7.
21. Mah JY, Otsuka NY. Scapular winging in young athletes. J Pediatr Orthop. 1992;12:245–7.
22. Makin GJ, Brown WF, Ebers GC. C7 radiculopathy: importance of scapular winging in clinical diagnosis. J Neurol Neurosurg Psychiatry. 1986;49:640–4.
23. Marin R. Scapula winger's brace: a case series on the management of long thoracic nerve palsy. Arch Phys Med Rehabil. 1998;79:1226–30.
24. Parsonage MJ, Turner JW. Neuralgic amyotrophy; the shoulder-girdle syndrome. Lancet. 1948;1:973–8.
25. Phillips LH II. Familial long thoracic nerve palsy: a manifestation of brachial plexus neuropathy. Neurology. 1986;36:1251–3.
26. Pugliese GN, Green RF, Antonacci A. Radiation-induced long thoracic nerve palsy. Cancer. 1987;60:1247–8.
27. Vastamäki M, Kauppila LI. Etiologic factors in isolated paralysis of the serratus anterior muscle: a report of 197 cases. J Shoulder Elb Surg. 1993;2:240–3.

28. Atasoy E, Majd M. Scapulothoracic stabilization for winging of the scapula using strips of autogenous fascia lata. J Bone Joint Surg Br. 2000;82:813–7.
29. Kauppila LI, Vastamäki M. Iatrogenic serratus anterior paralysis. Long-term outcome in 26 patients. Chest. 1996;109:31–4.
30. Perlmutter GS, Leffert RD. Results of transfer of the pectoralis major tendon to treat paralysis of the serratus anterior muscle. J Bone Joint Surg Am. 1999;81:377–84.
31. Sharp WJ, Nowak LR, Zamani T, Kresowik TF, Hoballah JJ, Ballinger BA, et al. Long-term follow-up and patient satisfaction after surgery for thoracic outlet syndrome. Ann Vasc Surg. 2001;15:32–6.
32. Friedenberg SM, Zimprich T, Harper CM. The natural history of long thoracic and spinal accessory neuropathies. Muscle Nerve. 2002;25:535–9.
33. Weisberger EC, Kincaid J, Riteris J. Cable grafting of the spinal accessory nerve after radical neck dissection. Arch Otolaryngol Head Neck Surg. 1998;124:377–80.
34. Gregg JR, Labosky D, Harty M, Lotke P, Ecker M, DiStefano V, et al. Serratus anterior paralysis in the young athlete. J Bone Joint Surg Am. 1979;61:825–32.
35. Klebe TM, Døssing KV, Blenstrup T, Nielsen-Ferreira J, Rejsenhus L, Aalkjaer G, et al. Scapulae alatae--englevinger. En opgørelse of 64 patienter behandlet med brace-bandage og fysioterapi på Viborg Sygehus [Scapulae alatae-angels' wings. A study of 64 patients treated with braces and physical therapy at the Viberg's hospital]. Ugeskr Laeger. 2003;165:1779–82.
36. Warner JJ, Navarro RA. Serratus anterior dysfunction. Recognition and treatment. Clin Orthop Relat Res. 1998;349:139–48.
37. Watson CJ, Schenkman M. Physical therapy management of isolated serratus anterior muscle paralysis. Phys Ther. 1995;75:194–202.
38. Wiater JM, Flatow EL. Long thoracic nerve injury. Clin Orthop Relat Res. 1999;368:17–27.
39. Berry H, MacDonald EA, Mrazek AC. Accessory nerve palsy: a review of 23 cases. Can J Neurol Sci. 1991;18:337–41.
40. Gordon SL, Graham WP III, Black JT, Miller SH. Accessory nerve function after surgical procedures in the posterior triangle. Arch Surg. 1977;112:264–8.
41. Mackinnon SE, Novak CB. Nerve transfers. New options for reconstruction following nerve injury. Hand Clin. 1999;15:643–66, ix.
42. Ogino T, Sugawara M, Minami A, Kato H, Ohnishi N. Accessory nerve injury: conservative or surgical treatment? J Hand Surg Br. 1991;16:531–6.
43. Saunders JR, Hirata RM, Jaques DA. Considering the spinal accessory nerve in head and neck surgery. Am J Surg. 1985;150:491–4.
44. Seckel BR. Enhancement of peripheral nerve regeneration. Muscle Nerve. 1990;13:785–800.
45. Fu SY, Gordon T. Contributing factors to poor functional recovery after delayed nerve repair: prolonged denervation. J Neurosci. 1995;15(5 Pt 2):3886–95.
46. Connor PM, Yamaguchi K, Manifold SG, Pollock RG, Flatow EL, Bigliani LU. Split pectoralis major transfer for serratus anterior palsy. Clin Orthop Relat Res. 1997;341:134–42.
47. Elhassan BT, Wagner ER. Outcome of transfer of the sternal head of the pectoralis major with its bone insertion to the scapula to manage scapular winging. J Shoulder Elb Surg. 2015;24:733–40.
48. Martinez J, Lovaglio A, Di Masi G, Mandolesi J, Zancolli P, Socolovsky M. Thoracodorsal to long thoracic nerve transfer in a patient with traumatic injury: a case report. Surg Neurol Int. 2024;15:163.

Part III

Nerve Transfers for Elbow Flexion

17 The "Ulnar-Biceps Median-Brachialis" Double Nerve Transfer

Belkheyar Zoubir, Cambon Adeline, and Oberlin Christophe

17.1 Principles of this Transfer

The goal of this transfer is to reinnervate the two most powerful elbow flexors using regional functioning donor nerves [1, 2]. The two muscles—biceps brachii and brachialis muscles—are innervated by motor branches arising from the musculocutaneous nerve. This nerve has also a sensory contingent, the lateral antebrachial cutaneous nerve. As a consequence, any nerve transfer on the main trunk of the musculocutaneous nerve will lead some scattering of regenerating nerves in sensory branches. Moreover, to achieve the shortest function recovery, the distance between regional donor motor branches and the recipient motor endplates has to be as short as possible. Oberlin first described the technique of nerve transfer from one fascicule of the ulnar nerve to the biceps motor branch in 1994 [1], and then added a transfer of one fascicule of the median nerve to the motor branch of the brachialis muscle [3]. Several authors showed that the double transfer gave better results in terms of elbow flexion strength [4, 5]. Patients that underwent the double transfer were more numerous than in the single transfer group to reach a MRC score ≥4 (83.0% vs. 63.3% in Donnelly systematic review) [4].

Selection of donor fasciculi is of utmost importance. They should be redundant motor branches for wrist flexion or forearm pronation, avoiding branches for intrinsic muscles of the hand and finger flexors. Alternatively, if the median nerve needs to be spared, two fasciculi may be harvested from the ulnar nerve for each elbow flexor [6].

17.2 Operative Technique

The patient is supine under general anesthesia with an arm table. Incision is on the anteromedial aspect of the proximal half of the arm. It descends 8–10 cm from the lower edge of the pectoralis major tendon along the bicipital sulcus. The fascia of the biceps muscle are open to retract the biceps muscle and expose the musculocutaneous nerve (MCN). The MCN lies between the bellies of the biceps muscle and brachialis muscle and is dissected from proximal to distal in order to identify its main terminal branches. In most of patients, those branches involve one (or two) for the biceps muscle, one for the brachialis muscle,

B. Zoubir · O. Christophe
Clinique du Mont Louis, Paris, France

C. Adeline (✉)
Orthopaedic and Traumatology Surgery Department, Sorbonne University, Saint-Antoine Hospital, Paris, France

F. Guedes et al. (eds.), *Nerve Transfers for Brachial Plexus Reconstruction after Trauma*,
https://doi.org/10.1007/978-3-031-92445-3_17

and the lateral antebrachial cutaneous nerve [7, 8]. In the case of several motor branches for the same muscle, dissection is continued proximally to a common trunk. Motor branches for the biceps exit from the MCN between 37% and 52% of the arm length, defined by distance between the coracoid process and the tip of the lateral epicondyle [7]. For the brachialis muscle, branches arise from 52% to 62% of the arm length.

The two identified main motor branches are dissected under microscope with microsurgical instruments. They are stimulated to confirm paralysis. Branches are separated proximally from the musculocutaneous nerve by approximately 2 cm before being sectioned.

The medial intermuscular septum of the arm is then opened to identify the ulnar nerve at the level of the biceps motor branch. The epineurium of the ulnar nerve is incised, and intraneural dissection is performed to isolate a motor fascicle of similar diameter to the biceps motor branch. Neurostimulation helps to select a motor branch supplying the flexor carpi ulnaris (FCU), which is frequently located on the anterolateral side of the ulnar nerve. Branches for intrinsic muscles of the hand should be avoided. Sufficient residual ulnar nerve function is verified via electrostimulation of the remaining fascicules. The chosen fascicle is then dissected distally for 2 cm, divided and turned laterally.

Internal neurolysis of the median nerve is performed as well at the level of the motor branch of the musculocutaneous nerve for the brachialis muscle in order to isolate a motor fascicle of similar diameter, dedicated to the pronator teres muscle and/or to the palmaris longus muscle.

Finally, direct ulnar-biceps and medial-brachial transfers are performed without tension using simple epi-perineural stitches of single-strand nonabsorbable 9.0 suture and coadapted with biological fibrin-based glue (Figs. 17.1 and 17.2).

Postoperatively, the shoulder is splinted in abduction with the elbow in flexion at 90° for 6 weeks when rehabilitation begins.

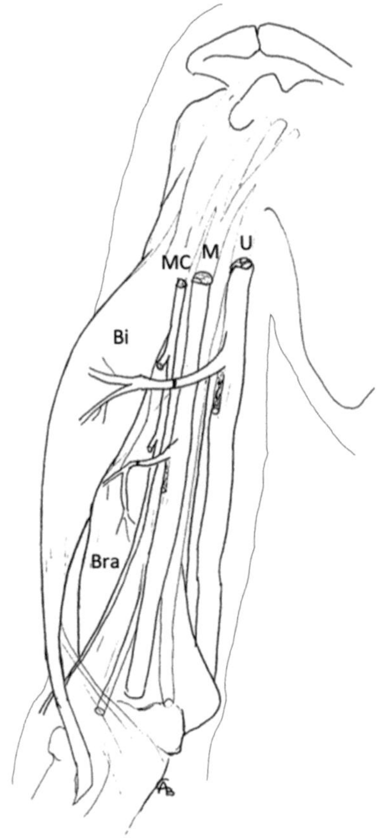

Fig. 17.1 Principle of the "Ulnar-Biceps Median-Brachialis" double transfer. Bi: biceps brachii; Bra: brachialis; MC: musculocutaneous nerve; M: median nerve; U: ulnar nerve

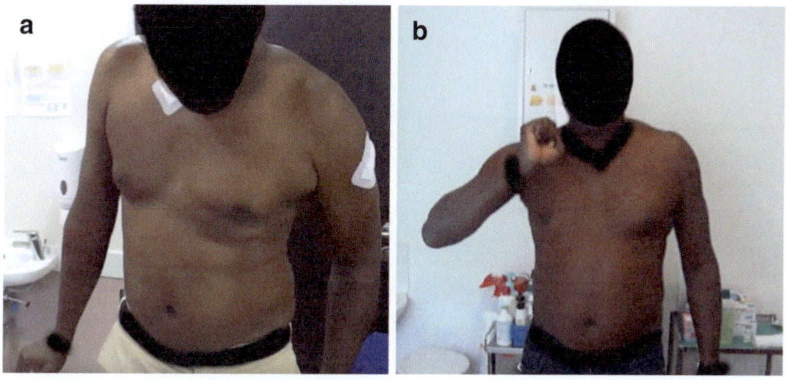

Fig. 17.2 Postoperative 36-year-old man with a C5–C6 brachial plexus palsy (**a**). Nerve surgery 5 months after the trauma included transfers from fascicules of the ulnar and median nerves, respectively, to the biceps motor branch and brachialis motor branch of the musculocutaneous nerve. On examination 24 months later, the patient had recovered 140° of elbow flexion (**b**)

References

1. Oberlin C, Béal D, Leechavengvongs S, Salon A, Dauge MC, Sarcy JJ. Nerve transfer to biceps muscle using a part of ulnar nerve for C5-C6 avulsion of the brachial plexus. Anatomical study and report of 4 cases. J Hand Surg Am. 1994;19(2):232–7.
2. Oberlin C, Ameur NE, Teboul F, Beaulieu JY, Vacher C. Restoration of elbow flexion in brachial plexus injury by transfer of ulnar nerve fascicles to the nerve to the biceps muscle. Tech Hand Up Extrem Surg. 2002;6:86–90.
3. Goubier JN, Teboul F. Technique of the double nerve transfer to recover elbow flexion in C5, C6, or C5 to C7 brachial plexus palsy. Tech Hand Up Extrem Surg. 2007;11(1):15–7.
4. Donnelly MR, Rezzadeh KT, Vieira D, Daar D, Hacquebord J. Is one nerve transfer enough? A systematic review and pooled analysis comparing ulnar fascicular nerve transfer and double ulnar and median fascicular nerve transfer for restoration of elbow flexion after traumatic brachial plexus injury. Microsurgery. 2020;40(3):361–9.
5. Sneiders D, Bulstra LF, Hundepool CA, Treling WJ, Hovius SER, Shin AY. Outcomes of single versus double fascicular nerve transfers for restoration of elbow flexion in patients with brachial plexus injuries: a systematic review and meta-analysis. Plast Reconstr Surg. 2019;144(1):155–66.
6. Kokkalis ZT, Bavelou A, Papanikos E, Konofaos P, Efstathopoulos DG, Soucacos PN. Reconstruction of elbow flexion with a modified Oberlin procedure: a comparative study. Injury. 2019;50(Suppl 5):71–6.
7. Cambon-Binder A, Leclercq C. Anatomical study of the musculocutaneous nerve branching pattern: application for selective neurectomy in the treatment of elbow flexors spasticity. Surg Radiol Anat. 2015;37(4):341–8.
8. Bhardwaj P, Venkatramani H, Sivakumar B, Graham DJ, Vigneswaran V, Sabapathy SR. Anatomic variations of the musculocutaneous nerve and clinical implications for restoration of elbow flexion. J Hand Surg Am. 2022;47(10):970–8.

18 Infraclavicular Intraplexual Transfers for Elbow Flexion

Stefano Ferraresi and Elisabetta Basso

Abbreviations

aUT Anterior (contribution) of the upper trunk
MC Medial cord
Mc Musculocutaneous nerve

18.1 Introduction

Much time has elapsed from the revolutionary technique popularized by Oberlin to reanimate elbow flexion from a motor fascicle of the ulnar nerve to the nerve branch(es) for the biceps [1–4].

Until then, plexus repair had always been planned as from a proximal stump reinnervating a recipient nerve in an "end-to-end" manner.

The evidence that a nerve can donate motor axons without losing its function gave rise to the "nerve transfer era" which is, by far, the major advance in the field of brachial plexus reconstructive surgery.

Since then, a variety of ingenious transfers have been introduced [5, 6], and the repair of a paralyzed nerve using an intact part of the plexus, without interposition of grafts, has gained worldwide acceptance.

The field of application obviously regards partial injuries, where selected fascicles of sound nerves (donors) may find their way into denervated targets (recipient nerves).

Before Oberlin's paper, several techniques had been attempted over the years to restore elbow flexion, but none of them, except for the medial pectoral nerves [7–9], offered constant and reliable results.

However, the risk of weakening the pectoralis muscle, with resultant loss of the thoraco-axillar pinch, prompted to investigate the role of other donors outside the brachial plexus in restoring elbow flexion, namely, the phrenic nerve [10, 11], the accessory nerve [12], the intercostal nerves [13, 14], the motor cervical rami [15], and the hypoglossal nerve [16]. All of them have been introduced with variable success.

The feasibility of intraplexual infraclavicular transfers requires that normal or quasi-normal functions are retained in the posterior and/or medial cords of the affected patients. *Complete palsies are obviously excluded.*

The ideal candidates are upper plexus (C5–C6 injury) injuries, although the upper-middle (C5–C6–C7 injury) palsies can obtain excellent results anyway. The one-root hand (C5–C6–C7–C8 injury) is very delicate to treat because the loss of an existing function sometimes ensuing after the transfer can strongly affect the quality of the overall result.

S. Ferraresi (✉) · E. Basso
Department of Neurosurgery, Ospedale Santa Maria della Misericordia, Rovigo, Italy

F. Guedes et al. (eds.), *Nerve Transfers for Brachial Plexus Reconstruction after Trauma*,
https://doi.org/10.1007/978-3-031-92445-3_18

In pure postganglionic infraclavicular injuries, i.e., with a normal supraclavicular plexus, an intraplexual transfer to the musculocutaneous nerve (Mc) can also be an option, but an anatomical repair (with grafts) of the musculocutaneous nerve is preferred in these cases because of the general good results obtainable without disturbing the sound nerves. Only when grafts exceed 10 cm length, one can resort to a direct transfer to the musculocutaneous (Mc) nerve using a different proximal nerve if a tension-free direct coaptation between the two can be carried out.

With time, the intraplexual nerve transfer strategy has increasingly become the first choice both in the case of a stretch and of an avulsive injury of the roots, since the results are generally better and, in addition, quicker and less invasive.

The main infraclavicular transfers available for reanimating the elbow flexion are the following:

- **The MC-Mc (medial cord-to musculocutaneous nerve transfer).**
- **The MC-aUT (medial cord to anterior contribution of the upper trunk transfer).**
- The pectoral nerve-Mc transfer.
- The thoracodorsal nerve-Mc transfer.

Each of them can attain a useful elbow flexion, but a very precise reason should support the utilization of the last two techniques because they entail a not negligible loss of function in the donor site.

Despite the good results still being obtained worldwide with the Oberlin's technique, there have been several reasons prompting the search for different techniques:

1. It is a "terminal" surgery: the recipient nerve cannot be prepared further distally. Therefore, in the case of failure caused by rupture of its fragile nerve suture, a new identification of the recipient fascicle is rendered extremely difficult by scar tissue. Consequently, the success of a second attempt is highly unpredictable and may end with a microvascular gracilis free flap.
2. Only the biceps is reinnervated. To add the brachialis muscle, a separate transfer of one fascicle from the median nerve to the brachialis nerve branch must be combined [4, 17]. This is also called a "double Oberlin" procedure [18].
3. In avulsive injury of C5 and C6, when a weak biceps (M1/M2) is sustained by C7, the Oberlin procedure cannot avoid the loss of this residual function.
4. Rarely, the interruption of a motor fascicle from the ulnar nerve can cause an imbalance between intrinsic and extrinsic muscles of the hand. This may be due to a loss of function but also to a spastic irritation, and this causes a typical hand posture characterized by metacarpophalangeal flexion with proximal and distal interphalangeal joint extension, called "intrinsic plus hand." It results in a very disabling condition.

On these grounds, in 2004 the first modification to the Oberlin's procedure was described [19], with a change in the recipient: the entire musculocutaneous nerve was sectioned and rerouted to receive one/two fascicles of the donor ulnar nerve.

Despite the considerable mismatch between donor and recipient, very good results have been obtained, owing to the involvement of the brachialis muscle in the reinnervation process.

Then the median nerve emerged as a more powerful donor than the ulnar nerve [20, 21] even if its lateral component is denervated in avulsive injuries of C5 and C6.

Following this observation, a change in the donor nerve was also introduced. The ulnar nerve was abandoned in favor of one large/two small fascicles selected from the medial cord at infraclavicular level, where the inner contributions of the median and the ulnar nerve diverge.

This procedure is known as the "medial cord to musculocutaneous (MC-Mc) nerve transfer" [22].

A technical variant, called medial cord to anterior upper trunk (MC-aUT) transfer, has been more recently published [23], but still is largely unknown. It has been introduced in agenesia of the musculocutaneous nerve from the lateral cord and when a residual function of the biceps is present because sustained by C7.

18.2 Surgical Technique of the MC-Mc (Medial Cord to Musculocutaneous Nerve) Transfer

The entire plexus is explored via the combined supraclavicular and infraclavicular approach. It is of utmost importance to assess the level and entity of the damage first, to exclude an unexpected integrity of the nerves and check for distal associated injuries, namely, the musculocutaneous nerve at the entrance into the coracobrachialis muscle and the axillary nerve at the quadrilateral space of Velpeau.

At the lateral cord, the musculocutaneous nerve is traced back with a gentle neurolysis and prepared to be cut as proximally as possible.

Then, an intraneural inspection of the medial compartment of the medial cord is undertaken. The procedure is painstaking, but it is imperative to accurately check at low intensity (0.2 and 0.3 mA) the area of division of the medial cord. Particular attention is focused on the medial contribution of the median nerve at the level of the take off with the ulnar nerve. Here, only the portion aimed at the flexor digitorum profundus or flexor carpi ulnaris is selected, usually consisting of one single voluminous fascicle or two smaller fascicles (Fig. 18.1).

Their diameter is smaller, but most of the time the coaptation accommodates well with the receiving musculocutaneous nerve. Stitches are done with 9–0 Nylon and fibrin glue.

This technique has been modified (**MC-aUT transfer**) in the presence of two circumstances:

- *Agenesia of the musculocutaneous nerve (5% of our series).*

In this anatomical variant, the lateral cord tapers directly into the external contribution of the median nerve and the branches for the biceps and the brachialis muscles take off distally, at the upper third of the arm (Fig. 18.2). This arrange-

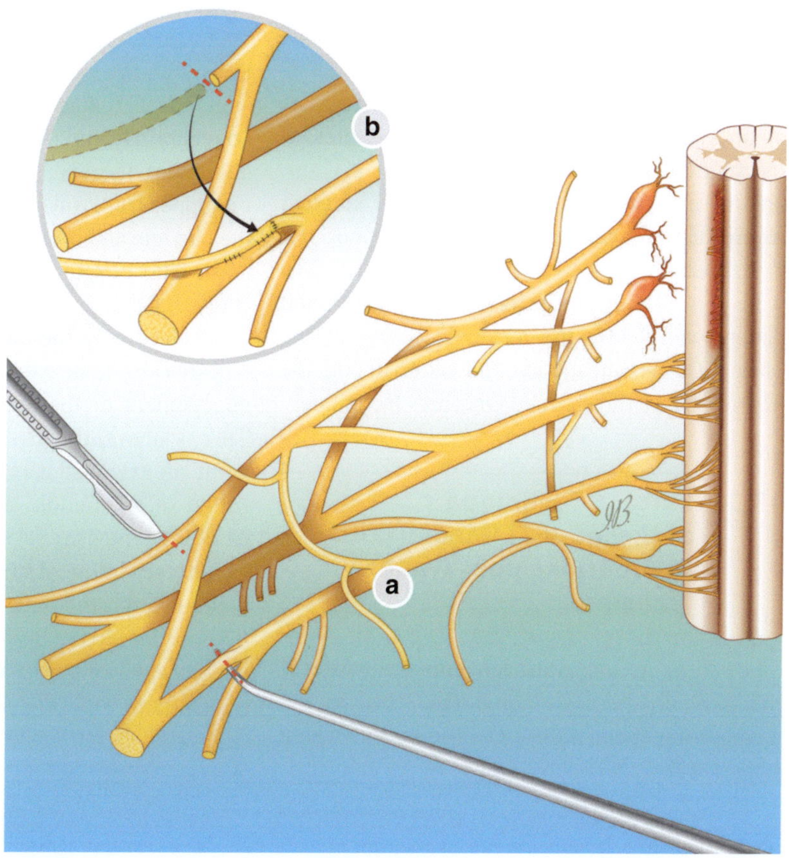

Fig. 18.1 The medial cord to musculocutaneous nerve transfer. (**a**) The tip of the scalpel indicates the recipient musculocutaneous nerve. The tip of the dissector points to the area of the donor fascicle. Tondo (**b**), a tensionless suture can be easily realized

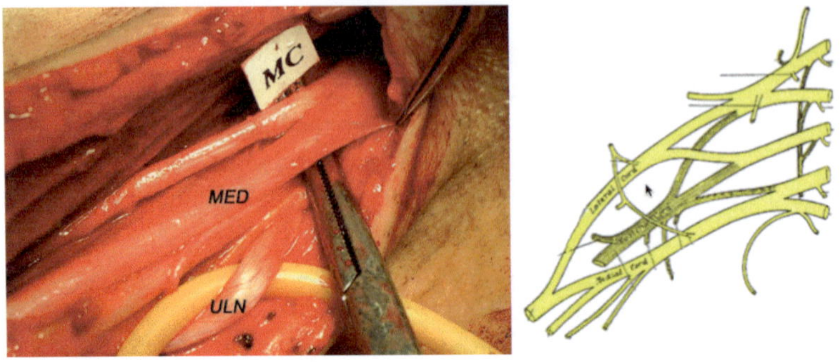

Fig. 18.2 Agenesia of the musculocutaneous nerve with direct confluence of the lateral cord into the medial compartment of the median nerve. Both continue as median nerve. *Surgical exposure*: a short musculocutaneous nerve emerging from the median nerve at the upper third of the arm

ment is hostile to the MC-Mc nerve transfer as it was originally conceived.

The problem can be solved by targeting, as the recipient nerve, the anterior contribution of the upper trunk, cut and rerouted under the clavicle to reach the medial cord.

– *Residual function of the musculocutaneous nerve due to a component from C7.*

Not infrequently (in 8% of our series), a biceps scoring M1 or sometimes M2 is present. In avulsive injuries of C5 and C6, such a function is obviously coming from C7. When it is present from the very early period after injury, it is not able to improve with time. Without a surgical reconstruction, the result would remain poor.

In such cases, if the musculocutaneous nerve were cut distally to receive the transfer, the patient would lose the residual activity of the biceps. This is a clear contraindication to both the MC-Mc nerve transfer and Oberlin's technique.

18.3 Surgical Technique of the MC-aUT (Medial Cord to Anterior Upper Trunk) Transfer

Since the axons innervating the motor function of the musculocutaneous nerve (Mc) run in the medial component of the upper trunk, from where they reach the upper pectoral loop and the lateral cord, the primary trunk is prepared, and the anterior contribution (aUT) is cut as it emerges from the trifurcation.

It is of paramount importance to focus on the correct branch to be reinnervated, namely, the most medial of the three (Fig. 18.3).

Beware that many two-dimensional anatomical drawings offer a misleading perspective and suggest its being the one in the middle.

An extensive dissection of the interconnections with the lateral cord, i.e., the anterior division of C7 and the afferent and efferent connection to and from the middle trunk, is mandatory. At the end, the anterior contribution of the upper trunk (aUT) is cut and rerouted under the clavicle and brought to the level of the medial cord. The coaptation must be without tension (Fig. 18.4).

Occasionally the anterior contribution of C7 requires also to be cut to allow the successful disengagement of the anterior upper trunk (aUT). This is uneventful if the C7 is clearly avulsed, while an extended careful dissection and mobilization of the middle trunk is mandatory in the case of its integrity.

The selection of the donor fascicles in the medial cord is the same as above. The square sections of the donor fascicle(s) in the medial cord and the anterior branch of the upper trunk usually match quite well (Fig. 18.4).

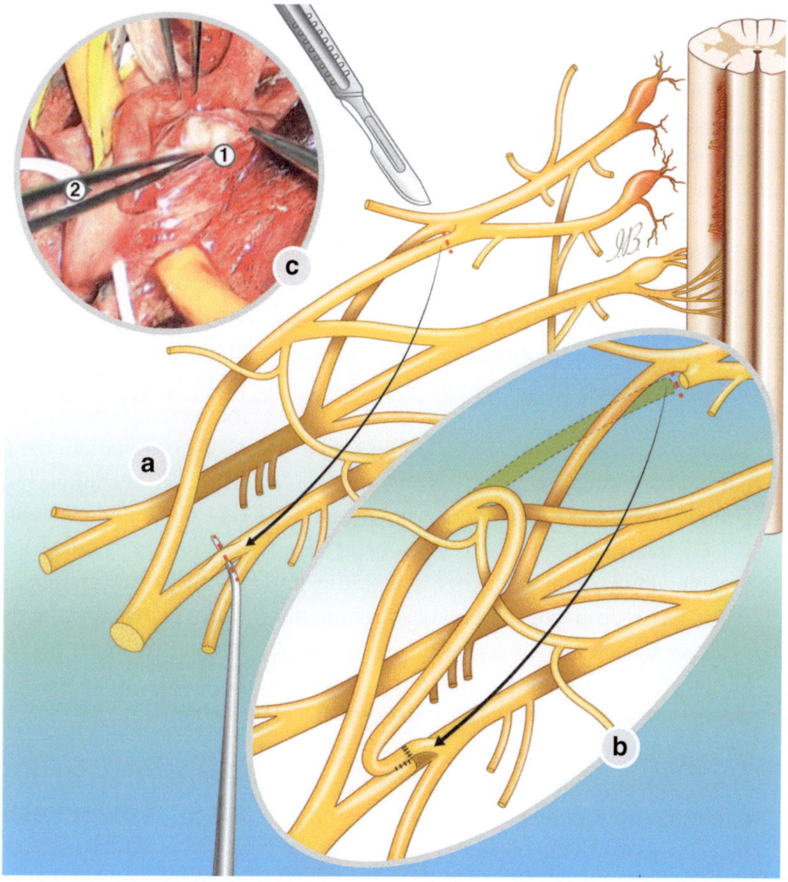

Fig. 18.3 The MC-aUT transfer. (A) Tip of the blade pointing to the anterior contribution of the upper trunk (red dotted line). Tip of the dissector indicating the donor fascicle in the medial cord. Black curved arrow indicates the intended rerouting. (B) Drawing representing the nerve transfer from the medial cord after section and rerouting of the anterior contribution of the upper trunk (curved black arrow). (C) Tip of the forceps (1) selecting the donor fascicle from the medial cord. Rerouted stump (2) of the anterior upper trunk visible below the branches of the forceps, halfway between 1 and 2

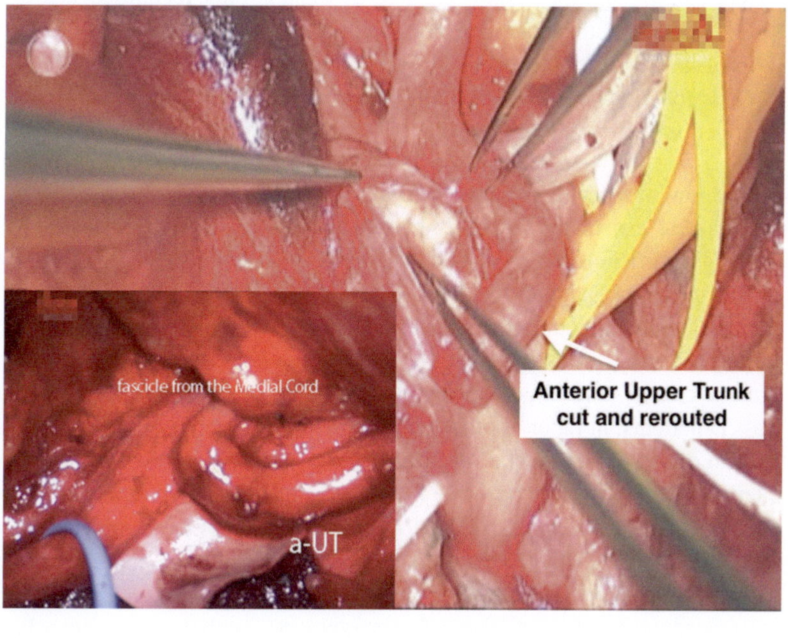

Fig. 18.4 Surgical detail: the MC-aUT nerve transfer. The tips of the forceps are selecting the donor fascicles from the medial cord. In the insert: the nerve suture has been realized without tension

18.4 Patients' Series

In almost 25 years, as many as 500 patients have been operated on with both techniques.

All of them were treated within 18 months after the trauma, with a peak incidence of 6 months.

Most were males (only 15 females). Their age at surgery ranged from the first to the seventh decade. Ten patients were over their 60s.

The patients are grouped into four classes according to their clinical pictures.

- Group A is the largest (75%), presenting a normal hand function.
- Group B includes a 20% patients having a C5–C6–C7 avulsive injury, with a powerful wrist flexion, normal finger flexors, and intrinsics but a wrist drop due to paralysis of all the extensor muscles in the forearm.
- Group C (8%) is represented by patients showing a remarkable loss of strength (M3) on wrist and finger flexors.
  Wrist and finger extensors muscles might or might not be functioning, but, when present, they are weaker than normal.
- For Group D (2%), only part of the T1 root is functioning, and the hand is capable of weak (M2) wrist and finger flexion along with some intrinsic function scoring rather poorly. Occasionally a weak wrist, thumb, and index finger extension are also retained.

The low number of patients forming the last two classes, especially the D, is biased by the ongoing experience.

Due to the several poor results observed in the course of time, in fact, transfers using the medial cord as a donor have been progressively discouraged in class C and almost always excluded in class D patients, in favor of other types of neurotization, mostly extraplexual (such as phrenic or intercostal nerves) or, more rarely, the pectoral nerves.

Presently, the MC-Mc transfer in type D patients is abandoned, while in type C patients, the procedure still is considered, but surgery is deferred after verification of a significant improvement in hand function.

Only quite recently (8 years ago), the MC-aUT technique was conceived: at the beginning it was prompted by the agenesia of the musculocutaneous nerve which obviously didn't permit the MC-Mc transfer.

In some of these patients, it was realized, serendipitously, that those retaining some function on the biceps before surgery had this function unaltered after the procedure, differently from what happened after section of the entire musculocutaneous nerve.

To summarize, the potential candidates to the MC-aUT technique are those with agenesia of the musculocutaneous nerve (5%) and those retaining a residual activity in the biceps (8%), for the overmentioned reasons. Nevertheless, its use is increasing after having observed reinnervation of the upper pectoralis nerve loop and, consequently, improvement in the upper part of the pectoralis major muscle.

18.5 Lower Pectoral Nerve to Musculocutaneous Nerve

This technique has been extensively published and doesn't need further description.

Usually, two nerve branches are available at the lower pectoral loop, and this is an important prerequisite since the function of the lower pectoral muscle can be retained after section of one of them.

In the presence of only one branch, instead, we discourage the use of this technique for fear of losing the axillary pinch, which is important in an heavily injured arm.

Provided that a tension-free direct suture is performed and that the selected branch is strongly reactive, the results are generally good, but not comparable to the procedures having the medial cord as a donor.

If the donor is weak, the procedure is not advisable. The "law of nerve transfer" requires a strongly reactive donor. The use of grafts also would end with poorer results when not complete failures.

This technique was commonly used in adult upper plexus injuries before the appearance of the Oberlin's technique. Nowadays, as we have seen, different techniques are preferred. Nevertheless, in pure infraclavicular injuries with complex and heavy scarring of the medial cord, where the pectoral loop has survived, the pectoral nerve remains a good neurotizer for the musculocutaneous nerve. To overcome the possible mismatch between donor and recipient, we use a small segment of vein as a neural tube covering the suture line, to avoid potential dispersion of axons.

18.6 Thoracodorsal Nerve to Musculocutaneous Nerve Transfer

This technique, described by Foster about a century ago, is also very easy to understand, and the surgical approach doesn't require to be described step by step. The thoracodorsal nerve is isolated from the posterior cord proximal to the division between radial and axillary nerve. Its function is checked with a nerve stimulator at low intensity (0.5 mA), and the muscle contraction must be brisk. Then, the nerve is followed as much distal as possible, cut and rerouted to join the musculocutaneous nerve. A direct suture without tension is the prerequisite. Grafting is highly discouraged. The use of its lateral branch only (with preservation of the latissimus dorsi muscle function) can be an option, but the results may suffer the paucity of motor axons [24].

As with the pectoral nerves, there is generally limited experience in adult injuries, because of the better choice offered by other techniques. Again, in extensively scarred injuries affecting the infraclavicular area of the medial cord, one can resort to this technique, which works properly and gives, despite the small series, a powerful elbow flexion.

Instead, considerable experience with this transfer has been gained in obstetrical palsies.

The realization of the MC-Mc transfer in babies, although possible, may be difficult, particularly during the phase of selection of donor fascicles. The extremely small dimensions of the neural structures would require magnification higher than that offered by the microscope, and the surgical instruments are sometimes felt frustratingly too big to manipulate the overly delicate nerve fascicles.

In those cases where there is no function in the biceps and the supraclavicular neuroma is not convincing (and a possible avulsion of C6 is likely), this kind of neurotization has been used with remarkable results (Fig. 18.5).

The ideal candidate is a baby with moderate to strong internal rotation contracture of the shoulder where the loss of an internal rotator would not be a problem and where an anterior release (section of the coracohumeral ligament and coracoidectomy) is deemed appropriate.

However, it must be kept in mind that a secondary Hoffer procedure (latissimus dorsi transfer) would become impossible. The use of half of the thoracodorsal nerve in the baby is hazardous due to the paucity of axons and the resultant limited mobility of the nerve: after the section of the recipient musculocutaneous nerve, a failure to reinnervate would leave the biceps completely floppy.

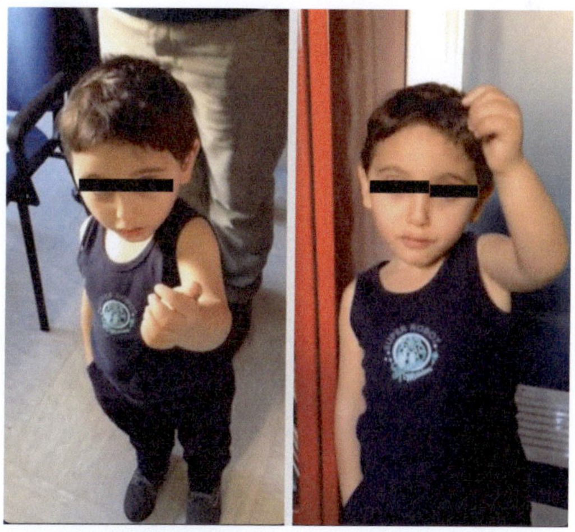

Fig. 18.5 Recovery of elbow flexion in a C5–C6–C7 obstetrical palsy: thoracodorsal to musculocutaneous nerve transfer

18.7 Results of the Medial Cord (MC-Mc and MC-aUT) Transfers

A British Medical Council (BMC) score of M5, i.e., normal strength, is considered impossible to attain after nerve repair, because fatigue is supposed to appear after prolonged and repetitive muscle contraction. Yet some of the best scores have a power and a muscle volume practically indistinguishable from normal.

However, to anticipate criticisms, the results from good to excellent will be all labeled as M4.

Results below M3 are considered failures, because ultimately unable to maintain elbow flexion.

During the intervening process of reinnervation, the flexion of the wrist and fingers initiates and then supports the contraction of biceps and brachialis. As muscle power increases, elbow flexion can be obtained without clenching the fist, with wrist and fingers completely outstretched and a supinated forearm (Fig. 18.6).

In most of the cases of Group A, the overall quality of the result is astonishing.

- Group A: The best results are obtained when a completely normal hand is present from the onset. In this group we have no failures.

A powerful biceps/brachialis complex (M4) has been obtained in 95% of the cases including the latest referral case (18 months) and in three patients older than 65.

A man aged 75 scored M3. None of them complained of loss of strength in the donor hand.

- Group B: The integrity of wrist/finger flexors and intrinsics, despite the lack of wrist and finger dorsiflexion, allows a powerful (M4) elbow flexion to be obtained in 70% of the patients, with a slight increase of M3 scores if compared to group A. Still there are no failures.

We think that the lack of extensor muscles (with a resultant reduced range of motion in wrist flexion and consequently a reduced use of the hand) might explain the worse results.

After the medial cord procedure, the ulnar wrist flexors and the pronator teres remain unchanged, and the tendon transfer procedures to restore wrist and finger dorsiflexion are always successful (Fig. 18.7).

- Group C: From the onset, these patients had intrinsics and wrist and finger flexors and extensors weaker than normal (M3). Out of them, 35% fail to regain a useful elbow flexion. Conversely, 65% recover, sometimes with risks for the integrity of the hand, as it happened in two cases (lately scoring M3 in the biceps/brachialis complex).

This happens for two reasons: (1) the surgeon is tempted to cut more than one fascicle to pro-

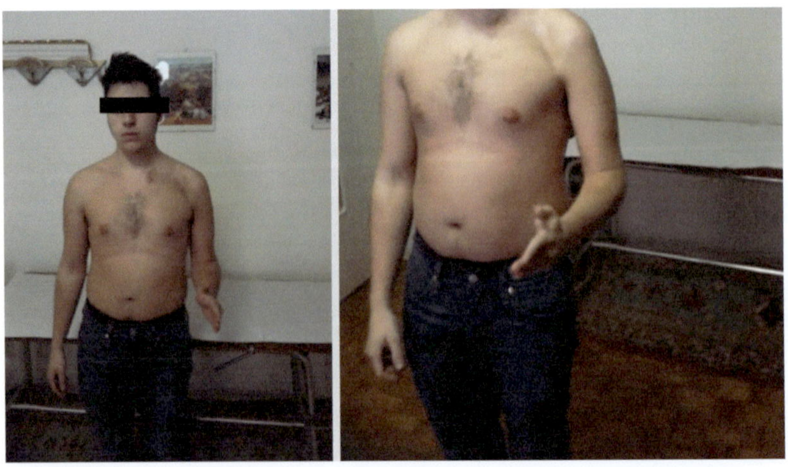

Fig. 18.6 Avulsive injury of C5 and C6: accessory to suprascapular nerve and flexion at the elbow after the MCMc transfer: the patient is maintaining with ease the position with wrist and finger outstretched and supinated forearm

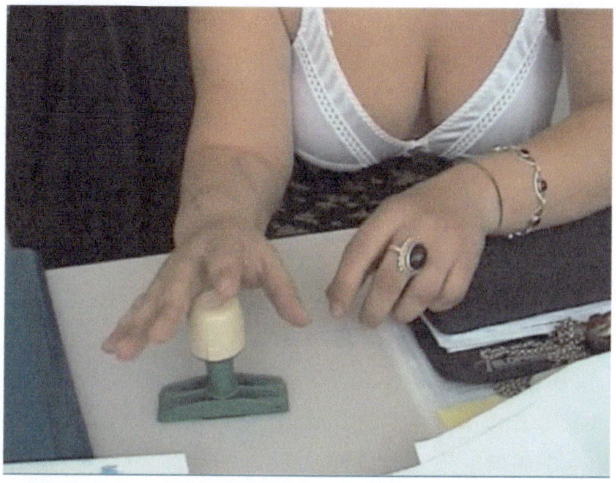

Fig. 18.7 Avulsive injury of C5, C6, C7, and MCMc transfer. Secondary surgery for finger and wrist dorsiflexion with excellent coordination

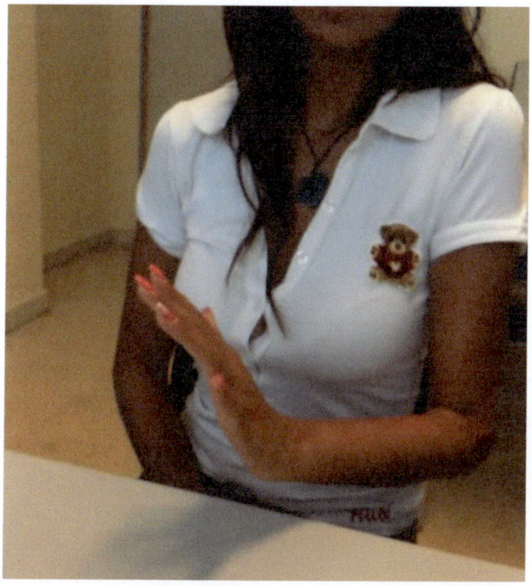

Fig. 18.8 Avulsive injury of C5–C6–C7 and partial damage of C8: good elbow flexion and a remarkable result of secondary surgery for wrist and finger drop. An MC-aUT transfer had been done 8 months after injury as soon as a weak wrist and finger flexion have improved to M4

vide more power, and (2) the electrical stimulation required to elicit muscle contraction is higher than 0,3 mA with resultant mass recruitment and less precise identification of the donor fascicles.

Experience has shown that *delayed surgery on a patient with a stronger hand is better than an early surgery in the presence of a weaker hand* (Fig. 18.8).

- Type D (the so-called T1 hand): In this group the results are highly unsatisfactory, and the medial cord procedure is no longer used in these patients.

An EMG performed in a sample of ten consecutive patients of group A confirms the recovery in both the biceps and the brachialis muscles.

The timing of recovery is somewhat longer than in the original Oberlin's technique.

The first signs are observed between the sixth to the ninth postoperative month, with a clear tendency toward an earlier recovery among the patients in group A.

The weaker the hand, the longer the period of recovery. Patients in group C never started their recovery before the nineth postoperative month.

The quickest onset was seen at 3 months after surgery, the slowest after 16 months.

At 18 months the patients in Group A and B show a well-developed biceps-brachialis complex, while C and D patients required 24 months or more to increase strength up to the final score.

Results of the MC-aUT Technique All the operated cases (7% of the whole series) had a preoperative normal hand, and the biceps and the brachialis regained an excellent function (M4).

The pectoralis major showed a recovery in half of the cases: this technique, due to the more proximal location of the recipient, has the possibility to reinnervate the upper pectoral nerve loop.

After the section of the upper trunk, those having a preoperative residual function of the biceps remain unaltered. This fact confirms the participation of the seventh root. Only on one occasion it was lost, but, in this case, the intraoperative stimulation of the anterior upper trunk had elicited a weak contraction of the biceps, which suggested an incomplete avulsion injury of the C6 root.

After the transfer, the patient fully recovered anyway.

Also, in the patients operated with this technique, who retain a normal wrist and finger function (Group A), the elbow flexion becomes independent from the movement of the hand around the first postoperative year.

On average, the activity in the biceps becomes visible a couple of months later than with the MC-Mc transfer, but in the long run, the results are the same.

18.8 Discussion

Some intraplexual nerve donors, such as medial pectoral nerves, subscapularis, and thoracodorsal nerves, require a complete sacrifice of their corresponding muscles.

The section of the thoracodorsal nerve, for example, is a questionable choice since it paralyzes the latissimus dorsi. This muscle could be alternatively transferred monopolar to stabilize and reinforce the shoulder muscles or bipolar as a support to elbow flexion or to elbow and wrist extension.

The subscapularis nerve, instead, would be good, since the sacrifice of the corresponding muscle is negligible. However, it works mainly as a neurotizer for the axillary nerve, and it is almost always affected in C5–C6–C7 avulsion injuries.

Similar considerations apply to the use of medial pectoral nerves (by far the most reliable procedure in C5–C6 avulsion injuries before the appearance of the technique described by Oberlin), since their section strongly weakens the lower pectoralis major and impairs the thoracobrachial pinch (useful to hold, e.g., a book under the armpit).

The accessory nerve, usually harvested distally after an intramuscular dissection in the anterior trapezius, would also be suitable, but its transfer to the suprascapular nerve is the preferred technique to restore a good shoulder abduction and external rotation [25].

Due to all these reasons, an intraplexual fascicular neurotization from the medial cord, which maintains the hand normal and saves the latissimus dorsi and low pectoralis major, was welcome as the best choice to reanimate elbow flexion.

Table 18.1 Highlights of the two medial cord procedures and the Oberlin's technique with their relevant indications

Comparing the techniques	Medial cord to musculocutaneous nerve (MCMc) transfer	Medial cord to anterior upper trunk (MC-aUT) transfer	Oberlin's technique (ulnar nerve fascicle to branch for the biceps)
Target muscles	Biceps, brachialis, and sensory branch of the musculocutaneous nerve that can be neurotized to the branch of brachioradialis	Biceps, brachialis, and upper pectoralis muscle loop	Biceps (to reinnervate the brachialis an associated procedure, a motor branch from the median nerve to the brachialis is required)
Second attempt at nerve repair upon failure of the first procedure	Oberlin's procedure as a second chance remains possible	Oberlin's procedure as a second chance still remains possible	Very unlikely, the tiny distal stump within the biceps muscle often cannot be recognized in the course of a second attempt
Preoperative residual activity in the musculocutaneous nerve (coming from C7)	Lost. As with the Oberlin procedure the section of the MC nerve also abolishes the contribution from C7	Very selective neurotization sparing the fibers coming from C7 and running within the musculocutaneous n. Best choice: the residual function is preserved	Oberlin procedure entails section of the distal nerve branch to the biceps with obvious loss of residual function
Timing of reinnervation	6 months on average	9 months on average	4–5 months on average

Due to its proximal position, the medial cord techniques offer distinct advantages, namely, the following (see Table 18.1 for more details):

- The technical procedure is delicate but does not require a special skill for an experienced plexus surgeon.
- Both variants of the procedure are straightforward in the course of a standard exploration of the plexus. Additional incisions in the arm are not needed.
- In the case of failure, they allow a "second chance." The Oberlin operation remains possible since the function in the ulnar-innervated muscles is not significantly weakened after the first procedure.
- The reinnervation of the entire MC nerve addresses both the biceps and the brachialis muscles, otherwise reinnervated with a painstaking double distal procedure from the ulnar and the median nerves (the so-called double Oberlin).
- In five cases a second surgery , done 6 months after the first procedure and consisting in a selective reinnervation of the branch directed to the brachioradialis muscle, was successful. The donor nerve was the cutaneous division of the Musculocutaneous nerve which, in the meanwhile, has hosted motor axons as a successful result of the former MC-Mc nerve transfer (Fig. 18.9).
  The description of this last procedure is beyond the scope of the present paper but confirms the plasticity of a sensory nerve branch as an "on site graft" for motor reinnervation.
- Denervation pain in the territory of the median or ulnar nerves has never been observed after the MC transfer. On the contrary, a severe reflex sympathetic dystrophy after a so-called double Oberlin (one fascicle from the ulnar nerve to the biceps and one fascicle from the median nerve to brachialis) has been observed.
- In the case of a weak ulnar nerve function, the medial cord technique offers a choice between mixed fascicles for flexor digitorum profundus (FDP) or flexor carpi ulnaris (FCU), while an Oberlin-type procedure can select only one nerve at the time, either the median or the ulnar (Fig. 18.10).

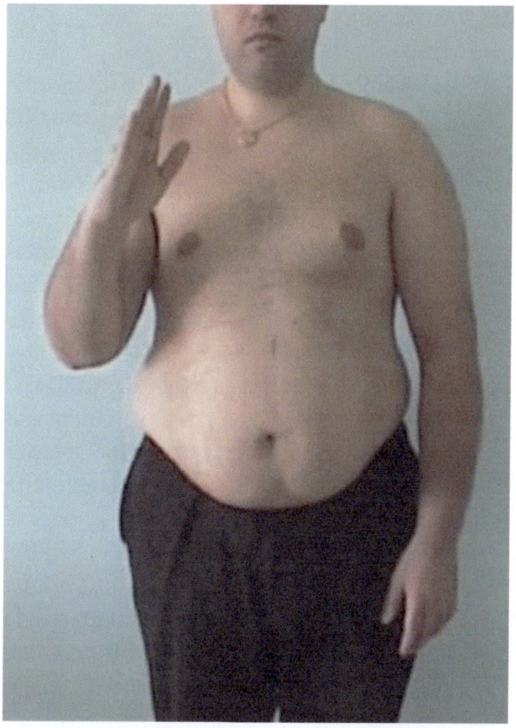

Fig. 18.9 MC-aUT transfer at 2-year follow-up: excellent endurance of elbow flexion with wrist in neutral position and fingers completely stretched out

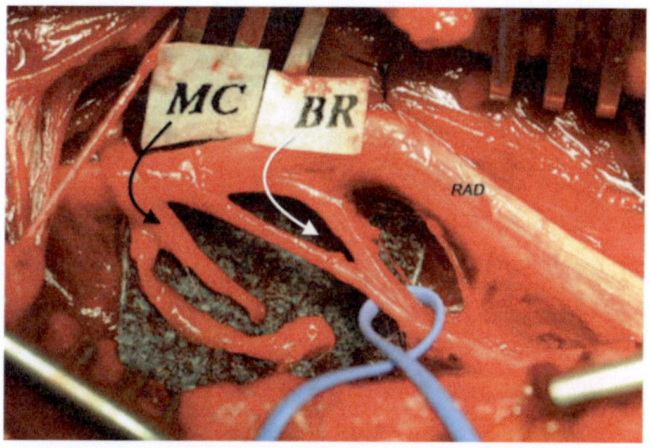

Fig. 18.10 Black arrow: the donor: two branches of the sensory musculocutaneous n. (reinnervated with motor axons after the MC-Mc procedure) cut and tunneled to approximate two recipient branches of the denervated brachioradialis muscle (white arrow)

18.9 Conclusion

- The medial cord technique (MC-Mc and the MC-aUT variant) is very effective, and the results are constant and reproducible when the hand function, or at least its flexor and intrinsic power, is completely retained. The absence of wrist and finger dorsiflexion doesn't interfere with a good outcome.
- A hostile anatomy of the lateral cord (absence of the musculocutaneous nerve) is the limitation of the MC-Mc transfer but the aUT-MC transfer technique overcomes the problem and shows similar results. As a target, the anterior upper trunk is more selective than the entire musculocutaneous nerve since it carries a smaller sensory component. The mobilization of the upper and middle plexus can be a little bit awkward, but it is very important to reroute loosely the anterior contribution of the upper trunk (aUT) and reach the medial cord without any tension.
- The medial cord-anterior upper trunk procedure (MC-aUT) appears to be the *technique of choice in the presence of a residual function of the musculocutaneous nerve, usually sustained by fibers coming from C7*. Under these conditions any type of nerve transfer to the distal Musculocutaneous (Mc) nerve would sacrifice that function, while the neurotization of the anterior upper trunk selectively replaces only the fibers coming from C5 and C6, leaving those from C7 intact.
- The endurance and the power of elbow flexion, thanks to both the biceps and the brachialis muscles, is stronger than with the classic Oberlin's technique.

Acknowledgments We are deeply indebted to Miss Ilaria Bondi, professional anatomical illustrator (www.illustrazionianatomiche.com) for her patient and dedicated work.

Conflicts of Interest None.

Disclosure of Funding None.

References

1. Bertelli JA, Ghizoni MF. Reconstruction of C5 and C6 brachial plexus avulsion injury by multiple nerve transfers: spinal accessory to suprascapular, ulnar fascicles to biceps branch, and triceps long or lateral head branch to axillary nerve. J Hand Surg Am. 2004;29:131–9.
2. Leechavengvongs S, et al. Nerve transfer to biceps muscle using a part of the ulnar nerve in brachial plexus injury (upper arm type): a report of 32 cases. J Hand Surg Am. 1998;23:711–6.
3. Oberlin C, Beal D, et al. Nerve transfer to biceps muscle using a part of ulnar nerve for C5-C6 avulsion of the brachial plexus: anatomical study and report of four cases. J Hand Surg Am. 1994;19:232–7.
4. Sungpet A, et al. Transfer of a single fascicle from the ulnar nerve to the biceps muscle after avulsions of upper roots of the brachial plexus. J Hand Surg Br. 2000;25:325–8.
5. Leechavengvongs S, et al. Nerve transfer to deltoid muscle using the nerve to the long head of the triceps, part II: a report of 7 cases. J Hand Surg Am. 2003;28:633–8.
6. Samardzic M, Rasulic L, et al. Results of nerve transfers to the musculocutaneous and axillary nerves. Neurosurgery. 2000;46:93–103.
7. Aszmann OC, Rab M, et al. The anatomy of the pectoral nerves and their significance in brachial plexus reconstruction. J Hand Surg Am. 2000;25:942–7.
8. Hansasuta A, Tubbs RS, Grabb PA. Surgical relationship of the medial pectoral nerve to the musculocutaneous nerve: a cadaveric study. Neurosurgery. 2001;48:203–7.
9. Samardzic M, Grujicic D, Rasulic L, et al. Transfer of the medial pectoral nerve: myth or reality? Neurosurgery. 2002;50:1277–82.
10. Luedemann W, Hamm M, Blomer U, et al. Brachial plexus neurotization with donor phrenic nerves and its effect on pulmonary function. J Neurosurg. 2002;96:523–6. Acta Neuroch (Wien) 2015; 157(6) 1077–86.
11. Sokolovsky M, Di Masi G, Bonilla G, et al. The phrenic nerve as a donor for brachial plexus injuries: is it safe and effective? Case series and literature analysis. Acta Neurochir (Wien). 2015;157(6):1077–86.
12. Waikakul S, Wongtragul S, Vanadurongwan V. Restoration of elbow flexion in brachial plexus avulsion injury: comparing spinal accessory nerve transfer with intercostal nerve transfer. J Hand Surg Am. 1999;24:571–7.
13. Malessy MJ, Thomeer RT. Evaluation of intercostal to musculocutaneous nerve transfer in reconstructive brachial plexus surgery. J Neurosurg. 1998;88:266–71.

14. Nagano A, Yamamoto S, Mikami Y. Intercostal nerve transfer to restore upper extremity functions after brachial plexus injury. Ann Acad Med Singap. 1995;24(Suppl 4):42–5.
15. Brunelli G, Monini L. Neurotization of avulsed roots of brachial plexus by means of anterior nerves of cervical plexus. Clin Plast Surg. 1984;11:149–52.
16. Ferraresi S, Garozzo D, Ravenni R, et al. Hemihypoglossal nerve transfer in brachial plexus repair: technique and results. Neurosurgery. 2002;50:332–5.
17. Mackinnon SE, Novak CB, Myckatyn TM, Tung TH. Results of reinnervation of the biceps and brachialis muscles with a double fascicular transfer for elbow flexion. J Hand Surg Am. 2005;30:978–85.
18. Tung TH, Novak CB, Mackinnon SE. Nerve transfers to the biceps and brachialis branches to improve elbow flexion strength after brachial plexus injuries. J Neurosurg. 2003;98:313–8.
19. Ferraresi S, Garozzo D, Buffatti P. Reinnervation of the biceps in C5-C7 brachial plexus avulsion injuries. Results after distal bypass surgery. Neurosurg Focus. 2004;16(5):E6.
20. Al Qattan MM, Al-Kharfy TM. Median nerve to biceps nerve transfer to restore elbow flexion in obstetric brachial plexus palsy. Biomed Res Int. 2014;2014:854084, 4 pages. https://doi.org/10.1155/2014/854084.
21. Sungpet A, et al. One-fascicle median nerve transfer to biceps muscle in C5 and C6 root avulsions of brachial plexus injury. Microsurgery. 2003;23:10–3.
22. Ferraresi S, Garozzo D, Basso E, et al. The medial cord to musculocutaneous (MCMc) nerve transfer: a new method to reanimate elbow flexion after C5-C6-C7-(C8) avulsive injuries of the brachial plexus—technique and result. Neurosurg Rev. 2014;37:321–9.
23. Ferraresi S, Basso E, Maistrello L, et al. The medial cord–anterior upper trunk (MC-aUT) nerve transfer in brachial plexus injuries. Technique and results. Austin Neurosurg Open Access. 2017;4(1):1055, 1–5.
24. Schusterman MA II, et al. Lateral branch of the thoracodorsal nerve (LaT branch) transfer for biceps reinnervation. Plast Reconstr Surg Glob Open. 2018;6:e1698. https://doi.org/10.1097/GOX.0000000000001698. Published online 19 March 2018.
25. Merrell GA, Barrie KA, Katz DL, et al. Results of nerve transfer techniques for restoration of shoulder and elbow function in the context of a meta-analysis of the English literature. J Hand Surg Am. 2001;26:303–14.

19 Medial Pectoral Nerve to Musculocutaneous Nerve

Lukas Rasulic and Miroslav Samardžić

Abbreviations

BP	Brachial plexus
MPN	Medial pectoral nerve
MCN	Musculocutaneous nerve
TDN	Thoracodorsal nerve

19.1 Introduction

The priorities in brachial plexus (BP) repair are to restore a full range and strong elbow flexion, shoulder stability, active arm abduction, and some external rotation. Simultaneous recovery of these functions is equally important since it enables elbow movements through a more functional range. The recovery of elbow flexion may be achieved through the reinnervation of the musculocutaneous nerve (MCN) using different technical methods, or separate reinnervation of the biceps and brachialis muscles to maximize the potential for recovery of strong function [1–10].

The medial pectoral (MPN) and thoracodorsal nerve (TDN) present the most used collateral BP branches in restoring the upper arm function following upper (C5-C6) and upper extended (C5-C7) BP injuries. As donors for infraclavicular intraplexal nerve transfers, they have several advantages over classical intraplexal and extraplexal transfers and could be a valuable method, especially in cases where other infraclavicular transfer methods are unavailable [11–15].

The history of these nerve transfers dates back almost 100 years, beginning in 1920 when Vulpius and Stoffel published about the use of the BP branches to the pectoral muscles as donors. In 1929, Foerster reported nerve transfer using the branches to the latissimus dorsi and subscapular muscles. Finally, in 1948 Lurja reported the use of the MPN and TDN in repair of the upper trunk injuries [16, 17]. Thereafter, there were no reports on this subject for several decades, until the late 1980s and early 1990s. Recently, results on the use of the MPN and the TDN as a donor in the reinnervation of the MCN were reported sporadically and with a limited number of cases. Possible reasons could be existing controversies and surgical problems [18–32].

In this chapter, we analyze the characteristics of MPN to MCN transfer (Fig. 19.1) and discuss some controversies, problems, and possible solutions based on personal experiences and published research.

The original version of the chapter has been revised. A correction to this chapter can be found at https://doi.org/10.1007/978-3-031-92445-3_31

L. Rasulic (✉) · M. Samardžić
Faculty of Medicine, University of Belgrade, Belgrade, Serbia

Department of Peripheral Nerve Surgery, Functional Neurosurgery and Pain Management Surgery, Clinic for Neurosurgery, University Clinical Centre of Serbia, Belgrade, Serbia

F. Guedes et al. (eds.), *Nerve Transfers for Brachial Plexus Reconstruction after Trauma*,
https://doi.org/10.1007/978-3-031-92445-3_19

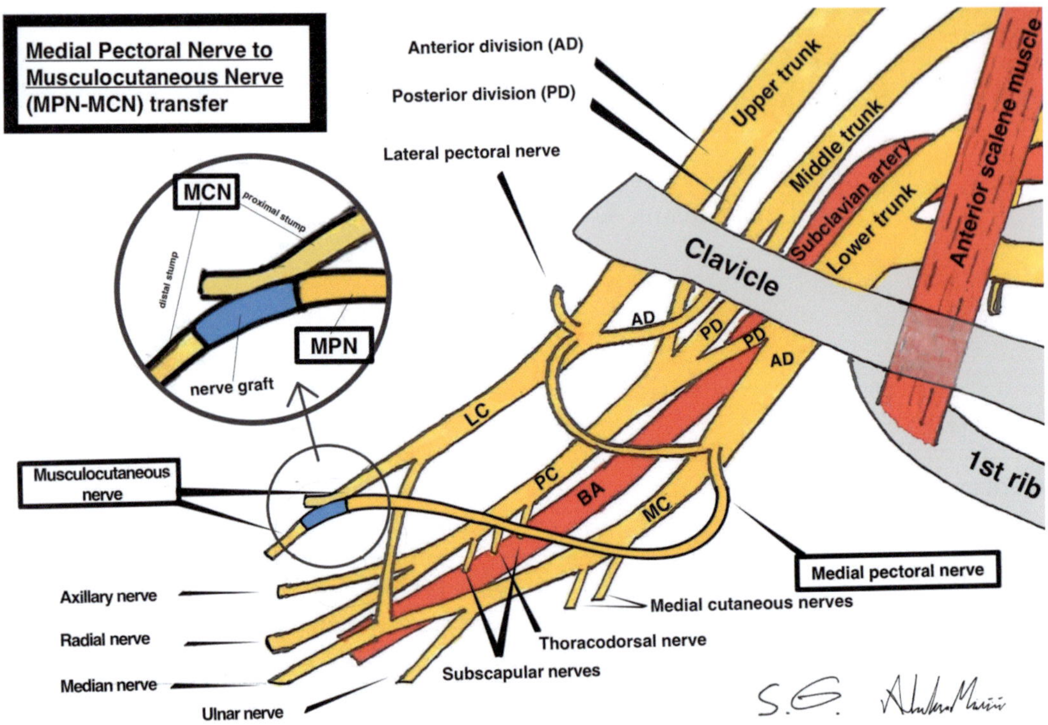

Fig. 19.1 Medial pectoral nerve (MPN) to musculocutaneous nerve (MCN) transfer. *LC* lateral cord, *PC* posterior cord, *MC* medial cord, *BA* brachial artery, *AD* anterior division, *PD* posterior division. Courtesy of Aleksa Mićić MD (University of Belgrade, Faculty of Medicine) and Strahinja Gligorijević BA (University of Belgrade, Faculty of Medicine)

19.2 Anatomy

- The MCN contains from 3,069 to 7,911 myelinated fibers. The average number of fibers in motor branches is 1,840 for the biceps and 1,826 for the brachialis muscle [16, 33].
- The MPN is a motor nerve that derives from the anterior division of the inferior trunk and receives nerve fibers from the eighth cervical and first thoracic spinal nerves. This nerve has cerebral centers that are integrated into the function of the upper extremity and innervate with several branches the sternal part of the pectoralis major muscle [34]. The surgically useable length of the MPN ranged from 30 to 78 mm [30]. However, this length may be increased by dissecting its terminal branches distally and their section close to the pectoral muscle.
- The anatomic relationship of the lateral and medial pectoral nerves is variable. Traditionally, they have been described as two distinct nerves linked with ansa that develop at the expense of the lateral nerve. Some authors, however, have described three distinct nerves: the superior, medial, and inferior The MPN ends in the pectoralis major muscle with two or three branches Occasionally, there were even four branches and one or two branches from the pectoral ansa [32, 35].
- The mean diameter of the nerve ranges from 1.5 to 2.5 or 2.7 mm. The number of motor fibers ranges from 1,170 to 2,140 in the main trunk and may reach 400–600 fibers in a muscular branch. The abovementioned branch of the pectoral ansa contains 330 to 440 nerve fibers. These numbers of motor fibers are especially favorable for nerve transfers [13, 31, 32].

19.3 General Principles

- Generally, there is no ideal donor nerve. Regardless, there are several important criteria which are important for a choice of the donor nerve [3, 5, 33]:
  1. Expendable nerve or nerve with duplicated function.
  2. Proximity to the recipient nerve facilitating a direct anastomosis.
  3. Proximity to the target muscle and its end plates to decrease the regeneration distance.
  4. Pure motor fiber composition, possibly with a few sensory fibers.
  5. A large number of motor fibers.
  6. Donor-recipient axon count ratio 0.7 or greater. However, a lower ratio should not be always a problem because only 20–30% of motor fibers are sufficient for the reinnervation of muscles with a simple function, such as the biceps muscle.
  7. Maximal nerve diameter matching enables more accurate coaptation.
  8. MRC grade at least M4 in the donor innervation zone.
  9. Synergistic function with the recipient nerve offers more effective and faster cortical reintegration.
- The MPN (as well as TDN) do not fulfill a few of the criteria for choosing the donor nerve, including the criterion that a motor nerve should be expendable or redundant, without significant diameter mismatching with the recipient nerve and preferably innervating synergistic muscles with the target muscle [13, 14, 17, 36]. These problems are especially important for the use of the MPN, but they may be overcome, at least partially (Fig. 19.2).
- There are general advantages to using the infraclavicular intraplexal nerve transfer (including the MPN) over the classical intraplexal and extraplexal transfers:
  1. The possibility for direct nerve anastomosis.

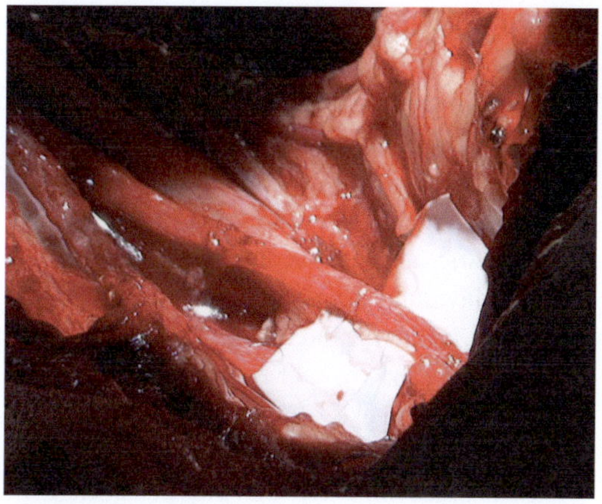

Fig. 19.2 An indirect coaptation of medial pectoral nerve (MPN) and musculocutaneous nerve (MCN), using cutanoeus nerve geraft without tension over the suture lines

  2. Anastomosis is closer to the target muscle.
  3. Shorter distance and time span for nerve regeneration with earlier reinnervation.
  4. Surgery outside zone of injury and scarred bed.
  5. Faster recovery with its higher quality.
  6. Surgical procedure that is more technically straightforward and can be performed with a significant gain in operative time [5, 37].
- In general, the ideal timing for nerve transfer has not been yet established. However, it is widely accepted that surgery should be done in a period between 3 and 5 months after injury if there are neither clinical nor electromyographic signs of recovery [2, 3, 11]. Target muscle should be reinnervated between 12 and 18 months to prevent muscle atrophy and loss of motor end plates [7]. The presence of fibrillation potentials after this period is an indication that denervated muscle is still viable. However, some authors do not recommend surgery after a postinjury period of 9 months, with a possible exception for the MPN and other donors for infraclavicular intraplexal nerve transfers including the TDN [10].

19.4 Surgical Procedure

- *Exploration*. The extent of surgical exploration should be adapted to the reliability of the preoperative diagnosis. In the majority of cases, BP is explored only infraclavicular. In diagnostically unclear cases, an additional supraclavicular exploration should be performed, limited to the C5 and C6 spinal nerves and upper trunk.
- *Surgical strategy*. Choosing the MPN as a donor for reinnervation of the MCN should be based predominantly on the possibility of direct nerve anastomosis. Identification of the MPN and confirmation of its functionality can be performed using direct nerve electrical stimulation and palpation of the corresponding muscle contractions. A compound muscular action potential recording after submaximal nerve stimulation during partial neuromuscular blockade with carefully titrated short-acting agents may also be used. In some cases, the MPN may be used as a donor in combination with the spinal accessory or intercostal nerves. The main reason for using additional donor nerves is the completion of the suture line in cases with recipient nerves of a considerably larger diameter. The choice of additional donor was also based on the anatomical relationship.
- *Microsurgical technique*. The MPN, either by itself or combined with a branch of pectoral ansa, or its two terminal branches, is joined in a common trunk by fibrin glue and anastomosed with the MCN directly or using short nerve grafts. The epifascicular epineurium of the MCN should be removed to reduce the occurrence of fibrosis over the suture line. Completion of the anastomosis may be done with two epiperineural sutures on the upper side of the nerve or with a circumferential suture using four to five stitches around the nerve. A combination of two sutures with a fibrine glue provides stabilization of the suture line, without tension and minimal damage to the tissue (Fig. 19.2).

19.5 Problems and Solutions

- Generally, there are several potential problems in the usage of the MPN and other infraclavicular intraplexal donors for the restoration of the upper arm function:

1. **Preexisting donor nerve injury**

   Different degrees of preexisting donor nerve injury may result in variations in obtained results and could be a contraindication for the transfer. There is always some damage to the functional nerves but located on the "edge" of the lesion. Notably, muscle weakness becomes apparent when 50% of the motor fibers are lost. Fibrillation potentials detected on electromyography indicate a potential injury and should be considered in the selection of a donor nerve [28].

2. **Donor nerve morbidity**

   Donor nerve morbidity is an important drawback, especially in cases with suboptimal, grade M3 or M4, function of the synergistic muscles. The potential functional loss could be avoided or diminished in several ways depending on the donor nerve. Generally, additional palsy of arm adduction and internal rotation should not be as significant in patients with severely disabled arm function. Moreover, the potential benefits exceed a relatively low rate of donor nerve morbidity. In the MPN transfer, some function of the pectoralis major muscle may be retained because of its multiple innervation patterns since the usual origin of the lateral pectoral nerve is from the C5 to C7 spinal nerves with a mean percentage of supply 50% from the C7 spinal nerve [14, 25, 32, 38].

   Furthermore, in cases of predominant innervation from the C7 spinal nerve, the function of synergistic muscles such as teres major may be sometimes partially preserved. Functional preservation is also possible by distal sectioning and sparing some of the branches. The remaining branch or branches usually produce strong contraction of the pectoralis major muscle. End-to-side anastomosis is another possibility for functional preservation of the donor nerves, but this is seldom used. Possible co-contractions could be very disabling, such as in intraplexal nerve transfers using spinal nerve stumps as donors because of massive cross-innervation of the synergistic and antagonistic muscles [13]. On the contrary, in the MPN to MCN transfer, contractions of the biceps muscle associated with arm adduction may be useful. Moreover, some authors favor this transfer rather than the fascicular transfers [5, 15, 33, 36, 39].

3. **Need for cortical re-education.**
4. **Possible co-contractions.**
5. **Muscle loss for musculo-tendinous transfer.**

- In the case of MPN to MCN transfer, the problems could be the following:
  1. **The large discrepancy in the diameter of the nerves**

     According to reported nerve dimensions, the cross-sectional area of the MPN usually covers between 60% and 70% of that of the recipient nerves. There are several methods in solving this problem of diameter mismatch including (1) suture of the MPN to the fascicle or fascicular group of the MCN, (2) anastomosis over the part of the MCN cross-sectional area [36], (3) epineurial fishmounting of the donor nerve, (4) epineurectomy of the recipient nerve with epi-perineurial anastomosis, (5) bundling of the externally neurolyzed MPN with the branch of the pectoral ansa, and (6) bundling of several nerve branches [13, 23, 40]. A possible option to overcome this problem is anastomosis with the biceps muscle nerve branch. In cases in which these procedures are insufficient, another option is the use of an additional donor (Fig. 19.3), usually one upper intercostal or spinal accessory nerve [15, 25, 26, 41–43]. Similarly, a combination of the MPN transfer and grafting from the anterior division of the lateral cord to the medial part of the MCN was used by Sulaiman et al. [27].

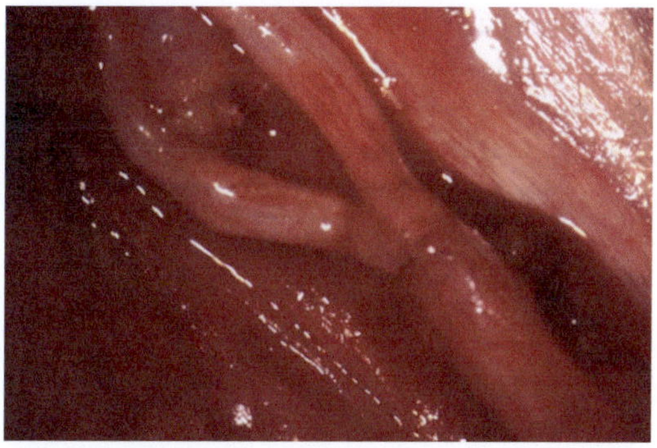

Fig. 19.3 Medial pectoral nerve (MPN) and intercostal nerve (ICN) combined transfer to the musculocutaneous nerve (MCN) to match the diameter of the recipient nerve

  2. **The insufficient length of the MPN for direct anastomosis**

     According to some investigations, the length of the MPN is insufficient for tension-free direct anastomosis with the MCN in approximately one-third of cases, and in all cases of anastomosis to the biceps muscle branch. The average length of this gap is 15 to 20 mm [14]. This problem may be overcome in several ways, such as (1) retrograde split of the MCN into the lateral cord, (2) distal dissection of the MPN branches, (3) dissection of the nerve from its branch to the pectoral ansa, and (4) sectioning of this arcade between two pectoral nerves [12, 13, 36].

19.6 Conclusion

The MPN to MCN transfer emerges as a valuable approach for restoring elbow flexion in cases of partial BP injuries. Positioned as a collateral BP branch and an infraclavicular intraplexal nerve donor, the MPN exhibits numerous advantages over classical intraplexal and extraplexal nerve donors. However, challenges inherent in infraclavicular intraplexal nerve transfers, including those applicable to the MPN, underscore the absence of ideal donor nerves. Notably, the significant drawbacks of using the MPN encompass the considerable diameter mismatch and the often insufficient length for direct anastomosis with the MCN. Ultimately, the choice of employing the MPN for MCN reinnervation should be meticulously based on intraoperative findings.

In conclusion, medial pectoral nerve (MPN) to musculocutaneous nerve (MCN) transfer is a valuable method in restoring upper arm function, particularly in cases of brachial plexus injuries. Despite challenges such as the need to overcome diameter discrepancies and potential donor nerve morbidity, the MPN, along with the TDN, presents advantages in infraclavicular intraplexal nerve transfers. The procedure's success relies on careful donor nerve selection based on specific criteria, emphasizing the importance of direct nerve anastomosis and proximity to the target muscle for optimal results in brachial plexus repair.

Acknowledgments The first author would like to express his gratitude to his Ph.D. student, Aleksa Mićić, for his contribution to the preparation of this chapter.

References

1. Borrero JL. Obstetrical brachial plexus paralysis. 2nd ed. Lake Mary: Design and Print Progressive Communications; 2007.
2. Narakas AO. Thoughts on neurotization or nerve transfers in irreparable nerve lesions. Clin Plast Surg. 1984;11(1):153–9.
3. Weber RV, MacKinnon SE. Nerve transfers in the upper extremity. Journal of the American Society for Surgery of the Hand. 2004;4(3):200–13.
4. Midha R. Nerve transfers for severe brachial plexus injuries: a review. Neurosurg Focus. 2004;16(5):E5.
5. Addas BM, Midha R. Nerve transfers for severe nerve injury. Neurosurg Clin N Am. 2009;20(1):27–38.
6. Colbert SH, Mackinnon S. Posterior approach for double nerve transfer for restoration of shoulder function in upper brachial plexus palsy. Hand (N Y). 2006;1(2):71–7.
7. Hussain T, Khan I, Ahmed M, Beg MSA. Neurotization of musculocutaneous nerve with intercostal nerve versus phrenic nerve—a retrospective comparative study. Surg Neurol Int. 2022;13:305.
8. Vekris MD, Beris AE, Johnson EO, Korobilias AV, Pafilas D, Vekris AD, et al. Musculocutaneous neurotization to restore elbow flexion in brachial plexus paralysis. Microsurgery. 2006;26(4):325–9.
9. Chuang DC. Brachial plexus injury: nerve reconstruction and functioning muscle transplantation. Semin Plast Surg. 2010;24(1):57–66.
10. Sakellariou VI, Badilas NK, Stavropoulos NA, Mazis G, Kotoulas HK, Kyriakopoulos S, et al. Treatment options for brachial plexus injuries. ISRN Orthop. 2014;2014:314137.
11. Samardzic MM, Grujicic DM, Rasulic LG, Milicic BR. The use of thoracodorsal nerve transfer in restoration of irreparable C5 and C6 spinal nerve lesions. Br J Plast Surg. 2005;58(4):541–6.
12. Wellons JC, Tubbs RS, Pugh JA, Bradley NJ, Law CR, Grabb PA. Medial pectoral nerve to musculocutaneous nerve neurotization for the treatment of persistent birth-related brachial plexus palsy: an 11-year institutional experience. J Neurosurg Pediatr. 2009;3(5):348–53.
13. Samardzic M, Grujicic D, Rasulic L, Bacetic D. Transfer of the medial pectoral nerve: myth or reality? Neurosurgery. 2002;50(6):1277–82.
14. Samardzić M, Rasulić L, Lakićević N, Bascarević V, Cvrkota I, Mićović M, et al. Collateral branches of the brachial plexus as donors in nerve transfers. Vojnosanit Pregl. 2012;69(7):594–603.
15. Janes LE, Crowe C, Shah N, Sasson D, Ko JH. Alternative nerve transfer for shoulder function: thoracodorsal and medial triceps to anterior axillary nerve. Plast Reconstr Surg Glob Open. 2022;10(10):e4614.
16. Narakas A. Neurotization in the treatment of brachial plexus injuries. In: Gelberman RH, editor. Operative nerve repair and reconstruction. Philadelphia: Lippincott Williams & Wilkins; 1991. p. 1258–329.
17. Vanaclocha-Vanaclocha V, Ortiz-Criado J, Sáiz-Sapena N, Vanaclocha N. Nerve transfers in the treatment of peripheral nerve injuries. Peripheral nerve regeneration-from surgery to new therapeutic approaches including biomaterials and cell-based therapies development. 1a ed. Croatia: IntechOpen; 2017. p. 67–98.
18. Dai SY, Lin DX, Han Z, Zhoug SZ. Transference of thoracodorsal nerve to musculocutaneous or axillary nerve in old traumatic injury. J Hand Surg Am. 1990;15(1):36–7.
19. Brandt KE, Mackinnon SE. A technique for maximizing biceps recovery in brachial plexus reconstruction. J Hand Surg Am. 1993;18(4):726–33.
20. Samardzic M, Rasulic LG, Grujicic DM, Bacetic DT, Milicic BR. Nerve transfers using collateral branches of the brachial plexus as donors in patients with upper palsy—thirty years' experience. Acta Neurochir. 2011;153(10):2009–19. discussion 19
21. Richardson PM. Recovery of biceps function after delayed repair for brachial plexus injury. J Trauma. 1997;42(5):791–2.
22. Novak CB, Mackinnon SE, Tung TH. Patient outcome following a thoracodorsal to musculocutaneous nerve

transfer for reconstruction of elbow flexion. Br J Plast Surg. 2002;55(5):416–9.
23. Samardzić M, Rasulić L, Grujicić D, Milicić B. Results of nerve transfers to the musculocutaneous and axillary nerves. Neurosurgery. 2000;46(1):93–101. discussion −3
24. Blaauw G, Slooff AC. Transfer of pectoral nerves to the musculocutaneous nerve in obstetric upper brachial plexus palsy. Neurosurgery. 2003;53(2):338–41. discussion 41–2
25. Tung TH, Novak CB, Mackinnon SE. Nerve transfers to the biceps and brachialis branches to improve elbow flexion strength after brachial plexus injuries. J Neurosurg. 2003;98(2):313–8.
26. Stockinger T, Aszmann OC, Frey M. Clinical application of pectoral nerve transfers in the treatment of traumatic brachial plexus injuries. J Hand Surg Am. 2008;33(7):1100–7.
27. Sulaiman OA, Kim DD, Burkett C, Kline DG. Nerve transfer surgery for adult brachial plexus injury: a 10-year experience at Louisiana State University. Neurosurgery. 2009;65(4 Suppl):A55–62.
28. Hems T. Nerve transfers for traumatic brachial plexus injury: advantages and problems. J Hand Microsurg. 2011;3(1):6–10.
29. Millesi H. Coordinated function oriented movements after multiple root avulsion. Acta Neurochir Suppl. 2007;100:117–9.
30. Hansasuta A, Tubbs RS, Grabb PA. Surgical relationship of the medial pectoral nerve to the musculocutaneous nerve: a cadaveric study. Neurosurgery 2001;48(1):203–6; discussion 6–7.
31. Namazi H, Sajadizadeh E, Dehghanian A, Fereidooni M, Akbarzadeh A. Feasibility of medial pectoral nerve to musculocutaneous nerve transfer using medial antebrachial cutaneous nerve of forearm graft: histopathologic and anatomical evaluation. Turk Neurosurg. 2021;31(6):913–7.
32. David S, Balaguer T, Baque P, Lebreton E. Transfer of pectoral nerves to suprascapular and axillary nerves: an anatomic feasibility study. J Hand Surg Am. 2010;35(1):92–6.
33. Schreiber JJ, Byun DJ, Khair MM, Rosenblatt L, Lee SK, Wolfe SW. Optimal axon counts for brachial plexus nerve transfers to restore elbow flexion. Plast Reconstr Surg. 2015;135(1):135e–41e.
34. Amr SM, Moharram AN. Repair of brachial plexus lesions by end-to-side side-to-side grafting neurorrhaphy: experience based on 11 cases. Microsurgery. 2005;25(2):126–46.
35. Cardenas-Mejia A, O'Boyle CP, Chen KT, Chuang DC. Evaluation of single-, double-, and triple-nerve transfers for shoulder abduction in 90 patients with supraclavicular brachial plexus injury. Plast Reconstr Surg. 2008;122(5):1470–8.
36. Samardzic M, Rasulic LG, Grujicic DM, Bacetic DT, Milicic BR. Nerve transfers using collateral branches of the brachial plexus as donors in patients with upper palsy—thirty years' experience. Acta Neurochir. 2011;153:2009–19.
37. Samardzic M, Joksimovic M, Antunovic V, Grujicic D. Regional donor nerves in the reinnervation of brachial plexus palsy due to upper spinal roots avulsion. Neurol Res. 1989;11(3):181–5.
38. Hinchcliff KM, Pulos N, Shin AY, Stutz C. Morbidity of nerve transfers for brachial plexus birth injury: a systematic review. J Pediatr Orthop. 2021;41(2):e188–e98.
39. Pavel H, Libor M. Ch. 4: Surgical treatment of brachial plexus injury. In: Ana Colette M, editor. Peripheral nerve regeneration. Rijeka: IntechOpen; 2017.
40. Samardzic M, Grujicic D, Antunovic V. Nerve transfer in brachial plexus traction injuries. J Neurosurg. 1992;76(2):191–7.
41. Bertelli JA, Ghizoni MF. Transfer of the accessory nerve to the suprascapular nerve in brachial plexus reconstruction. J Hand Surg Am. 2007;32(7):989–98.
42. Terzis JK, Kostas I. Suprascapular nerve reconstruction in 118 cases of adult posttraumatic brachial plexus. Plast Reconstr Surg. 2006;117(2):613–29.
43. Suzuki K, Doi K, Hattori Y, Pagsaligan JM. Long-term results of spinal accessory nerve transfer to the suprascapular nerve in upper-type paralysis of brachial plexus injury. J Reconstr Microsurg. 2007;23(06):295–9.

20 Long Thoracic Nerve to Musculocutaneous Nerve

Lukas Rasulic and Miroslav Samardžić

Abbreviations

BP	Brachial plexus
LTN	Long thoracic nerve
MPN	Medial pectoral nerve
MCN	Musculocutaneous nerve
TDN	Thoracodorsal nerve

20.1 Introduction

Similar to the other collateral brachial plexus (BP) branches (the medial pectoral (MPN) and the thoracodorsal (TDN) nerves), the long thoracic nerve (LTN) may be used as an infraclavicular intraplexal nerve donor for the musculocutaneous nerve (MCN) reinnervation in treatment of patients with partial BP lesions. However, regarding to the literature, the LTN was less frequently used, compared to the MPN and TDN, and up to date, there is a small number of studies concerning outcomes, advantages, and disadvantages of this procedure.

Lurje used the LTN distal to its innervation for the superior two digitations of the serratus anterior muscle for reinnervation of the transected suprascapular nerve in 1948 [1, 2]. Narakas and Hentz [3] used the LTN in the reinnervation of the different parts of the BP in seven patients, with good recovery in only two of them. More recently, Haninec et al. [4] obtained a useful functional recovery in all three cases for the MCN.

20.2 Anatomy

- The MCN contains from 3,069 to 7,911 myelinated fibers [5]. The average number of fibers in motor branches is 1,840 for the biceps and 1,826 for the brachialis muscle [2, 6].
- The LTN arises from the ventral rami of the fifth, sixth, and seventh spinal nerves. The eighth cervical spinal nerve may contribute in 8% of cases. The mean surgically useable length is 22.0 cm with a range from 18.0 to 27.0 cm. The overall mean diameter of the nerve is 3.0 mm, with a range of 2.2–3.5 mm The number of motor fibers ranges from 1,600 to 1,800, but only half of them can be used in patients with upper brachial plexus palsy [7, 8].

The original version of the chapter has been revised. A correction to this chapter can be found at https://doi.org/10.1007/978-3-031-92445-3_31

L. Rasulic (✉) · M. Samardžić
Faculty of Medicine, University of Belgrade, Belgrade, Serbia

Department of Peripheral Nerve Surgery, Functional Neurosurgery and Pain Management Surgery, Clinic for Neurosurgery, University Clinical Centre of Serbia, Belgrade, Serbia

F. Guedes et al. (eds.), *Nerve Transfers for Brachial Plexus Reconstruction after Trauma*, https://doi.org/10.1007/978-3-031-92445-3_20

20.3 Surgical Procedure

- There are three main approaches to the LTN: the distal axillary/thoracic approach, the proximal or supraclavicular approach, and the two-level proximal and distal approach. The distal approach has been more commonly described in the literature [9] and may be performed together with the standard infraclavicular approach to the BP and MCN (Fig. 20.1). The epineurial suture is used to secure the transfer (Fig. 20.2). Sural nerve grafts may be used in cases of insufficient LTN length, such as in cases of using the proximal approach.

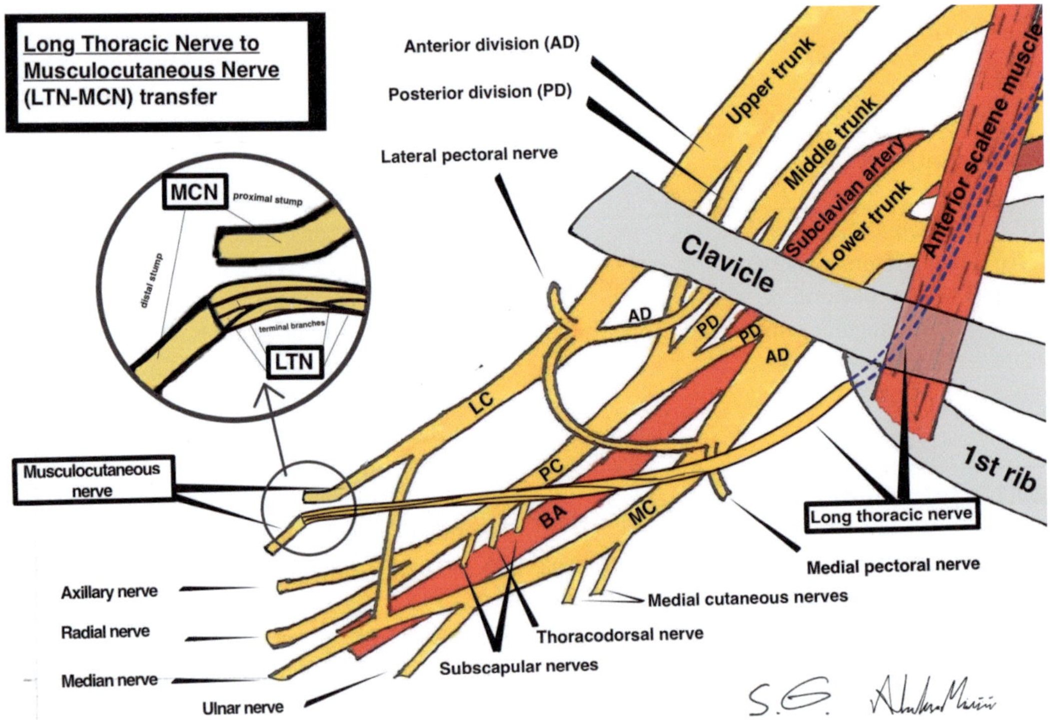

Fig. 20.1 Long thoracicc nerve (LTN) to musculocutaneous nerve (MCN) transfer. *LC* lateral cord, *PC* posterior cord, *MC* medial cord, *BA* brachial artery, *AD* anterior division, *PD* posterior division. Courtesy of Aleksa Mićić MD (University of Belgrade, Faculty of Medicine) and Strahinja Gligorijević BA (University of Belgrade, Faculty of Biology)

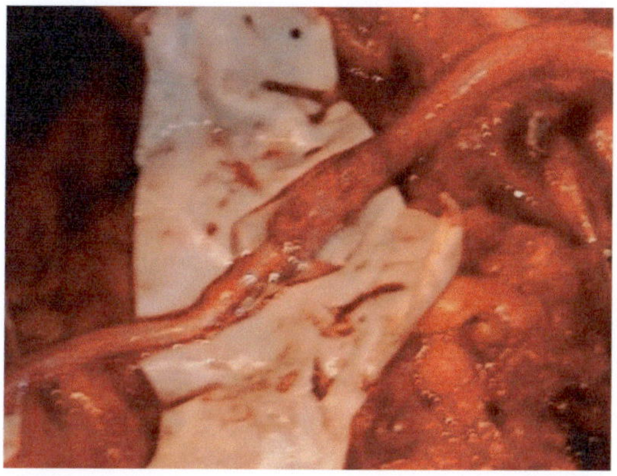

Fig. 20.2 A direct end-to-end coaptation of long thoracic nerve (LTN) and musculocutaneous nerve (MCN), without tension over the suture line

20.4 Problems and Solutions

- The sacrifice of LTN function leads to serratus anterior muscle weakness and consequential deficit called the "winged scapula".
- The LTN may be divided into multiple terminal branches innervating the serratus muscle, which presents a greater surgical challenge. More time is needed to explore every one of the LTN terminal branches and merge them into the solitary donor stump. This could be prevented by transecting the LTN more proximally before the branching and using the longer sural nerve grafts.
- The diameter of the LTN is insufficient for total neurotization of the MCN, and combined transfers may be used to overreach this problem.

20.5 Outcomes

The literature is scarce on the outcomes of LTN to MCN transfer. Haninec et al. [4] obtained a useful functional recovery in all three cases. Klumper et al. [10] revealed satisfying results in the treatment of children with brachial plexus injury while emphasizing that the best use of the LTN may be for delayed neurotization of a free functioning muscle transfer after failure of the initial plexus reconstruction and there are no other donors are available.

20.6 Conclusion

The LTN to MCN nerve transfer remains controversial. It may be used in cases where there are no other possible donors and when the consequential motor deficit due to LTN sacrifice is acceptable.

Acknowledgments The first author would like to express his gratitude to his Ph.D. student, Aleksa Mićić, for his contribution to the preparation of this chapter.

References

1. Lurje A. Concerning surgical treatment of traumatic injury to the upper division of the Brachial Plexus (Erb's Type). Ann Surg. 1948;127(2):317–26.
2. Narakas A. Neurotization in the treatment of brachial plexus injuries. In: Gelberman RH, editor. Operative nerve repair and reconstruction. Philadelphia: Lippincott Williams & Wilkins; 1991. p. 1258–329.
3. Narakas AO, Hentz VR. Neurotization in brachial plexus injuries. Indication and results. Clin Orthop Relat Res. 1988;237:43–56.
4. Haninec P, Sámal F, Tomás R, Houstava L, Dubovwý P. Direct repair (nerve grafting), neurotization, and end-to-side neurorrhaphy in the treatment of brachial plexus injury. J Neurosurg. 2007;106(3):391–9.
5. Weber RV, MacKinnon SE. Nerve transfers in the upper extremity. J Am Soc Surg Hand. 2004;4(3):200–13.
6. Schreiber JJ, Byun DJ, Khair MM, Rosenblatt L, Lee SK, Wolfe SW. Optimal axon counts for brachial plexus nerve transfers to restore elbow flexion. Plast Reconstr Surg. 2015;135(1):135e–41e.
7. Tubbs RS, Loukas M, Shoja MM, Shokouhi G, Wellons JC, Oakes WJ, et al. The contralateral long thoracic nerve as a donor for upper brachial plexus neurotization procedures: cadaveric feasibility study. J Neurosurg. 2009;110(4):749–53.
8. Brandt KE, Mackinnon SE. A technique for maximizing biceps recovery in brachial plexus reconstruction. J Hand Surg Am. 1993;18(4):726–33.
9. Noland SS, Krauss EM, Felder JM, Mackinnon SE. Surgical and clinical decision making in isolated long thoracic nerve palsy. Hand (N Y). 2018;13(6):689–94.
10. Kluemper C, Aversano M, Kozin S, Zlotolow DA. Long thoracic nerve transfer for children with brachial plexus injuries. J Pediatr Orthop. 2021;41(6):374–8.

21 Thoracodorsal Nerve to Musculocutaneous Nerve

Lukas Rasulic and Miroslav Samardžić

Abbreviations

BP	Brachial plexus
MPN	Medial pectoral nerve
MCN	Musculocutaneous nerve
TDN	Thoracodorsal nerve

21.1 Introduction

The thoracodorsal nerve (TDN) is one of the collateral brachial plexus (BP) branches that may be used as an infraclavicular intraplexal nerve donor to restore elbow function in patients with partial BP lesions. The restoration of elbow function is one of the first priorities in the treatment of these patients and may be achieved by reinnervation of the musculocutaneous nerve (MCN). In this chapter, we analyze the characteristics of TDN to MCN transfer and discuss some controversies, problems, and possible solutions based on personal experiences and published research.

The original version of the chapter has been revised. A correction to this chapter can be found at https://doi.org/10.1007/978-3-031-92445-3_31

L. Rasulic (✉) · M. Samardžić
Faculty of Medicine, University of Belgrade, Belgrade, Serbia

Department of Peripheral Nerve Surgery, Functional Neurosurgery and Pain Management Surgery, Clinic for Neurosurgery, University Clinical Centre of Serbia, Belgrade, Serbia

21.2 Anatomy

- The MCN contains from 3,069 to 7,911 myelinated fibers. The average number of fibers in motor branches is 1,840 for the biceps and 1,826 for the brachialis muscle [1].
- The TDN is a motor nerve that originates from the posterior cord of the BP and receives nerve fibers from the seventh, eighth, and sometimes sixth cervical spinal nerves. More than 52% of motor fibers originate from the C7 nerve. This nerve also has cerebral centers integrated into the function of the upper extremity and innervates the latissimus dorsi muscle. The mean surgically useable length of the nerve is 12.3 cm with a range between 8.9 and 19.0 cm [2, 3].
- The number of motor axons in the TDN is sufficient for reinnervation of the biceps and brachialis muscles without a need for neurolysis and exclusion or redirection of the lateral antebrachial cutaneous nerve. Similarly, there is no need for augmentation by additional transfer to the brachialis muscle as proposed by Tung et al. [4]. The diameter of the nerve ranges from 2.1 to 3.0 mm. The number of myelinated fibers ranges from 1,530 to 2,479 or up to 3,496. The mean length of its lateral branch up to its first intramuscular branch is

F. Guedes et al. (eds.), *Nerve Transfers for Brachial Plexus Reconstruction after Trauma*,
https://doi.org/10.1007/978-3-031-92445-3_21

8.14 cm with a range between 5.99 and 12.29 cm. The mean number of motor fibers in this branch is 1,453 and ranges between 1,016 and 2,414 which presents a donor-recipient biceps nerve branch axon count ratio 0.85:1. According to these characteristics, the TDN may be considered as an excellent donor for the MCN reinnervation [5–7].

21.3 General Principles

- Similar to the MPN, the TDN does not fulfill a few criteria for choosing the donor nerve [2]. However, it is of lesser importance when compared to the MPN.
- The fact that there is no ideal time for performing the nerve transfer applies to the usage of TDN. As well as the MPN, the TDN is exempted from the recommendations of some authors not to carry out transfers after a postinjury period of 9 months [6, 8].

21.4 Surgical Procedure

The surgical strategy and principles of the TDN exploration are the same as in the case of the MPN. The BP is explored only infraclavicular, except in the diagnostically unclear cases (Fig. 21.1). Choosing the TDN as a donor should be based on the possibility of direct nerve anastomosis, while its identification and integrity confirmation can be performed using direct nerve stimulation or muscular action potential recording. In cases when the MCN diameter is significantly larger compared to the TDN, it can be used in combination with the subscapular, long tho-

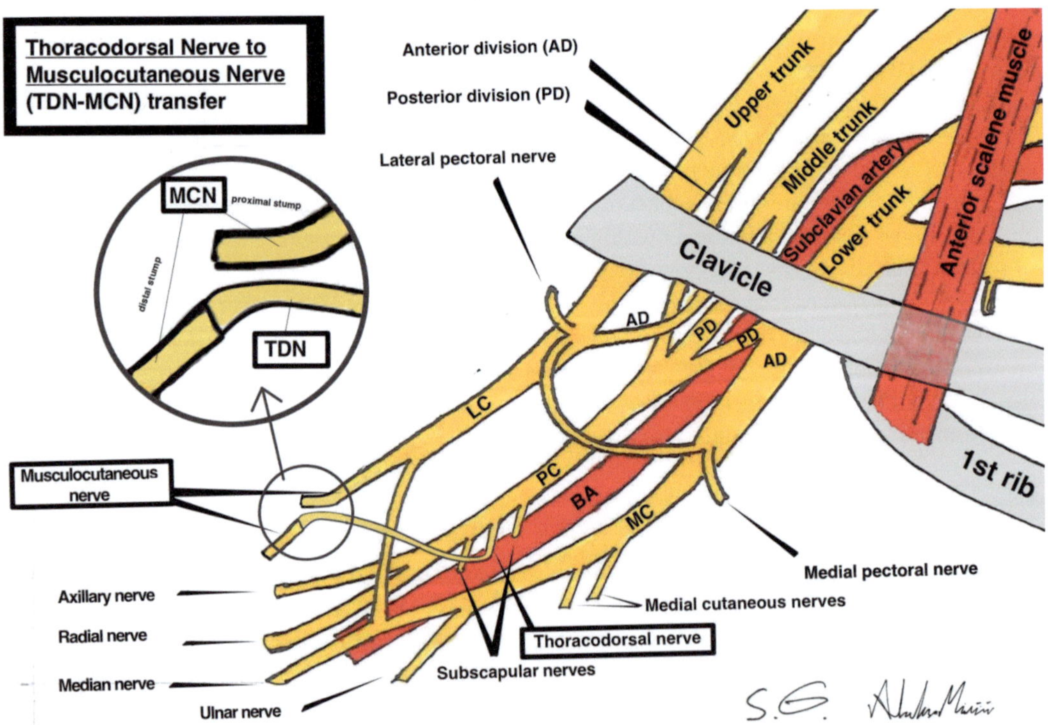

Fig. 21.1 Thoracodorsal nerve (TDN) to musculocutaneous nerve (MCN) transfer. *LC* lateral cord, *PC* posterior cord, *MC* medial cord, *BA* brachial artery, *AD* anterior division, *PD* posterior division. Courtesy of Aleksa Mićić MD (University of Belgrade, Faculty of Medicine) and Strahinja Gligorijević BA (University of Belgrade, Faculty of Biology)

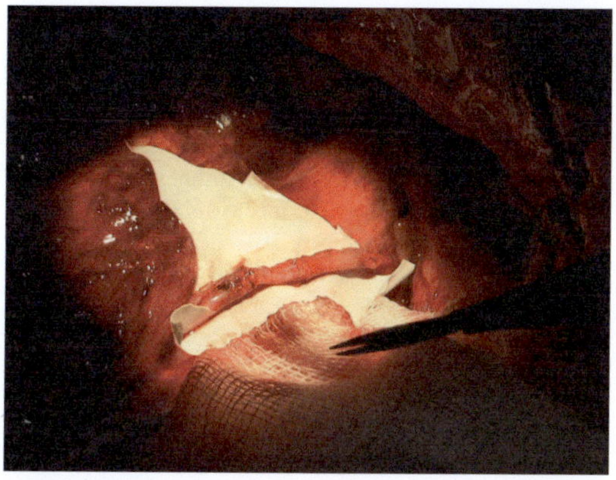

Fig. 21.2 An indirect coaptation of thoracodorsal nerve (TDN) and musculocutaneous nerve (MCN) nerve, using cutaneous nerve graft, without tension over the suture line

racic, or intercostal nerves. Contrary to the MPN, the direct anastomosis of TDN with the MCN is usually feasible. However, the cases of extensive MCN lesions may require longer nerve grafts (Fig. 21.2).

21.5 Problems and Solutions

- The general problems of using infraclavicular intraplexal nerve transfer to restore the upper arm function may be applied to the TDN.
- Regarding the TDN transfer, several authors did not register ill effects from the denervation of the latissimus dorsi muscle. Similarly to the MPN transfer, the partially preserved function of the teres major muscle may be a contributing factor to arm adduction. Finally, some functions could be retained using one of two TDN branches to the latissimus dorsi muscle owing to a large number of motor fibers.
- The loosing of the muscle from the donor innervation zone for musculotendinous transfer is especially important for the latissimus dorsi muscle transfer. Therefore, a balance of potential risks and benefits should be carefully estimated in individual cases.
- The main disadvantage of TDN usage in MCN reinnervation is that in most cases with extended upper brachial plexus injury (involving the C7 spinal nerve), the TDN is not functional [4, 9–12].

21.6 Conclusion

The TDN to MCN transfer is a valuable method for the restoration of elbow flexion in the treatment of patients with partial BP lesions. The main advantage of using the TDN as a donor compared to the MPN is the fact that its length and number of motor axons are sufficient for the MCN reinnervation, without a need for neurolysis and exclusion or redirection of the lateral antebrachial cutaneous nerve, or for augmentation by additional transfer to the brachialis muscle. The main disadvantage of TDN use compared to MPN is that the TDN is not viable in most patients with upper BP injury, more precisely the extended ones, that involve the root C7.

Acknowledgments The first author would like to express his gratitude to his Ph.D. student, Aleksa Mićić, for his contribution to the preparation of this chapter.

References

1. Schreiber JJ, Byun DJ, Khair MM, Rosenblatt L, Lee SK, Wolfe SW. Optimal axon counts for brachial plexus nerve transfers to restore elbow flexion. Plast Reconstr Surg. 2015;135(1):135e–41e.
2. Samardzić M, Rasulić L, Lakićević N, Bascarević V, Cvrkota I, Mićović M, et al. Collateral branches of the brachial plexus as donors in nerve transfers. Vojnosanit Pregl. 2012;69(7):594–603.
3. Lee KS. Variation of the spinal nerve compositions of thoracodorsal nerve. Clin Anat. 2007;20(6):660–2.
4. Tung TH, Novak CB, Mackinnon SE. Nerve transfers to the biceps and brachialis branches to improve

elbow flexion strength after brachial plexus injuries. J Neurosurg. 2003;98(2):313–8.
5. Chu B, Bordoni B. Anatomy, Thorax, Thoracodorsal Nerves. StatPearls. Treasure Island (FL) ineligible companies. Disclosure: Bruno Bordoni declares no relevant financial relationships with ineligible companies.: StatPearls Publishing. Copyright © 2023, StatPearls Publishing LLC.; 2023.
6. Samardzic MM, Grujicic DM, Rasulic LG, Milicic BR. The use of thoracodorsal nerve transfer in restoration of irreparable C5 and C6 spinal nerve lesions. Br J Plast Surg. 2005;58(4):541–6.
7. Theeuwes HP, Gosselink MP, Bruynzeel H, Kleinrensink G-J, Walbeehm ET. An anatomical study of the length of the neural pedicle after the bifurcation of the thoracodorsal nerve: implications for innervated free partial latissimus Dorsi flaps. Plast Reconstr Surg. 2011;127(1):210–4.
8. Narakas AO. Thoughts on neurotization or nerve transfers in irreparable nerve lesions. Clin Plast Surg. 1984;11(1):153–9.
9. Lu W, Xu JG, Wang DP, Gu YD. Microanatomical study on the functional origin and direction of the thoracodorsal nerve from the trunks of brachial plexus. Clin Anat. 2008;21(6):509–13.
10. Schusterman MA 2nd, Jindal R, Unadkat JV, Spiess AM. Lateral branch of the thoracodorsal nerve (LaT branch) transfer for biceps reinnervation. Plast Reconstr Surg Glob Open. 2018;6(3):e1698.
11. Wellons JC, Tubbs RS, Pugh JA, Bradley NJ, Law CR, Grabb PA. Medial pectoral nerve to musculocutaneous nerve neurotization for the treatment of persistent birth-related brachial plexus palsy: an 11-year institutional experience. J Neurosurg Pediatr. 2009;3(5):348–53.
12. Janes LE, Crowe C, Shah N, Sasson D, Ko JH. Alternative nerve transfer for shoulder function: thoracodorsal and medial triceps to anterior axillary nerve. Plast Reconstr Surg Glob Open. 2022;10(10):e4614.

22 Intercostal Nerve to Musculocutaneous Nerve Transfer

Willem Pondaag, Justus L. Groen, and Martijn J. A. Malessy

22.1 Introduction

The first ICN-MCN nerve transfer, performed in 1961, is attributed to Seddon and Yeoman [1]. The third and fourth intercostal nerves were connected to the musculocutaneous nerve using the ulnar nerve as an interposed graft. Tsuyama and Nagano, in 1965, improved the surgical technique by direct coaptation of the ICNs to the MCN using a fish-mouth technique. The technique was labeled "nerve crossing" (instead of the current "nerve transfer") and resulted in 70% of their patients regaining voluntary elbow flexion [2]. For several decades the ICNs were the prime source of axons for extraplexal to intraplexal nerve transfer, together with the spinal accessory nerve. The use of ICN-MCN transfer decreased after intraplexal nerve transfers had shown more favorable results. One favored alternative was the medial pectoral nerve transfer, but especially the ulnar fascicle to biceps branch of the MCN described by Oberlin in 1994 proved very successful [3]. In patients without the possibility for nerve grafting or intraplexal nerve transfer, ICN-MCN remains a useful option in the toolbox of the nerve surgeon. Alternative extraplexal sources for axons are the spinal accessory nerve, phrenic nerve, and the contralateral C7. To restore elbow flexion for patients with a total avulsion injury who are referred late, another option is a free functioning gracilis muscle transfer innervated either by intercostal nerves or by the spinal accessory nerve; this treatment options is the first choice in some centers [4].

W. Pondaag (✉) · J. L. Groen · M. J. A. Malessy
Department of Neurosurgery | Leiden Nerve Center, Leiden University Medical Center, Leiden, The Netherlands
e-mail: W.Pondaag@lumc.nl; J.L.Groen@lumc.nl; Malessy@lumc.nl

22.2 Surgical Anatomy and Histology

22.2.1 Anatomy of the Intercostal Nerves

Intercostal nerves (ICNs) are the anterior rami of the thoracic spinal nerves. Each ICN enters the corresponding intercostal space between the posterior intercostal membrane and the parietal pleura. The nerve then travels forward with the intercostal vessels in or below the costal groove of the corresponding rib, between the internal and innermost intercostal muscles. The lateral cutaneous branch generally branches from the main nerve mid-rib between the vertebrae and the sternum, usually at the midaxillary line. This lateral cutaneous nerve further divides into anterior and posterior branches. The lateral cutaneous branch of the second intercostal nerve does not branch; it is known as the intercostobrachial nerve. This nerve joins the medial brachial

F. Guedes et al. (eds.), *Nerve Transfers for Brachial Plexus Reconstruction after Trauma*,
https://doi.org/10.1007/978-3-031-92445-3_22

cutaneous nerve to supply the skin of the upper half of the medial and posterior arm.

The first six intercostal nerves innervate nearby intercostal muscles, the cutaneous territory on the side of the thoracic wall, the thoracic pleura, and end as terminal branches (anterior cutaneous branch) to innervate the skin near the midline of the chest [5]. The anterior cutaneous branch and lateral cutaneous branch of the fourth ICN supply the largest area of the breast skin and nipple/nipple-areola complex [6].

22.2.2 Surgical Anatomy of the Musculocutaneous Nerve

According to "classic anatomy," the lateral cord divides at the level of the axilla into the musculocutaneous nerve and the lateral contribution to the median nerve. The MCN usually pierces the coracobrachialis muscle, then provides one or two branches to the biceps muscle, and finally divides in the brachialis muscle branch and the lateral cutaneous nerve of the forearm. This textbook anatomy was encountered in approximately 90% of patients that underwent nerve transfers to the MCN [7]. Nerve surgeons must be aware that anatomical variants have been described where different types of connections exist between median nerve and MCN; in some case the nerves to the biceps and brachialis directly branch from the median nerve. To be able to perform a direct coaptation with the ICNs, extra length of the MCN has to be obtained. This can be done by dissecting intraneural MCN fascicles out of the lateral cord in a proximal direction. In cadaver dissection studies, it appeared even possible to dissect the specific muscular branches proximally up to this level [8].

22.2.3 Axonal Counts in ICN and MCN

A consistent account of the axonal content of the ICN is difficult to obtain from the literature, as the number of axons differs among various publications, probably due to methodological differences. To our knowledge, there is not one paper that examined axonal content of both ICN and MCN with the same methodology. In a study on ICN to axillary transfer, the average number of myelinated nerve fibers of the third, fourth, and fifth intercostal nerves were 742, 830, and 1353, respectively [9]. Others quoted that each ICN contains 520–720 axons, which would result in 1500–2000 motor axons available when transferring three ICNs [10]. The number of motor axons decreases gradually along the course of the ICN, as it gives off branches to the intercostal muscles along its way. Distal to the cutaneous branch, the ICN was shown to contain 30–40% motor axons [11].

The MCN contains around 7000 motor axons, and distal to the coracobrachialis muscle 5000 [12]. The terminal branches of the MCN were found to contain a mean of 1826 axons for the musculocutaneous biceps branch and 1840 for the brachialis branch [13]. Others reported that the biceps branch contains 882 motor axons and the brachialis branch 1072 [14]. Most recently, the number of efferent axons in the MCN was determined as only 1600 ± 160; the majority of fibers in the MCN (24,300 ± 5870) were categorized as afferent axons [15].

Combining axon counts for donor and recipient in nerve transfer options has thus resulted in an unfavorable donor-recipient ratio of the ICNs as compared to the ulnar or median fascicle transfer [13]. Additionally, in a morphometric study of the upper intercostal nerves, the mean surface area of the ICNs at the parasternal level was measured as 0.23 mm^2, while that at the axillary level was 0.34 mm^2. When three ICNs are attached to the MCN (mean surface area of 2.64 mm^2), only 26% of the MCN was covered [16]. The imbalance in axonal count and size may be one factor in the diminished motor recovery after ICN-MCN transfer compared to other transfers for biceps function.

22.3 Indication for Intercostal to Musculocutaneous Nerve Transfer

The main indication for ICN-MCN transfer in adult patients is a brachial plexus injury comprising multiple root avulsions, when both a proximal stump is unavailable for grafting and intraplexal nerve transfer is not a valid option. Given the superior results of intraplexal nerve transfers in upper lesions, these intraplexal transfers (specifically of ulnar and/or median nerve fascicle) have become the first choice to reanimate elbow flexion in most patients. Obviously, intraplexal nerve transfers can only be applied if the function of at least C8 and T1 is maintained. In traumatic brachial lesions in adults with five avulsions, or with incomplete function of ulnar and/or median nerves, the intercostal nerves have remained the appropriate donor for restoration of elbow flexion, as alternative reconstruction options are limited.

One alternative extraplexal source of axons is the contralateral C7. Cerebral plastic adaptation, a requirement for independent control of the reinnervated muscle, is inadequate following this transfer. Therefore, we would not apply this technique in adults [17]. Inadequate plastic adaptation was also for the hypoglossal nerve transfer—the reason we have abandoned this technique [18]. The phrenic nerve has proven to be a reliable source of donor axons, but little is known about long-term (20 years or more) limitations of pulmonary function. The spinal accessory nerve has proven a poor donor to reanimate the biceps brachialis muscle. This may be caused by the need to use a nerve graft because direct coaptation to the MCN is not possible. The final alternative to restore elbow flexion is a free functioning gracilis muscle transfer innervated either by intercostal nerves or by the spinal accessory nerve. The benefit of this technique is that there is a direct coaptation possible from SAN to recipient nerve [4].

In children with a C5-T1 brachial plexus birth injury, ICN-MCN transfer is an option to restore elbow flexion. The ICN-MCN transfer may even be used even in the presence of a viable proximal root. In these cases, the C5 spinal nerve is entirely used as lead-out for grafts reanimate hand function, while nerve transfers (ICN-MCN and spinal accessory-suprascapular) are employed for shoulder and elbow flexion [19]. Another indication for ICN-MCN nerve transfers in children is incomplete recovery after acute flaccid myelitis. In these children, due to their patchy neurological deficit, intraplexal nerve transfers may not be reliable.

22.4 Surgical Technique

We have described our surgical technique previously [20]. In all cases we expose the entire trajectory of the brachial plexus, and root avulsions are confirmed by empty intervertebral foramen in addition to imaging. The MCN is identified and followed as proximally as possible by interfascicular dissection in the lateral cord until fascicular intermingling is encountered.

The third through the fifth ICNs are dissected free by means of an undulating skin incision, starting at the inferior border of the major pectoral muscle, continuing beneath the nipple (or breast in women), and extending medially up to the costosternal junction (Fig. 22.1a). The inferior part of the major pectoral muscle is shifted upward, sometimes necessitating partial cutting of its costal and sternal insertion. The main branch of the ICN is identified in the anterior axillary line at the bone groove of the lower costal border and dissected free over its anterior course (Fig. 22.1b). The ICNs can be most easily identified by dissecting the intercostal muscles in their fiber direction. The external and internal intercostal muscles are cut stepwise over a length of about 2 cm. The different layers of intercostal muscles cannot always be clearly identified by their fiber direction. The nerve stimulator is used to identify the course of the ICN. Care must be taken to ensure that contractions that are observed are actually due to ICN stimulation, and not due to direct muscle stimulation. The ICN is usually located several millimeters below the rib on the parietal pleura or a very thin layer of innermost intercostal muscles. Care has to be taken not to damage the parietal pleura. The use of a little nerve hook to lift the nerve form the parietal pleura has proven very helpful. Subsequently, the entire course of the ICN is dissected free by cutting the intercostal muscles. Care has to be taken not to divide the ICN before the needed length is dissected free. A little tension on the nerve facili-

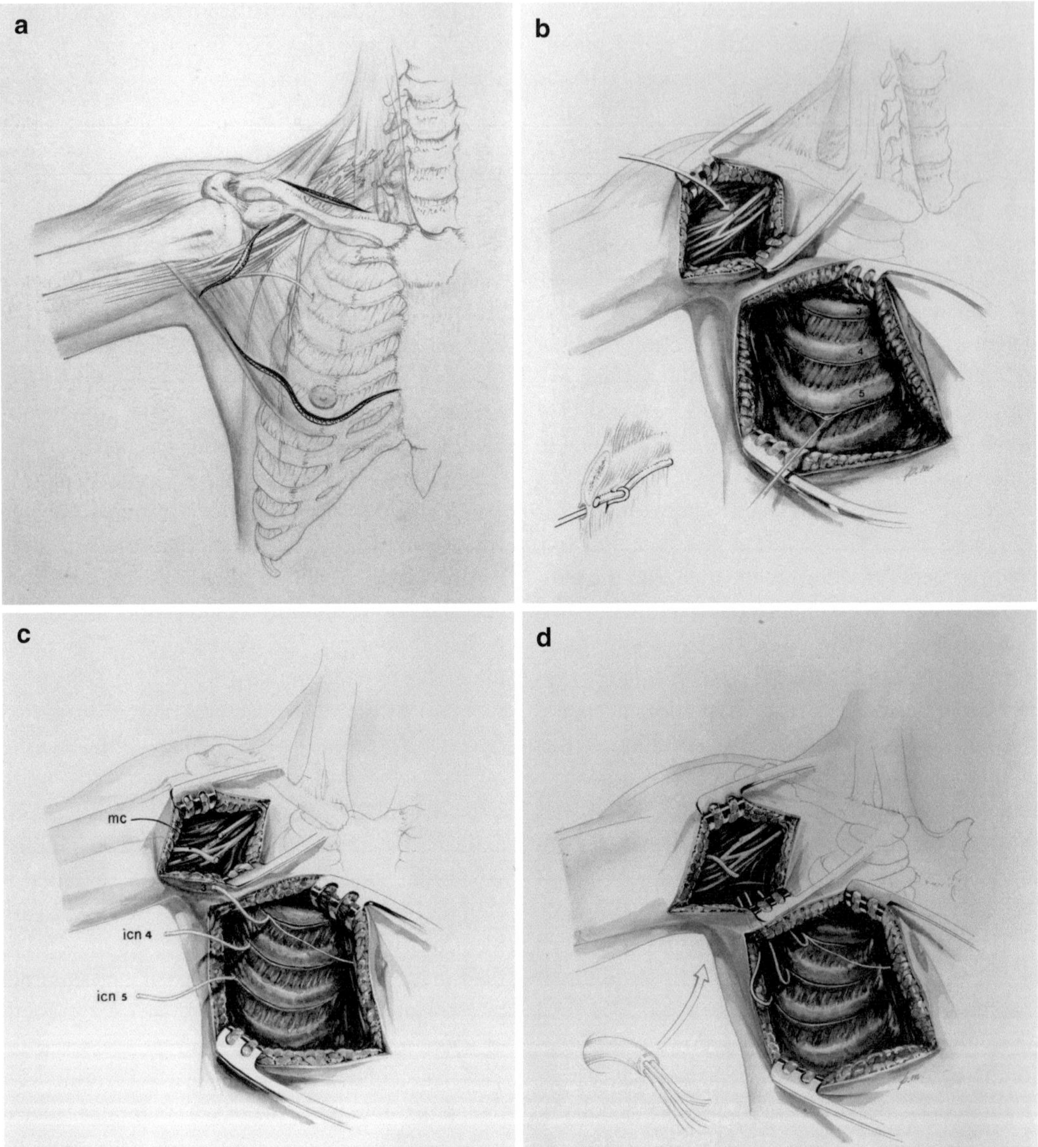

Fig. 22.1 Drawings depicting the operative technique of direct coaptation of ICNs to the MC nerve. (**a**) Skin incisions. (**b**) Identification of the main branch of the ICN in its course at the lower costal border. (**c**) The ICNs were transected as close as possible to the sternum. The MCN is cut as proximally as possible after freeing it from the lateral cord until fascicular intermingling is encountered. (**d**) The ICNs are tunneled underneath an intact skin area between the infraclavicular and intercostal wounds, and direct ICN-MC nerve coaptation is performed with the patient's arm abducted 90°. (Figures from [20], reproduced by permission)

tates the dissection. Some authors advocate opening and detaching the periosteum from the rib to identify the nerve, but this is not the optimal way to identify the nerve.

Motor responses are assessed by using electrical nerve stimulation. If feasible, sensory branches are identified by their course toward the skin and are kept intact after they had been dissected interfascicularly from the main ICN in proximal direction. Special care is taken to spare these sensory branches in order to preserve sensory innervation to the nipple (specifically ICN4). To assess the required length of the ICN, a vessel loop or suture can be hinged around the proximal pivot point to check if the MCN can be reached for direct coaptation. The ICNs are then transected at the required length or as close as possible to the sternum and are tunneled to the axilla (Fig. 22.1c). The infraclavicular and intercostal wounds remain separated from each other by an area of intact skin at the anterior axilla, facilitating later wound closure. The MCN is cut as proximally as possible after freeing it from the lateral cord (Fig. 22.1b). No attempt is made to identify the motor branches within the MC nerve. Before coaptation, the patient's arm is abducted 90°, and proximal and distal stump fascicles were carefully trimmed. The ICNs are coapted centrally to the MCN fascicles by means of 10-0 sutures and/or fibrin glue (Fig. 22.1d).

In children we employ the same surgical technique, but special care is taken to keep the periosteum of the ribs intact. Since they are not yet full grown, damage may cause rib cage deformity.

22.5 Results of ICN-MCN Nerve Transfers

22.5.1 Adults

The results regarding ICN-MCN transfer that have been published so far from different centers are difficult to compare. The number of patients in each study is relatively small, and differences exist in several factors known to affect outcome, such as age, body mass index, patient selection, interval between trauma and nerve reconstruction, and divergences in technique. The largest series from Nagano et al. was published in 1989. They described their results of 156 cases: 10 children and 146 adults. In 146 patients (over 16 years of age), MRC4 or better was obtained in 38 patients (26.0%), MRC 3 in 64 (43.8%), MRC 1 or 2 in 37 (25.3%), and MRC 0 in 7 (4.8%) [2]. The authors found that younger age (younger than 30 years) and shorter delay after trauma (less than 6 months) were determining factors for success.

In a publication from 1998, we reported our experience in 25 patients. From these, 14 patients (56%) achieved MRC Grade 4, 2 (8%) gained MRC Grade 3, and 9 (36%) had MRC Grade 2 or lower [20]. When we analyzed the results of the past 10 years (2009–2019, data not published, Table 22.1), we employed the ICN-MCN transfer in 22 patients. In our treatment algorithm, we strive to operate as early as possible. We analyzed the effect of timing of surgery on outcome. Both patients that we operated within 14 days after trauma recovered to MRC3 or MRC4 of elbow flexion. Nine of 12 patients (75%) who were operated after 2 weeks, but within 3 months, recovered MRC 3 ($n = 4$) or MRC 4 ($n = 5$). After a 3-month delay, only 2/8 patients recovered MRC 3. In this contemporary series, surgical delay proved a strong predictor of outcome, with interval longer than 3 months likely leading to failure of the procedure.

Two recent papers pooled results from literature. The first paper defined successful outcome

Table 22.1 LUMC contemporary series (2009–2019) of results In MRC grading after ICN-MCN transfer in adult traumatic brachial plexus injury

	Interval between lesion and surgery				
		<2 w	2 w–3 m	3 m–6 m	>6 m
		($n = 2$)	($n = 12$)	($n = 5$)	($n = 3$)
MRC	0–1	0	1	2	0
	2	0	2	2	2
	3	1	4	1	1
	4+	1	5	0	0
	Total > 3	100%	75%	20%	33%
Timing (dichotomized)		<3 m		>3 m	
% >3		79%		25%	

as MRC4 or better. This was obtained in 134/372 patients (36%) for transfer of 2 ICNs and in 93/213 patients (44%) for 3 ICNs [13]. The second review included 12 studies for a total of 196 patients. Either 2 (n = 113), 3 (n = 69), or 4 (n = 11) ICNs were transferred to the MCN. In this pooled analysis, elbow flexion ≥MRC3 was achieved in 71.3% of patients with two ICNs, 67.7% of patients with three ICNs, and 77.0% of patients with four ICNs. Elbow flexion ≥M4 was achieved in 51.1% of patients with two ICNs, 42.1% of patients with three ICNs, and 48.4% of patients with four ICNs. As the groups did not statistically differ, the optimal number of intercostal nerves was considered to be two ICNs [21]. In our own practice, we routinely use three ICNs for transfer. All in all, these analyses show that a good biceps recovery can be obtained in part of the patients with total or subtotal brachial plexus traction injuries in adults.

There is a paucity of literature describing sensory outcomes. Anecdotally an unpleasant "phantom sensation" on the chest was reported when the patient was touched on the lateral forearm in the distribution of the lateral antebrachial cutaneous nerve [22]. We have asked patients where they locate touch if stroked over the area of the lateral antebrachial cutaneous nerve. Patients locate touch in this area over the thoracic wall. None of our patients reported this as problematic. Other authors have reported successful late intercostal nerve transfer for pain relief from preganglionic injury, targeting the lateral or median cord [23]. It is unknown in this context whether successful ICN-MCN nerve transfer results in useful sensation or pain reduction.

22.5.2 Children

We have published our own results (from 1995 to 2008) of nerve transfers for elbow flexion in children with brachial plexus birth injury [24]. In the first part of the study period (1995–2000), we only used the ICN-MCN transfer, which was at that time the preferred technique in the treatment of traumatic brachial plexus lesion in adult patients. We routinely used three ICNs. After 2001 our preference shifted toward intraplexal nerve transfers, if possible. From 2001 onward the medial pectoral nerve-MCN transfer was the preferred procedure in C5-C6 or C5-C6-C7 lesions. In the ICN-MCN transfer group (n = 17), successful elbow flexion against gravity was obtained in 14 patients (82%). Three failures occurred; one failure could potentially be explained by the need to interpose a nerve graft. Another ICN-MCN patient had a chromosome abnormality with developmental cognitive problems, which might be associated with impaired central control.

Other authors have reported similar results with the ICN-MCN transfer in brachial plexus birth injury. In Kawabata's series of 31 transfers, 94% reached MRC Grade ≥ 3 [25]. Two ICNs were used in 26 cases and 3 ICNs in 5 cases. The strength of the biceps muscle was rated Grade M4 in 26 (84%) patients. In the 12 patients who underwent surgery when they were younger than 5 months of age, all exhibited a grade of M4 (100%) in their biceps muscle power.

Luo et al. described 24 children, in whom 2, 3, or 4 ICNs were transferred [26]. Of 14 transfers with 4 intercostals, biceps gained M4 strength in 8, M3 in 4, and M2 in 2. Of nine transfers with three intercostals, biceps obtained M4 strength in eight and M3 in one. One transfer with two intercostals got M4 strength of biceps. Twelve patients whose intercostals were transferred to MCN, gained M4 strength of biceps in 11 and M3 in 1, whereas the other 12 patients with intercostals transferred to anterior division of the upper trunk, obtained M4 strength of biceps in 6, M3 in 4, and M2 in 2. The rate of M3 strength or more was 92% and that of M4 was 71%. These 24 children were followed up for 24 to 79 months, with an average of 53 months. No complications were found in the respiratory system.

El-Gammal et al. employed the Active Movement Score as outcome measure for ICN-MCN transfer after brachial plexus birth injury. He reported a 94% success rate in 31 patients (Active Movement Score of 6 or 7) [27]. A particular feature is that in their series, nine children had preoperative and postoperative chest CT scans. All these nine children developed basal pulmonary atelectasis postoperatively, which was mostly ipsilateral, although this was not related to clinical respiratory problems.

We did not note any adverse effects in the ICN-MCN group, and in particular we did not see any rib cage deformity. Such deformities have been anecdotally mentioned, but we are not aware of any published reports. Kawabata et al. investigated all patients a with radiographs at final follow-up (after a mean of 5 years, range 3–12 years) and found mild growth retardation in ribs corresponding to the sites of donor ICNs in 7 of 31 patients, although no thoracic cage deformity could be detected clinically [25].

Apart from brachial plexus birth injuries, we employed the ICN-MCN nerve transfer in two children (age 6 and 7) after acute flaccid myelitis. Both regained elbow-flexion MRC4.

22.6 Cerebral Plasticity

The first signs of recovery after ICN-MCN transfer are characterized by involuntary contraction of the biceps that is linked to breathing. Subsequently, after several weeks, patients become aware that they can contract their biceps but only by sustained inspiration or expiration. In time, voluntary contraction of the biceps and brachialis ultimately becomes independent of respiration. Flexion can then be maintained while breathing normally. The control over elbow flexion is experienced as before the brachial plexus lesion. These changes from respiratory to volitional control require brain plasticity, which has been studied in different ways. Complete independence between the two functions, however, is never actually achieved [28].

A way to explore the mechanisms behind cerebral plastic changes is to study the facilitatory effects of respiration and voluntary contraction on cortical motor-evoked potentials of the biceps muscle. The time course of the facilitatory effect of respiration and voluntary contraction differed significantly. In the end stage of nerve regeneration, the facilitatory effect of voluntary contraction was significantly larger than that of respiration, indicating that the CNS control network over the muscle comes to resemble that of the recipient nerve (MCN) rather than that of the donor nerve (ICN) [29].

Elbow flexion is initially controlled by the sagittal region of the primary motor cortex. This area is related to the intercostal muscles active in respiration. After a few months, however, the original more laterally located area for voluntary biceps control becomes involved. This shift in cortical activity from medial to lateral is most likely based on the activation of a preexisting inter neuronal network with low-activity connections between the two involved cortical areas. Such connections seem logical as intercostal muscles contract simultaneously with the biceps when, for instance, a heavy object is lifted. This movement, after all, requires not only biceps contraction but also, although less obvious, stabilization of the thorax and torso posture. From plasticity studies it was concluded that to achieve successful voluntary control after nerve transfer, the donor and acceptor must have some central nervous system connection between the two motor areas (i.e., horizontal intrinsic connections) before transfer [17]. These central connections are present in the case of ICN-MCN transfer and become activated by the peripheral nerve transfers.

References

1. Seddon HJ. Nerve grafting. J Bone Joint Surg Br. 1963;45:447–61.
2. Nagano A, Tsuyama N, Ochiai N, Hara T, Takahashi M. Direct nerve crossing with the intercostal nerve to treat avulsion injuries of the brachial plexus. J Hand Surg Am. 1989;14(6):980–5.
3. Oberlin C, Beal D, Leechavengvongs S, Salon A, Dauge MC, Sarcy JJ. Nerve transfer to biceps muscle using a part of ulnar nerve for C5-C6 avulsion of the brachial plexus: anatomical study and report of four cases. J Hand Surg Am. 1994;19(2):232–7.
4. Maldonado AA, Kircher MF, Spinner RJ, Bishop AT, Shin AY. Free functioning gracilis muscle transfer versus intercostal nerve transfer to musculocutaneous nerve for restoration of elbow flexion after traumatic adult brachial pan-plexus injury. Plast Reconstr Surg. 2016;138(3):483e–8e.
5. Ostrowska M, Mamede de Carvalho M. Injuries of the nerves of the thorax. In: Tubbs RS, Rizk EB, Shoja M, Loukas M, Barbaro N, Spinner RJ, editors. Nerves

and nerve injuries: Vol 2: Pain, treatment, injury, disease and future directions. Academic Press; 2015.
6. Smeele HP, Bijkerk E, van Kuijk SMJ, Lataster A, van der Hulst R, Tuinder SMH. Innervation of the female breast and nipple: a systematic review and meta-analysis of anatomical dissection studies. Plast Reconstr Surg. 2022;150(2):243–55.
7. Bhardwaj P, Venkatramani H, Sivakumar B, Graham DJ, Vigneswaran V, Sabapathy SR. Anatomic variations of the musculocutaneous nerve and clinical implications for restoration of elbow flexion. J Hand Surg Am. 2022;47(10):970–8.
8. Fleury M, Lepage D, Pluvy I, Pauchot J. Nerve transfer between the intercostal nerves and the motor component of the musculocutaneous nerve. Anatomical study of feasibility. Ann Chir Plast Esthet. 2017;62(3):255–60.
9. Malungpaishrope K, Leechavengvongs S, Uerpairojkit C, Witoonchart K, Jitprapaikulsarn S, Chongthammakun S. Nerve transfer to deltoid muscle using the intercostal nerves through the posterior approach: an anatomic study and two case reports. J Hand Surg Am. 2007;32(2):218–24.
10. Samardzic M, Antunovic V, Joksimovic M, Bacetic D. Donor nerves in the reinnervation of brachial plexus. Neurol Res. 1986;8(2):117–22.
11. Freilinger G, Holle J, Sulzgruber SC. Distribution of motor and sensory fibers in the intercostal nerves. Significance in reconstructive surgery. Plast Reconstr Surg. 1978;62(2):240–4.
12. Aszmann OC, Rab M, Kamolz L, Frey M. The anatomy of the pectoral nerves and their significance in brachial plexus reconstruction. J Hand Surg Am. 2000;25(5):942–7.
13. Schreiber JJ, Byun DJ, Khair MM, Rosenblatt L, Lee SK, Wolfe SW. Optimal axon counts for brachial plexus nerve transfers to restore elbow flexion. Plast Reconstr Surg. 2015;135(1):135e–41e.
14. Cheah A, Lee EY, Lim AYT. Upper extremity axon counts and clinical implications for motor nerve transfer. Plast Reconstr Surg. 2019;144(6):1044e–50e.
15. Gesslbauer B, Hruby LA, Roche AD, Farina D, Blumer R, Aszmann OC. Axonal components of nerves innervating the human arm. Ann Neurol. 2017;82(3):396–408.
16. Asfazadourian H, Tramond B, Dauge MC, Oberlin C. Morphometric study of the upper intercostal nerves: practical application for neurotizations in traumatic brachial plexus palsies. Chir Main. 1999;18(4):243–53.
17. Socolovsky M, Malessy M. Brain changes after peripheral nerve repair: limitations of neuroplasticity. J Neurosurg Sci. 2021;65(4):421–30.
18. Malessy MJ, Hoffmann CF, Thomeer RT. Initial report on the limited value of hypoglossal nerve transfer to treat brachial plexus root avulsions. J Neurosurg. 1999;91(4):601–4.
19. Pondaag W, Malessy MJ. Recovery of hand function following nerve grafting and transfer in obstetric brachial plexus lesions. J Neurosurg. 2006;105(1 Suppl):33–40.
20. Malessy MJ, Thomeer RT. Evaluation of intercostal to musculocutaneous nerve transfer in reconstructive brachial plexus surgery. J Neurosurg. 1998;88(2):266–71.
21. Leland HA, Azadgoli B, Gould DJ, Seruya M. Investigation into the optimal number of intercostal nerve transfers for musculocutaneous nerve reinnervation: a systematic review. Hand (N Y). 2018;13(6):621–6.
22. Mlaver E, Keifer O Jr, Tora MS, Campbell M, Boulis NM. Phantom sensation-underreported sensory outcome following intercostal-to-musculocutaneous nerve transfer. World Neurosurg. 2019;122:303–7.
23. Berman J, Anand P, Chen L, Taggart M, Birch R. Pain relief from preganglionic injury to the brachial plexus by late intercostal nerve transfer. J Bone Joint Surg Br. 1996;78(5):759–60.
24. Pondaag W, Malessy MJ. Intercostal and pectoral nerve transfers to re-innervate the biceps muscle in obstetric brachial plexus lesions. J Hand Surg Eur. 2014;39(6):647–52.
25. Kawabata H, Shibata T, Matsui Y, Yasui N. Use of intercostal nerves for neurotization of the musculocutaneous nerve in infants with birth-related brachial plexus palsy. J Neurosurg. 2001;94(3):386–91.
26. Luo PB, Chen L, Zhou CH, Hu SN, Gu YD. Results of intercostal nerve transfer to the musculocutaneous nerve in brachial plexus birth palsy. J Pediatr Orthop 2011;31(8):884–8.
27. El-Gammal TA, Abdel-Latif MM, Kotb MM, El-Sayed A, Ragheb YF, Saleh WR, et al. Intercostal nerve transfer in infants with obstetric brachial plexus palsy. Microsurgery. 2008;28(7):499–504.
28. Malessy MJ, van Dijk JG, Thomeer RT. Respiration-related activity in the biceps brachii muscle after intercostal-musculocutaneous nerve transfer. Clin Neurol Neurosurg. 1993;95(Suppl):S95–102.
29. Malessy MJ, Thomeer RT, van Dijk JG. Changing central nervous system control following intercostal nerve transfer. J Neurosurg. 1998;89(4):568–74.

Part IV

Nerve Transfers for Elbow Extension

Nerve Transfers for Elbow Extension

23

Ellen Y. Lee and Alexander Y. Shin

23.1 Background

Active elbow extension by the triceps allows for overhead reach and stabilizes the hand in space, increasing the functional workspace of the hand. In a brachial plexus injury (BPI) patient, loss of elbow extension can be facilitated by gravity. Triceps function is imperative for overhead activity if patients have shoulder function with abduction and forward flexion greater than horizontal. Patients with C5–C7 or upper and middle trunk injuries may have triceps recovery by C8 reinnervation. Patients with complete pan plexus injuries are unlikely to have spontaneous triceps recovery. Elbow flexion and shoulder function are the primary goals in brachial plexus reconstruction. However, when reconstructing prehension for complete pan BPI patients with a gracilis free functioning muscle transfer (FFMT), it is important to restore active elbow extension so that the gracilis excursion will result in distal function, such as wrist extension or finger flexion, instead of just flexing the elbow [1].

E. Y. Lee (✉)
Department of Hand and Reconstructive Microsurgery, National University Health System, Singapore, Singapore

A. Y. Shin
Mayo Clinic Brachial Plexus Clinic, Departments of Orthopedics and Neurosurgery, Rochester, MN, USA
e-mail: shin.alexander@mayo.edu

Triceps neurotization options in these patients include nerve grafting from available ruptured roots or nerve transfers from intercostal nerves (ICN) or spinal accessory nerve, and less commonly from phrenic nerve, cervical plexus, or contralateral C7 [2–5]. In patients with C5–C7 injuries, nerve transfer to triceps was shown to improve active elbow extension when compared to a control group who did not undergo triceps neurotization [6]. Partial BPI patients have more donor nerve options that include medial pectoral nerve, fascicles/branches from ulnar or median nerves, extensor carpi radialis longus (ECRL) or extensor digitorum communis (EDC) branches of radial nerve, thoracodorsal nerve, levator scapulae motor branch, or posterior axillary nerve branch to deltoid [6–11].

23.2 Preoperative Assessment and Counseling

Triceps reinnervation is the third priority after elbow flexion and shoulder function reconstruction in a patient with a flail upper limb interested in regaining prehension. Careful cataloguing of available donors facilitates nerve economics in these situations where there are more desired functions to restore than available donor nerves. Patients will likely have a graftable C5 root if they have a supraclavicular Tinel sign, a functioning rhomboid muscle, symmetric diaphragm

F. Guedes et al. (eds.), *Nerve Transfers for Brachial Plexus Reconstruction after Trauma*,
https://doi.org/10.1007/978-3-031-92445-3_23

excursion, and no paraspinal fibrillations on electromyography (EMG). Spinal accessory nerve function is seen in the symmetry of trapezius muscle bulk on shoulder shrug and the ability to maintain shrug against resistance. The diaphragmatic function is evaluated by inspiratory and expiratory chest radiographs or a fluoroscopic sniff test. Symmetric diaphragm excursion indicates phrenic nerve availability. For surgeons who do not routinely use the phrenic nerve, it helps reassure patients about the low likelihood of respiratory complications after harvesting intercostal nerves (ICN). Chest radiographs will also show displaced rib fractures that may limit the use of ICN as donors. In cases of healed rib fractures, ICNs are tested with a handheld stimulator before harvest. Our current practice uses cervical root grafting for shoulder function, spinal accessory nerve to power the gracilis FFMT for elbow and finger flexion, and intercostal nerves for elbow extension. Patients are advised that if there is no available cervical root for grafting, shoulder reinnervation will be abandoned, and shoulder stability will later be achieved by glenohumeral fusion.

Some patients with complete pan plexus injury may spontaneously recover upper trunk function. This allows for the use of the posterior branch of the axillary nerve (PBAN) to restore elbow extension via a direct nerve transfer [8]. Strength of the posterior deltoid is tested by assessing shoulder extension in the swimmers position and has been also called the swallow tail test [12]. The PBAN is deemed fit for transfer if the patient's active range of shoulder extension is the same as the passive range and the shoulder can be extended against resistance (Medical Research Council or MRC grade 4 or 5). The PBAN can also serve as a donor for elbow extension in patients with C7-T1 injuries [9]. It is a synergistic donor that does not require interposition nerve grafting.

In C5–C7 injury patients, the clinical examination should evaluate the range of motion and strength of wrist flexors, ECRL, EDC, lower pectoral muscles, and latissimus dorsi. Donor nerve selection depends on muscle strength, planned incisions considering other procedures being performed, the patient's choice of acceptable donor morbidity, and the surgeon's experience. Direct end-to-end transfers are preferred over those requiring interposition nerve grafts. Electromyogram is used to confirm the absence of motor unit potentials in the triceps and status of motor unit recruitment in the donor nerve's muscle [13].

23.3 Surgical Techniques

23.3.1 Intercostal Nerves (ICN) to the Triceps Branch of the Radial Nerve

This transfer is performed as previously described [14] with some modifications from incorporating it into our pan brachial plexus reconstruction, including supraclavicular exploration, root grafting to shoulder targets, and FFMT innervated by spinal accessory nerve for elbow flexion and finger flexion. The patient is supine under general anesthesia without neuromuscular blockade so that intraoperative nerve stimulation can be performed. The deltopectoral incision used to identify the thoracoacromial trunk for FFMT is extended with a transverse incision across the anterior wall of the axilla, curving it distally on the lateral chest wall crossing toward the anterior midline distal to the nipple and then curving slightly proximally over the sternum and costal cartilage. The skin and pectoral muscles are elevated from the underlying ribs through this incision. The pectoralis major tendon insertion on the humerus is divided for further exposure. Ribs 3-6 are identified, and the ICNs at the mid-anterior line of the rib are harvested by carefully reflecting the periosteum from each rib and incising the deep surface of the periosteum along the under surface of the rib to expose the ICN. This is performed under 3.5-4x loupe magnification. Each motor ICN is then stimulated to confirm its identity and function. The stimulation must result in vigorous contraction of the intercostal muscles for the nerve to be considered for use as donors, especially in cases where there are healed rib fractures. Each ICN is dissected distally to the

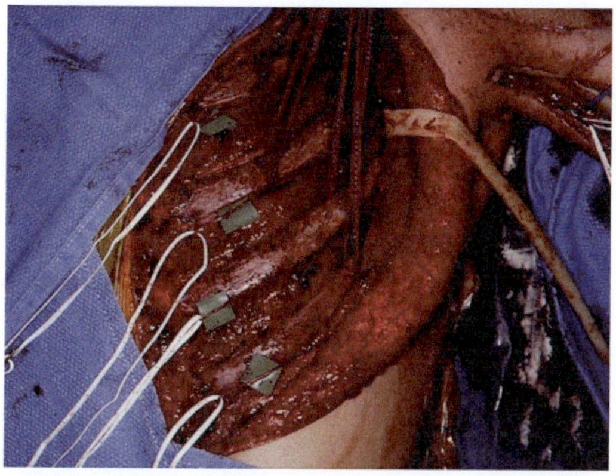

Fig. 23.1 Intercostal nerves harvested for transfer. Motor ICNs are in white vessel loops and green backgrounds. (Used with permission of the Mayo Foundation for Medical Education and Research)

costochondral junction and laterally to the anterior axillary line (Fig. 23.1).

The triceps branches of radial nerve are identified in the distal deltopectoral incision. The pectoralis minor tendon is released from the coracoid, and the axillary sheath is identified. The lateral cord, lateral cord contribution of the median nerve, musculocutaneous nerve, and posterior cord with its axillary and radial branches were progressively identified around the axillary artery. The first large radial nerve branch distal to the take-off of the axillary nerve is identified. Its identity is confirmed by tracing it distally into the triceps. This triceps branch is then dissected proximally, carefully splitting it from the remainder of the radial nerve as proximally as possible to create a long distally based triceps motor branch.

The operating microscope is then brought into the field and the ICNs are glued together to create a cable that has a good size match with the triceps branch. The ICN cable and the triceps motor branch are repaired with the shoulder positioned in 90° of abduction and maximum external rotation to ensure a tension-free nerve transfer (Fig. 23.2). The repair is performed with orienting 9-0 nylon epineurial microsutures and completed with a split collagen tube to maintain the ICN cable shape and fibrin glue. The patient is placed in a shoulder immobilizer with the elbow flexed 90° for 3 weeks.

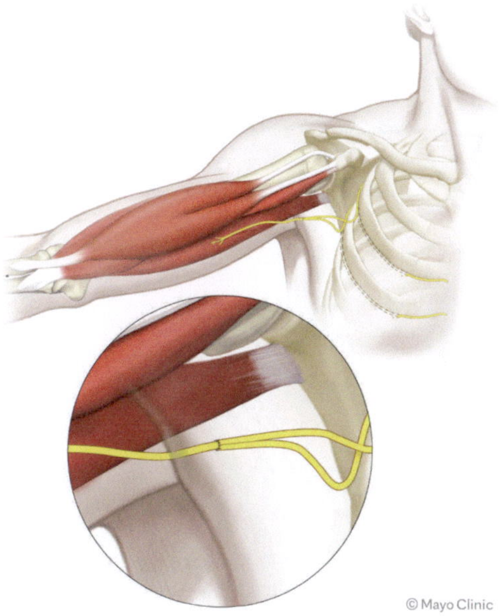

Fig. 23.2 Diagram of intercostal nerves to triceps branch transfer. (Used with permission of the Mayo Foundation for Medical Education and Research)

23.3.2 Posterior Deltoid Branch of the Axillary Nerve (PBAN) to the Triceps Branch of the Radial Nerve

This transfer is performed as previously described [9]. Patient is positioned supine under general anesthesia with the arm draped across the chest. A longitudinal incision is.made over the quadrilateral and triangular interval. The posterior border of the deltoid is identified and elevated. The sensory branch of the axillary nerve is identified and traced back to the quadrilateral space where the PBAN to the posterior deltoid is located. Nerve stimulation is used to confirm strong contractions from both anterior and posterior axillary nerve branches to the deltoid before harvesting. The PBAN branch is harvested distally (Fig. 23.3a). The triceps motor branch (Fig. 23.3b) is next identified in the triangular interval. The teres minor branch can be harvested (Fig. 23.3a) with the PBAN if there is a considerable size mismatch with the triceps branch. Epineural repair is performed under a microscope (Fig. 23.3c). The patient is placed in a shoulder immobilizer for 3 weeks.

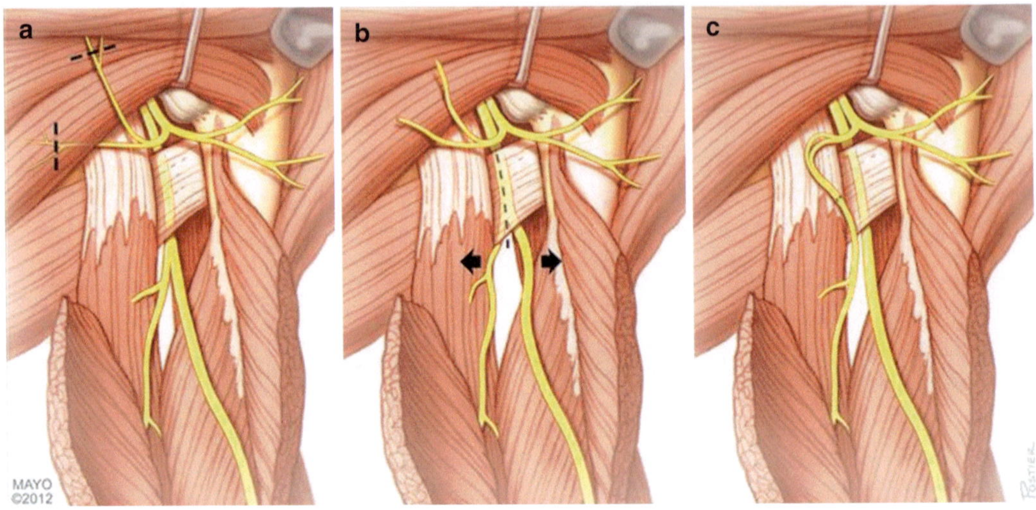

Fig. 23.3 Diagrams for the posterior deltoid branch of axillary nerve transfer to the triceps. (**a**) Posterior branch of axillary nerve and teres minor branch. (**b**) Triceps motor branch in triangular interval. (**c**) Repair after transfer. (Used with permission of the Mayo Foundation for Medical Education and Research)

23.3.3 Levator Scapulae to the Long Head of the Triceps Branch of the Radial Nerve

The levator scapulae is innervated by the dorsal scapular nerve and branches from C3 and C4 via the cervical plexus. The C4 root can be identified on the anterior scalene muscle during supraclavicular exploration by tracing the phrenic nerve proximally. The nerve to the levator scapulae is identified by following the C4 root distally [15, 16]. The long head of the triceps branch is identified in the triangular interval at the shoulder and dissected proximally until its branching point. The gap is bridged by sural nerve autografts.

23.3.4 Flexor Carpi Ulnaris (FCU) to the Triceps Branch of the Radial Nerve

Transfers of the ulnar nerve fascicle innervating FCU have been described [7, 10]. We position the patient supine and use a 10-cm proximal medial arm incision. The radial nerve is identified posterior to the brachial artery, anterior to the long head of the triceps muscle. One or more triceps branches are selected as they enter the muscle without targeting a specific branch. The absence of triceps contraction is confirmed with a handheld nerve stimulator. Multiple triceps branches are selected and combined by careful proximal dissection to form a single recipient motor nerve. The ulnar nerve is identified at the level of the divided triceps motor branches. The ulnar nerve fascicles are dissected distally from this level, and the nerve stimulator is used to identify fascicles producing mostly FCU contraction. The stimulation of the remaining ulnar nerve fascicles confirms strong contraction of hand intrinsic muscles. FCU fascicles matching the diameter of the triceps branch are isolated and divided distally with a length measured to permit their rotation to meet the triceps motor branches without tension (Fig. 23.4). The patient is placed in a shoulder immobilizer for 3 weeks.

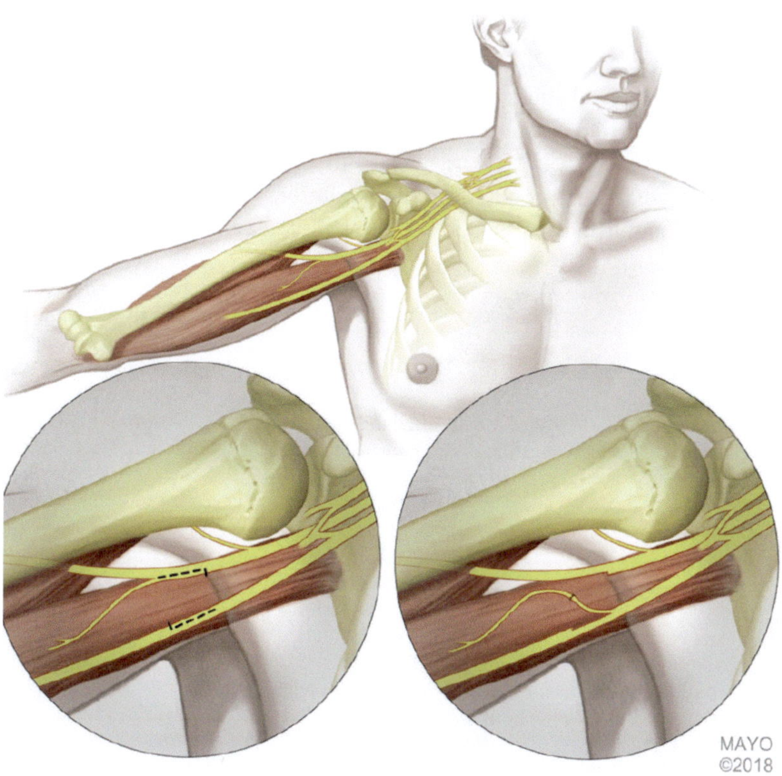

Fig. 23.4 Diagram of the FCU fascicle to triceps branch transfer. A triceps nerve branch is identified and carefully separated from the radial nerve proximally to obtain additional length. The ulnar nerve is identified and the FCU fascicle is intraneurally dissected. (lower left) An FCU fascicle of the ulnar nerve is coapted to a triceps nerve branch without tension. (lower right) (Used with permission of the Mayo Foundation for Medical Education and Research)

23.4 Outcomes

Terzis reported 31.65% MRC grade 3 or stronger elbow extension in 162 BPI patients who underwent various elbow extension reconstruction over a 28-year period [3]. In this cohort, 33.33% patients ($n = 30$) with direct ICNs transfer had stronger than MRC grade 3 elbow extension recovery [3]. The authors recommended ICN as a preferred donor in patients with multiple avulsions. Doi reported useful triceps muscle recovery in 14 of 26 (53.8%) complete avulsion patients with intercostals to triceps transfer performed as part of prehension reconstruction with double FFMT [17]. In another cohort of 39 patients with total plexus palsy, 27 patients (69%) recovered MRC grade 3 or stronger elbow extension after transfer of third to fifth ICNs to long head of triceps [4]. Smaller cohorts had conflicting results. Transfer of three ICN to the long head of triceps branch in seven complete plexus and three C5–C7 palsy resulted in eight patients (80%) recovering MRC grade 3 or stronger elbow extension [14]. Seven of ten (70%) complete avulsion patients with three ICNs to the long head of triceps reconstruction recovered antigravity elbow extension [18] compared to none of seven (0%) complete avulsion patients who had two to three ICN to triceps branch transfers [19].

The levator scapulae nerve was used to reconstruct elbow extension by grafting to the long head of triceps branch in 12 pan plexus avulsion injury patients [11]. The nerve grafts were 16.8 cm in length on average. All 12 recovered active elbow extension with MRC grade 4 in 3 and MRC grade 3 in 9 patients after an average of 27 months [11].

Results of PBAN and FCU transfers are described in case reports of five or less patients [6–10]. Transfer of FCU ulnar nerve fascicles to triceps yielded MRC grade 4 or 5 elbow extension [6–8, 10]. Similar results were reported for three patients who had PBAN transfer to triceps [8, 9].

23.5 Conclusion

Elbow extension reconstruction is necessary when reconstructing prehension in complete pan brachial plexus injuries. ICN transfer to triceps branch of radial nerve resulted in antigravity or stronger elbow extension in 33.3–69% of these patients.

References

1. Doi K, Shigetomi M, Kaneko K, et al. Significance of elbow extension in reconstruction of prehension with reinnervated free-muscle transfer following complete brachial plexus avulsion. Plast Reconstr Surg. 1997;100(2):364–74.
2. Shin AY, Socolovsky M, Desai K, Fox M, Wang S, Spinner RJ. Differences in management and treatment of traumatic adult pan brachial plexus injuries: a global perspective regarding continental variations. J Hand Surg Eur. 2022;47(1):40–51.
3. Terzis JK, Barmpitsioti A. Our experience with triceps nerve reconstruction in patients with brachial plexus injury. J Plast Reconstr Aesthet Surg. 2012;65(5):590–600.
4. Kittithamvongs P, Leechavengvongs S, Malungpaishrope K, Pongpinyopap W, Anantavorasakul N, Uerpairojkit C. The intercostal nerves transfer to the radial nerve branch to the long head triceps muscle: influencing factor and outcome of 55 cases. J Hand Surg Am. Published online. 2022;
5. Bulstra LF, Rbia N, Kircher MF, Spinner RJ, Bishop AT, Shin AY. Spinal accessory nerve to triceps muscle transfer using long autologous nerve grafts for recovery of elbow extension in traumatic brachial plexus injuries. J Neurosurg. 2018;129(4):1041–7.
6. Flores LP. Results of surgical techniques for reinnervation of the triceps as additional procedures for patients with upper root injuries. J Hand Surg Eur. 2013;38(3):248–56.
7. Pet MA, Ray WZ, Yee A, MacKinnon SE. Nerve transfer to the triceps after brachial plexus injury: report of four cases. J Hand Surg Am. 2011;36(3):398–405.
8. Alolabi N, Lovy AJ, Kircher MF, Spinner RJ, Bishop AT, Shin AY. Distal nerve transfers to the triceps Brachii muscle: surgical technique and clinical outcomes. J Hand Surg Am. 2020;45(2):155.e1–8.
9. Klika BJ, Spinner RJ, Bishop AT, Kircher MF, Shin AY. Posterior branch of the axillary nerve transfer to the lateral triceps branch for restoration of elbow extension: case report. J Hand Surg Am. 2013;38(6):1145–9.
10. Bertelli J, Soldado F, Ghizoni MF, Rodríguez-Baeza A. Transfer of a terminal motor branch nerve to the flexor carpi Ulnaris for triceps reinnervation: anatomical study and clinical cases. J Hand Surg Am. 2015;40(11):2229–2235.e2.
11. Bertelli JA, Ghizoni MF. Reconstruction of complete palsies of the adult brachial plexus by root grafting using long grafts and nerve transfers to target nerves. J Hand Surg Am. 2010;35(10):1640–6.
12. Nishijima N, Yamamuro T, Fujio K, Ohba M. The swallow-tail sign: a test of deltoid function. J Bone Joint Surg Br. 1995;77(1):152–3.
13. Schreiber JJ, Feinberg JH, Byun DJ, Lee SK, Wolfe SW. Preoperative donor nerve electromyography as a predictor of nerve transfer outcomes. J Hand Surg Am. 2014;39(1):42–9.
14. Goubier JN, Teboul F. Transfer of the intercostal nerves to the nerve of the long head of the triceps to recover elbow extension in brachial plexus palsy. Tech Hand Up Extrem Surg. 2007;11(2):139–41.
15. Martins RS, Siqueira MG, Heise CO, Foroni L, Neto HS, Teixeira MJ. The nerve to the levator scapulae muscle as donor in brachial plexus surgery: an anatomical study and case series. J Neurosurg. 2021;135(4):1223–30.
16. Saltzman EB, Krishnan K, Winston MJ, Das De S, Lee SK, Wolfe SW. A cadaveric study on the utility of the Levator scapulae motor nerve as a donor for brachial plexus reconstruction. J Hand Surg Am. 2021;46(9):812.e1–5.
17. Doi K, Muramatsu K, Hattori Y, et al. Restoration of prehension with the double free muscle technique following complete avulsion of the brachial plexus. Indications and long-term results. J Bone Joint Surg Am. 2000;82(5):652–66.
18. Malungpaishope K, Leechavengvongs S, Ratchawatana P, et al. Simultaneous phrenic and intercostal nerves transfer for elbow flexion and extension in total brachial plexus root avulsion injury. J Hand Surg Asian Pac. 2018;23(4):496–500.
19. Zheng MX, Xu WD, Qiu YQ, Xu JG, Gu YD. Phrenic nerve transfer for elbow flexion and intercostal nerve transfer for elbow extension. J Hand Surg Am. 2010;35(8):1304–9.

Transfers from the Ulnar Nerve for Restoration of Elbow Extension

24

Belkheyar Zoubir, Cambon Adeline, and Oberlin Christophe

24.1 Transfer of a Branch of the Ulnar Nerve Onto One Nerve to the Triceps Brachii Muscle

24.1.1 Principles of the Transfer

Patients with lesions of posterior cord of the brachial plexus suffer from palsy of deltoid, triceps muscle, and all muscles innervated by radial nerve. Contrary to the adage that restoration of active extension of the elbow is useless because it may be replaced by the action of gravity, a patient with voluntary elbow extension will be able to push, pull, and stabilize objects. The restoration of active elbow extension is of major importance.

As most of posterior cord lesions are in continuity (grade III or IV of Sunderland classification), waiting spontaneous recovery is recommended.

If there is no recovery 5 months after the injury, our strategy is to operate on these patients using a combination of nerve and tendon transfers. For the axillary nerve, a neurotization is usually performed using two or three intercostal nerves. Wrist, thumb, and finger extension are restored using conventional tendon transfers. For elbow extension, our usual technique is the transfer of one fascicule of the ulnar nerve dedicated to the flexor carpi ulnaris (FCU) muscle to the nerve of the long head of the triceps [1].

Bertelli and al. showed in an anatomical study that the mean number of ulnar nerve branches to the FCU muscle was 2.9 [2]. Moreover, mean FCU nerve length and diameter were 50 and 1.0 mm, respectively. Histological analysis revealed that the number of myelinated fibers in the FCU branch and the triceps upper medial head motor branch were similar (818 and 743, respectively). In a short patient series, he showed that in spite of FCU branch harvesting, patients retained a functional FCU with a British Medical Research Council score of M4.

In 2013, we reported the results of five patients with a posterior cord lesion, who underwent the transfer of FCU branch to one of the nerves to the triceps brachii (medial or lateral head) at a mean delay of 6 months after their accident [3]. All of them recovered triceps strength M4 according to the BMRC grading system, against a resistance of 5 kg (range, 3.8 to 7 kg), which represented approximatively 50% of the contralateral extension strength. Of note, elbow extension strength may easily be tested with the elbow flexed at 90°, by asking the patient to push with the wrist on a kitchen scale. Interestingly, no cocontraction was observed between ulnar-innervated muscles and

B. Zoubir · O. Christophe
Clinique du Mont Louis, Paris, France

C. Adeline (✉)
Orthopaedic and Traumatology Surgery Department, Sorbonne University, Saint-Antoine Hospital, Paris, France

F. Guedes et al. (eds.), *Nerve Transfers for Brachial Plexus Reconstruction after Trauma*,
https://doi.org/10.1007/978-3-031-92445-3_24

triceps muscle. Since then, we preserve the branches to the lateral and medial heads of the triceps in the case of some additional spontaneous recovery occurs. Other authors observed similar good functional results of this nerve transfer, without noticeable donor muscle weakness [4, 5].

Goubier et al. showed that the transfer of one fascicule of ulnar nerve to the branch of the long head of the triceps was also reliable for active elbow extension recovery in C5, C6, and C7 brachial plexus palsies [6].

24.1.2 Operative Technique

Under general anesthesia, the patient is placed on supine position. The skin incision is done along the medial border of the proximal arm and extended in the armpit. The radial nerve is identified above the latissimus tendon, and a branch to the triceps brachii is identified thanks to electrostimulation. This branch is the first to arise from the radial nerve at the distal end of the axilla. In recent years we select the branch to the long head of the triceps brachii. It is cut as proximal as possible. The ulnar nerve is approached, and a motor branch responding in the FCU on electrostimulation is harvested. Tensionless direct suture with a conventional epiperineural suture is finally performed between the two nerve endings (Fig. 24.1). The arm is immobilized in a thoracobrachial sling for 6 weeks. Then, physiotherapy is begun.

24.1.3 Common Outcomes

In our experience, this transfer leads in more than 70% of cases to a useful elbow extension (Fig. 24.2).

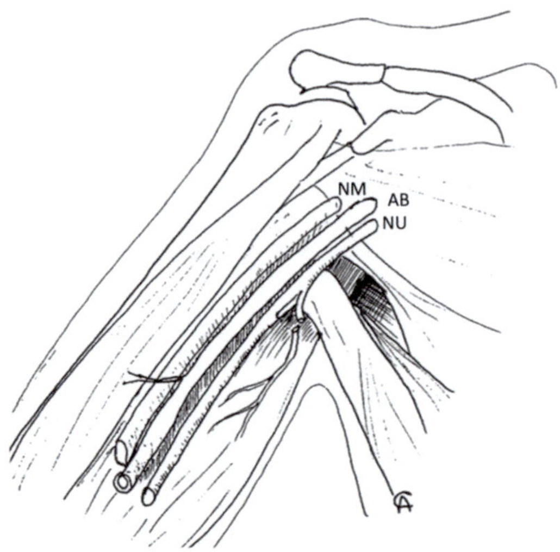

Fig. 24.2 Surgical technique of the transfer of one fascicule of the ulnar nerve to the radial nerve branch of the long head of the triceps brachii

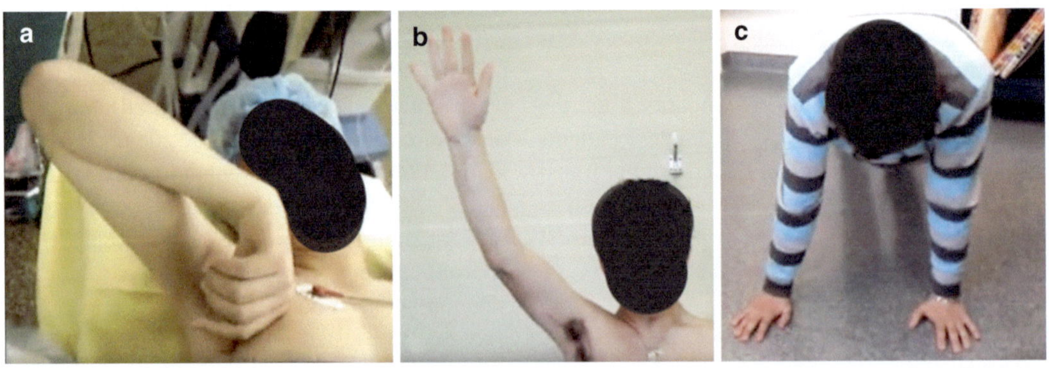

Fig. 24.1 Complete palsy of the triceps in a 17-year-old boy with a lesion of posterior cord of the brachial plexus (**a**). On examination 25 months after the transfer of one fascicule of the ulnar nerve onto one branch of triceps brachii muscle, active elbow extension was restored (**b**) with enough strength to do push-ups (**c**)

References

1. Oberlin C, Durand S, Belheyar Z, Shafi M, David E, Asfazadourian H. Nerve transfers in brachial plexus palsies. Chir Main. 2009;28:1–9.
2. Bertelli J, Soldado F, Ghizoni MF, Rodríguez-Baeza A. Transfer of a terminal motor branch nerve to the Flexor Carpi ulnaris for triceps reinnervation: anatomical study and clinical cases. J Hand Surg Am. 2015;40(11):2229–35.
3. Oberlin C, Chino J, Belkheyar Z. Surgical treatment of brachial plexus posterior cord lesion: a combination of nerve and tendon transfers, about nine patients. Chir Main. 2013;32(3):141–6.
4. Pet MA, Ray WZ, Yee A, Mackinnon SE. Nerve transfer to the triceps after brachial plexus injury: report of four cases. J Hand Surg Am. 2011;36(3):398–405.
5. Alolabi N, Lovy AJ, Kircher MF, Spinner RJ, Bishop AT, Shin AY. Distal nerve transfers to the triceps brachii muscle: surgical technique and clinical outcomes. J Hand Surg Am. 2020;45(2):155e1–155.e8.
6. Goubier JN, Maillot C, Asmar G, Teboul F. Partial ulnar nerve transfer to the branch of the long head of the triceps to recover elbow extension in C5, C6 and C7 brachial plexus palsy. Injury. 2019;50(Suppl 5):S68–70.

Anterior Interosseous Nerve Transfers for Restoration of Pinch and Grip

25

Jasmine Thum, Stanley Bazarek, Margaret Sten, and Justin M. Brown

Abbreviations

AIN	anterior interosseous nerve
BB	biceps brachii
BPI	Brachial plexus injury
BR	brachioradialis
BRA	brachialis
ECRB	extensor carpi radialis brevis
ECRL	extensor carpi radialis longus
FCU	flexor carpi ulnaris
FDP	flexor digitorum profundus
FDS	flexor digitorum superficialis
FPL	flexor pollicis longus
IP	interphalangeal joint
LABC	lateral antebrachial cutaneous nerve
MABC	medial antebrachial cutaneous nerve
MCN	musculocutaneous nerve
MN	median nerve
PIN	posterior interosseous nerve
PQ	pronator quadratus
PT	pronator teres
RN	radial nerve
SCI	spinal cord injury
SSRN	superficial sensory radial nerve
SUP	supinator

J. Thum
Department of Neurosurgery, University of California San Francisco, San Francisco, CA, USA

S. Bazarek
Department of Neurosurgery, Harvard Medical School, Boston, MA, USA
e-mail: sbazarek@bwh.harvard.edu

M. Sten
Georgetown University School of Medicine, DC, Washington, USA

J. M. Brown (✉)
Department of Neurosurgery, Massachusetts General Hospital Boston, Boston, MA, USA
e-mail: jmbrown@mgh.harvard.edu

25.1 Introduction

Grasp function can be lost due to a cervical spinal cord injury (SCI), brachial plexus injury (BPI) that includes the lower trunk, or peripheral nerve damage affecting the median and ulnar nerves. Recovering grasp is critical in these populations so that patients can carry out activities of daily living such as independent feeding, writing, operating a phone, self-catheterization, and interacting with assistive devices such as motorized wheelchairs in the case of tetraplegic patients. Recovery of arm/hand function is consistently rated as the most important function to improve the quality of life in cervical SCI [1]. As such, in SCI, restoration of hand function (grasp and release) is prioritized, followed by triceps function [2]. Preserved active wrist extension can often provide a passive tenodesis grasp and release, but active grasp and release are prioritized when it is an option.

F. Guedes et al. (eds.), *Nerve Transfers for Brachial Plexus Reconstruction after Trauma*,
https://doi.org/10.1007/978-3-031-92445-3_25

Historically, tendon transfers were primarily used to restore pinch and grip strength after loss of grasp function, often utilizing extensor carpi radialis longus (ECRL) to flexor digitorum profundus (FDP) (when strong wrist extension was preserved) and brachioradialis (BR) to flexor pollicis longus (FPL) tendon transfer [3, 4]. It has been demonstrated that nerve transfers can also achieve these goals, with less postoperative immobilization and therapy requirements, and can provide options for patients who might not have tendon transfer options [5, 6]. When grasp function is lost, the AIN (innervated by C8 and T1) becomes the primary nerve target for recovering prehension [7]. The anterior interosseous nerve (AIN) innervates the flexor pollicis longus (FPL), the radial two flexor digitorum profundus (FDP), and the pronator quadratus (PQ). It is a motor branch of the median nerve (MN) primarily responsible for the index finger-thumb pinch and grasp function.

25.2 Nerve Transfers: Overview

Four nerve transfers are outlined in this chapter: pronator teres (PT) to AIN, supinator (SUP) to AIN, extensor carpi radialis brevis (ECRB) to AIN, and brachialis to AIN. While outcomes have been reported to be favorable in SCI and BPI, there are currently no adequately powered studies to compare nerve transfer and tendon transfer options to recover grasp. There may be cases in which one option is preferred over the other. It is important to note that some nerve transfers may preclude future tendon transfer options, and this should be considered if planning surgery in a less-than-optimal scenario. Of the transfers listed, ECRB is the only one that will necessarily eliminate the option of an ECRL tendon transfer. The PT nerve transfer often requires only one of the nerve branches to the muscle, leaving this muscle functional but weaker and, therefore, a less optimal tendon transfer candidate. Transfer of the brachialis nerve branch eliminates the option of tendon transfer of biceps to triceps as elbow flexion would then be lost [8]. Finally sacrifice of the SUP for AIN or PIN function would also make the biceps to triceps transfer less appealing as utilizing these together would eliminate active supination. Nonetheless, these are important surgical techniques for any peripheral nerve surgeon to be familiar with, given that nerve and tendon transfers have different advantages and indications. Selecting one reconstruction solution over the other should be patient-specific, driven by the individual's needs, the likelihood of success given the clinical context, and the patient's ability to adhere to the required postoperative therapy.

Optimal nerve transfers utilize a donor near close to the recipient to minimize reinnervation time. The most common distal nerve donors include the PT branch of the MN and the ECRB or SUP branches of the radial nerve (RN). If no distal options are available because they are either (1) considered to be a poor donor (MRC < 4 or significantly reduced motor units on EMG) or (2) conflict with another reconstructive plan as discussed above, a proximal donor such as the brachialis (BRA) may be used. The BRA to AIN transfer can be done directly with lengthy intraneural neurolysis of the AIN proximally. However it is our preference to do a two-stage approach utilizing an intervening nerve graft. The ease of technique drives this preference as there is a risk of loss of tone to other median nerve muscles with this lengthy intraneural dissection and a dramatic size mismatch of the AIN at the level of the BRA branch. As in any nerve repair requiring an intervening graft, not only does nerve regeneration take longer due to the much larger distance to target with greater axon loss across an additional coaptation site, but the rehabilitation can be more challenging and less intuitive than the other donor sources.

This chapter will discuss the three primary distal transfers (PT, ECRB, and SUP) and the two-stage proximal BRA-AIN transfer. Relevant donor anatomy and function, indications for the transfer, and the surgical technique will be detailed. A brief discussion of less common nerve transfers to the AIN that have been proposed is briefly discussed at the end of the chapter.

25.3 Distal Nerve Transfers

These three nerve transfers, Sup (high C6), ECRB (lower C6), and PT (C7), are all located in the forearm and provide for direct end-to-end repair of the donor nerve to the AIN (C8-T1) [9]. The PT to AIN transfer is favored by the authors of this chapter for AIN restoration as it can be completed through a single volar forearm incision (Fig. 25.1), is typically tension-free, and is surgically straightforward. In addition, patients requiring grasp and release reconstruction are typically candidates for supinator to PIN for finger extension. When exchanging supination for finger extension, adding the agonist function (pronation) to provide finger flexion, makes rehabilitation much more straightforward for both the therapist and the patient. The two radial nerve transfers are reasonable; however, they are sometimes more easily performed with a second dorsal incision (Fig. 25.1), although this is unnecessary. Determining whether ECRL (C6–C7) is present and strong before transferring the ECRB nerve branch is critical. These patients will typically not have an extensor carpi ulnaris (ECU, C8 innervation through the posterior interosseous nerve), and therefore, if ECRL is weak, the transfer may result in a critical deficit in wrist extension. Of note, this would be uncommon as the typical recovery of function progresses to the ECRL before the ECRB is present. Thus, it is rare (in SCI) to have a strong ECRB without also having a strong ECRL.

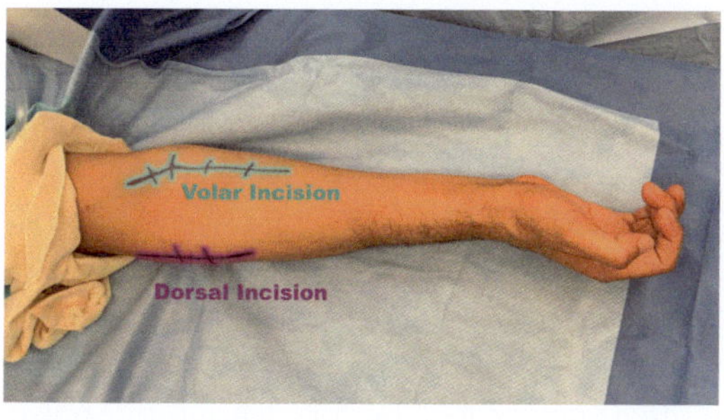

Fig. 25.1 Incisions used for distal nerve transfers. Via the dorsal incision, the interval between the BR and wrist extensors (ECRL/ECRB) provides a direct approach to the RN for more facile neurolysis. The volar incision is used to access the MN but can also be used alone without the dorsal incision to access both the MN and RN

25.4 Median Nerve (Pronator Teres) to AIN (Fig. 25.2)

25.4.1 Median Nerve Anatomy

The MN provides innervation to critical superficial and deep flexors of the forearm and hand and key functional movements for the hand [10]. It provides finger flexion to the radial three digits, thumb opposition, pinch, forearm pronation, and critical sensation to the hand, including the thumb, index, and middle finger which are critical for fine manipulation.

The MN has contributions from the lateral and medial cords of the brachial plexus and contains axons from the roots of C6-T1, but it can also even have contributions from C5. The MN forms in the center of the arm, just lateral to the brachial artery, and maintains a relatively superficial course as it continues distally, eventually coursing medial to the brachial artery. Before passing under the flexor retinaculum to enter the forearm, the MN passes between the biceps brachii (BB) and BRA tendons and then travels between the deep and superficial heads of the PT muscle to gain access to the forearm. The MN has no branches in the arm, but as soon as it begins to cross the antecubital fossa, it sends off its first muscular branch to the PT. Next, a second branch of the PT emerges on the superficial surface of the nerve. Following, on the deep side of the nerve, branches to the flexor carpi radialis and palmaris longus muscles emerge. As it dives deeper and passes between the flexor digitorum superficialis (FDS) and FDP muscles, it bifurcates into a two-thirds and one-third caliber nerve. The AIN is the smaller of these, typically diverging to the radial side. Shortly after this, and typically on the opposite side of the nerve, two or more branches will be found that innervate the FDS. Finally, the MN emerges distally between the FDS and FPL muscles before entering the hand via the carpal tunnel, where it gives off motor branches to the first and second lumbri-

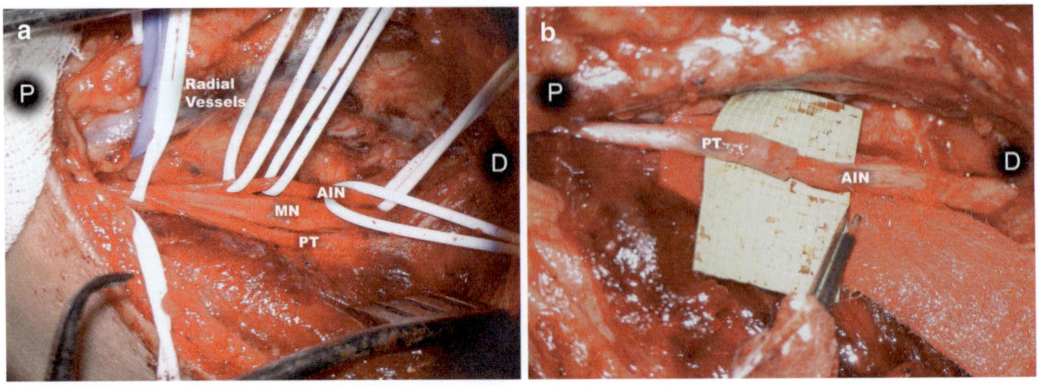

Fig. 25.2 Pronator teres to AIN transfer. (**a**) Neurolysis of the MN demonstrating the distal PT branch lying superficial and the AIN on the radial side of the MN trunk. (**b**) Coaptation of the PT to the AIN is an easy repair. The coaptation is protected within a collagen sleeve sutured to the epineurium. Distal (D), proximal (P)

cals, the opponens pollicis, abductor pollicis brevis, and flexor pollicis brevis.

25.4.2 AIN Exposure

The entire course of the MN is in the anterior compartment of the arm and forearm. The AIN can, therefore, be accessed through a proximal volar incision. The hockey stick incision begins distally about 3–4 inches beyond the crease of the antecubital fossa, between the BR laterally and flexor-pronator mass medially, and extends proximally into the antecubital fossa, where we typically angle the incision radially at about the level of the biceps tendon. This provides access radially, under the BR and avoids a straight line incision across the elbow flexion crease (Fig. 25.1). Care should be taken in the proximal aspect of this incision to avoid dividing the cephalic or accessory cephalic veins and to avoid injuring branches of the lateral antebrachial cutaneous nerve (LABC). After subcutaneous dissection, the forearm fascia is exposed and divided distally to proximally. This should expose the radial vessels and provide access to the space between the flexor-pronator mass and the BR. As the fascial opening moves proximally, the lacertus fibrosus is also divided, allowing retraction of the flexor pronator mass medially.

To access the MN, the forearm can be partially pronated to relax the PT and a self-retaining retractor is placed to mobilize the PT ulnarly. Alternatively, the BR can be mobilized laterally to expose the tendon of the superficial head of the PT as it approaches its radius insertion. This tendon can then be step-lengthened to augment the exposure [9], allowing for greater retraction of the PT more proximally without requiring forearm pronation. Lateral retraction of the radial vessels more proximally also provides exposure of the MN deeper in the antecubital fossa as it dives under the deep head of the PT. The deep head of the PT can be divided, if necessary, to provide additional exposure. Similarly, the tendinous arch of the FDS muscle is typically divided, to gain better access to the distal branches, including AIN and FDS.

The AIN is usually readily visible as a distinct fascicle and can have a longitudinal vessel demarcating the cleavage plane between the main MN trunk and the AIN. The AIN can then be neurolyzed, separated, and looped. Proximal neurolysis of the AIN parallel to the MN can typically be performed over a significant length, at least to the antecubital fossa before interfascicular connections are encountered. This intraneural dissection is often required to allow for a tension-free repair to any of the proposed source nerves, particularly the supinator branches. This PT transfer requires the least intraneural dissection. This is the same basic exposure that is used in each of the following AIN nerve transfers.

25.5 PT to AIN

The PT, innervated predominantly by C7, is one of two muscles that pronates the forearm and hand along with the PQ (innervated by AIN; C8/T1). Therefore, when PT is used as a donor for the AIN, there is potential for it to reinnervate PQ, restoring its strength. We do not count on this and prefer to simply use the second branch to the PT, preserving the first branch and thus the proximal one-third to one-half of the PT muscle innervation.

Technical aspects: The PT to AIN nerve transfer can easily be accomplished through a single volar incision as described in the "AIN Exposure" section above. This is a particularly straightforward nerve transfer as the PT and AIN are both easily exposed within the same incision, and are nearby, exiting off the MN in the proximal half of the anterior compartment of the forearm (Fig. 25.2a). The PT is the first muscular nerve branch off the MN, near the level of the antecubital fossa. Exposure of the AIN also readily provides access to the PT branches. The proximal PT branch is usually less apparent than the distal branch and requires additional proximal dissection to identify. We typically lift using an army navy retractor and loop this branch to ensure that adequate strength will be maintained following sacrifice of the distal branch. The distal branch courses on the superficial surface of the median nerve before it innervates the PT muscle, eventually dividing into two branches (to the deep and superficial heads). Care must be given to placing deep self-retaining retractors as retraction of the flexor-pronator mass will often result in direct pressure to the distal PT nerve as it enters the muscle and can confound its assessment. The nerve will not stimulate well if it has been compressed under a retractor. Once the proximal branch is identified and stimulated to confirm adequate strength, the distal branch is looped and followed distally and then divided, with about 4 cm of available length. This usually provides good overlap of the takeoff of the AIN. Of note, as is true of nerves in general, they become larger in caliber the more distally they are followed and smaller when progressing proximally. The PT and AIN should both be neurolyzed to a location where their caliber matches nicely and then divided with some redundancy. The AIN is looped distally and followed proximally, freeing it from the main trunk of the MN and well overlapping the PT nerve. It is then divided as well. The coaptation (Fig. 25.2b) is carried out in a similar fashion for all nerve transfers discussed in this chapter: (1) trimming of nerve ends, sizing, and placement of nerve protector; (2) apposition of the donor and recipient nerve ends without tension on a green background; (3) 3–4 perineural sutures placed across the coaptation site with 9-0 nylon microsuture; (4) translation of the nerve protector tube over the coaptation site, with tension relieving 8-0 nylon microsutures placed from the tube to the epineurium; and (5) fibrin sealant glue placed over the entire nerve protector to reinforce the repair. Closure is also carried out in a similar fashion for all nerve transfers discussed: (1) copious irrigation of the surgical bed with hemostasis (and repair of the step-lengthened pronator teres if required) (2) closure of the skin with inverted subcutaneous 3-0 vicryl suture with skin glue placed over the incision (assuming skin edges are well-apposed).

25.6 Radial Nerve Transfers (Fig. 25.3)

25.6.1 Radial Nerve Anatomy

The RN provides innervation to muscles of the posterior compartment of the arm and forearm, along with sensory innervation to the posterior arm and forearm, dorsal radial hand, and dorsal three and a half digits of the hand [11]. These muscles are primarily involved in extension of the arm, hand, and fingers and supination for reaching and interacting with the space in front of, around, or above a patient (with the triceps function particularly important). These muscles are critical for opening the hand and extending the wrist in preparation for grasp, especially posterior interosseous nerve (PIN) innervated muscles such as the extensor digitorum communis, extensor pollicis longus, and abductor pollicis

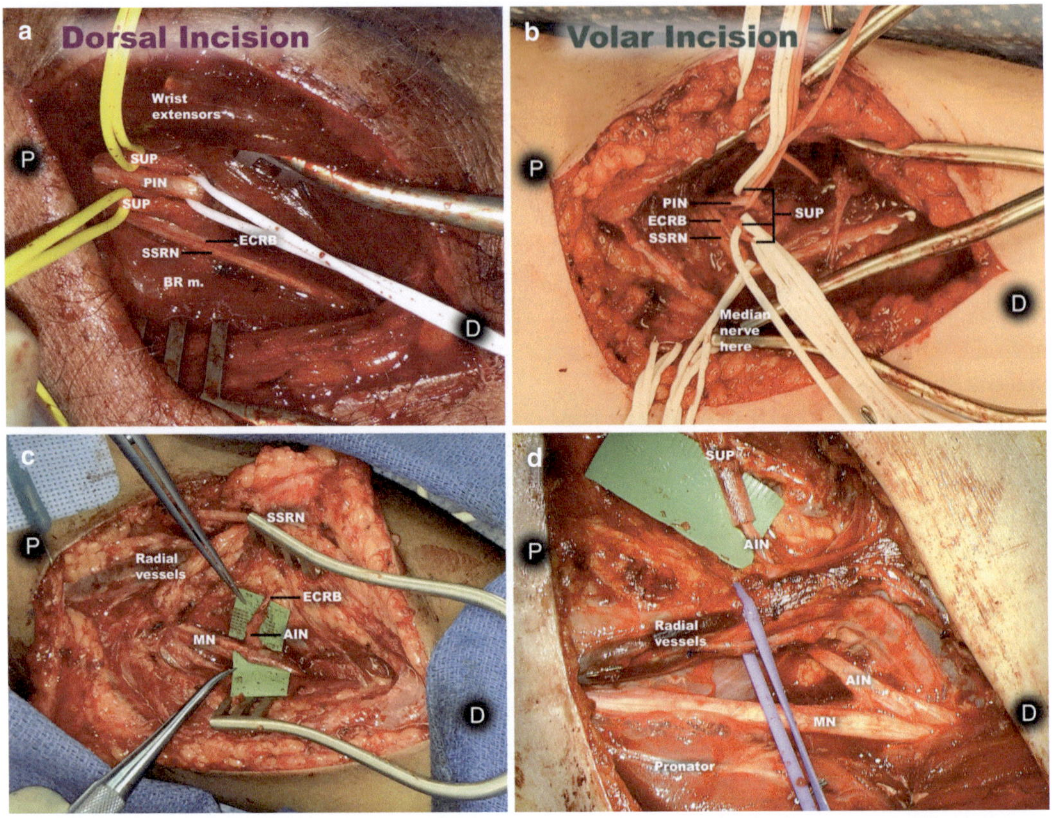

Fig. 25.3 Radial nerve to AIN transfers. (**a**) Neurolysis of the RN from the dorsal approach. (**b**) Neurolysis of the RN from the volar approach. In this view, the MN and radial vessels are retracted to the ulnar side and the BR muscle radially to expose the RN and its branches. (**c**) The ECRB is tunneled under the radial vessels for coaptation with the AIN (viewed through the volar approach). (**d**) The AIN requires more extensive neurolysis, and it is tunneled under the radial vessels to reach the short SUP branches. Distal (D), proximal (P)

longus, as well as the wrist extensors, respectively.

The RN arises from the posterior cord of the brachial plexus, with contributions from the posterior division of each trunk, and contains nerve root fibers from the entire brachial plexus from C5-T1. The RN is the largest terminal branch of the brachial plexus and originates from the posterior cord in the axilla, where is splits from the axillary nerve just posterior to the axillary artery, between the coracobrachialis and teres major muscles. It then enters the arm's posterior compartment, innervating the triceps brachii, along with the skin of the posterior arm via the posterior cutaneous branches. It then courses between the medial and lateral heads of the triceps along the radial groove on the humerus, adjacent to the brachial artery and pierces the lateral intermuscular septum. Just distal to this, it gives off motor branches to the BR muscle and a posterior cutaneous branch to the forearm. It continues its course, wrapping anterior to the lateral humeral condyle, giving off a motor branch to ECRL. After crossing the cubital fossa into the posterior compartment of the forearm, it terminates into the superficial sensory RN (SSRN) branch along with the ECRB nerve, which both deviate from the rest of the PIN in the interval between the BR and ECRL muscles. The PIN then gives off the SUP branches, which innervate the SUP muscle, and the rest of the PIN then travels under this same muscle [12].

The interval between the BR and ECRB muscles on the dorsal forearm is an interval through which the ECRB and SUP nerve donors can be accessed [13]. In this interval, a branch to ECRB comes off the RN along with the SSRN. ECRB is always the smaller caliber of the two. The rest of the PIN represents a separate but immediately adjacent bundle. The SUP branches are often closely associated with the PIN and on either side of it as it approaches the SUP muscle. There are typically two SUP branches coming from either side of the PIN, but there can be up to four. After passing under the SUP muscle, the PIN courses in a plane between the superficial and deep extensor muscles and provides the primary motor supply to the muscles of the forearm posterior compartment used for finger, and thumb extension as well as ulnar wrist extension.

25.7 ECRB to AIN

As discussed above, the ECRB arises from the RN [14]. It is one of the three primary muscles involved in wrist extension (in addition to the ECRL, arising from the RN more proximally, and the extensor carpi ulnaris, which arises from the PIN). The ECRB nerve branches off the RN in the proximal volar forearm near the antecubital fossa in the BR/ECRL interval discussed previously and is innervated primarily by the C6 nerve root. The ECRB branches off the RN just distal to the takeoff of the SSRN and runs immediately adjacent to this nerve. While this nerve is easily accessed dorsally, as described above, it can also be accessed from a volar incision.

Technical aspects: Due to its location just deep to the BR muscle, the ECRB to AIN transfer can be approached through either a two-incision approach with a dorsal incision to access ECRB and volar incision to access AIN, or through a single volar incision as described above for the PT to AIN transfer with adequate mobilization of BR.

Single incision approach (Fig. 25.3b): The authors prefer the single incision approach for this transfer. Once the MN dissection is complete, we carefully move to the other side of the radial vessels and identify the BR muscle. The muscle is followed to its inferior surface, and once the connective tissue is released, the SSRN is usually readily apparent. This nerve is looped and then followed proximally to about the level of the antecubital fossa. At that level, the ECRB nerve will be found immediately adjacent to the SSRN and can be stimulated to confirm its identity. This nerve is usually less than half of the caliber of the sensory branch. As is customary with nerve transfers, obtaining enough distal length on the ECRB is important so that the distal nerve end can be mobilized into the volar space adjacent to the AIN to allow for a tensionless repair. Therefore, the ECRB is looped at this level and then followed distally alongside the sensory nerve. Usually several centimeters can be harvested. It is important to note that the greater length achieved may result in losing side branches and thus the ultimate number of axons transferred. Thus, we typically only take as much length as is required to perform a tenson-free repair (Fig. 25.3c) and include any identified side branches. These branches are then passed under the radial vessels to easily reach the AIN.

Two incision approach: A two-incision approach can also be used (Fig. 25.1), as the dorsal incision provides direct access to the RN for easier neurolysis (Fig. 25.3a). Furthermore, the SUP-PIN transfer is also typically performed to restore finger extension; therefore, this corridor has been developed in most cases. The dorsal incision should start at the lateral edge of the skin crease of the antecubital fossa, just lateral to the BR muscle mass and medial to ECRL muscle mass, and extend as a linear incision in this interval to about one-third of the way down the forearm. The lateral antebrachial cutaneous nerve (LABC) branches should be avoided during subcutaneous dissection. The fascial layer to the posterior compartment of the forearm is opened, and the interval between the BR and ECRL can be gently developed with blunt finger dissection. To confirm the correct interval, the wrist can be passively flexed and extended; the ECRL/ECRB muscles will move with this action, while the BR muscle will not. The SSRN is often the first nerve identified during this blunt dissection. As discussed before, once identified and looped, it can be traced proximally to the RN, and the

ECRB nerve will be identified running alongside it and should exit just distal to its origin. Because the ECRB nerve is deep to the BR, the BR will have to be gently mobilized and retracted to follow the ECRB to its distal penetration into the ECRB muscle, where is it can be divided and mobilized for transfer. In general, though, the distal dissection of the ECRB is better accessed through the volar incision. Therefore, if the ECRB is accessed through the dorsal approach, the nerve is dissected free proximally to gain optimal length and then looped. That loop should be passed under the BR to ensure that the full length is delivered into the volar incision. Then, the nerve is followed distally and divided from the volar incision, including its side branches. These are then typically passed under the radial vessels to the AIN to achieve the shortest distance between these branches. The steps followed for nerve coaptation and closure are the same as discussed previously in the PT to AIN transfer.

25.8 Supinator to AIN

The SUP is one of two muscles that supinates the forearm and hand, the other being the BB muscle (innervated primarily by C5 via the musculocutaneous (MCN) nerve). The SUP nerve branches come off the RN as discussed in the "Radial Nerve Anatomy" section above, and usually consists of at least two, and often more, distinct branches which exit the RN just proximal to the where the posterior interosseous nerve (PIN) passes under the supinator muscle [13]. This is the best donor nerve for finger extension, so this will only be used for finger flexion if there are no other good nerve transfer options available for finger flexion or if finger extension function has been retained [15].

Technical aspects: Due to the deeper anatomic location of the supinator branches, and their intimate association with the PIN, this nerve transfer is typically more easily performed with a two-incision approach—a volar AIN incision and a dorsal incision to access the SUP nerve branches as discussed above.

Two incision approach: The dorsal approach is similar to that discussed in the ECRB dissection above (Fig. 25.3a); however, once the ECRB and RN are identified, the RN continues to be followed distally until it passes under the arcade of Frohse/supinator fascia. Just proximal to this, the supinator branches can be found running with the PIN. When needed, the leading edge of the supinator muscle can be carefully lifted and divided to provide additional distal exposure of the PIN to be sure to separate it from any late emerging supinator branches. Typically, a SUP branch is found on either side of the PIN, but one may also be deep to the PIN. Branches are separated from the PIN and looped. Nerve stimulation differentiates between supinator branches (which should result in forearm supination) and the PIN (which should result in wrist extension via the ECU, and thumb/finger extension). Of note, the ECRB may also send a proximal branch that can be confused with a supinator branch right at the level of the Arcade. This can be avoided or even included if additional axons appear to be required. It is important to identify all branches of the supinator, so that as many axons can be available for the nerve transfer into the AIN as possible and to avoid a persistent synkinesis of finger flexion and supination long after the transfer is learned. Once all SUP branches are identified, the nerve branches can be brought together and glued with fibrin sealant and then trimmed together to make a single, larger donor nerve which is technically easier to repair to the AIN. For these transfers, proximal neurolysis of the AIN from the MN on the volar aspect is particularly important, so that it can be mobilized well enough to pass under the radial vessels and BR to reach these shorter branches (Fig. 25.3d). Technical aspects of coaptation and closure are the same as previously discussed.

Single incision approach: As discussed in the ECRB section, a volar-only approach can also be used for this transfer (Fig. 25.3b). In this case, the SSRN is followed proximally as described above until we reach the proximal radial nerve. Crossing vessels are divided and the PIN is exposed. We find the angle of dissection a bit more cumbersome for harvesting all of the supinator branches than is the case with the dorsal approach, but it is feasible. In either case, the AIN must be dissected quite proximally to reach the SUP for the repair given the limited length of these donor branches (Fig. 25.3d). In this case, the AIN is passed under the radial vessels and brought adjacent to the PIN for a tension-free repair to the supinator branches.

25.9 Brachialis Motor Branch to AIN (Fig. 25.4)

Particularly when considering SCI, where many target nerves remain innervated but lack volitional control from injured upper motor neuron fibers, a two-stage nerve graft approach may be utilized to recruit proximal nerve sources. In these cases, a graft is interposed at a first stage with no distal hookup. Later, after sufficient time has transpired for those axons to traverse the graft, the distal end can be coapted to the target nerve. The second stage allows the target muscle to remain innervated, preventing neuromuscular degeneration during axon regeneration. The graft selected is up to the surgeon's (and patient's) preference. In most cases, we have used the sural nerve from the leg or the immediately available medial antebrachial cutaneous (MABC) nerve graft in the arm through an extension of the same medial arm incision used to expose the musculocutaneous nerve. In the case of C5 SCI patients, the first stage of the procedure usually takes place at the same time as the triceps nerve transfer and the graft is hooked up to the BRA nerve branch and its distal end is tunneled into the forearm where it can simply be left in the subcutaneous space. If a temporary target is preferred, the distal end of the graft can be tucked into a local muscle or sutured end-to-side into the ulnar nerve. A few months [4–9] are allowed to transpire, while the proximal donor axons grow through the nerve graft. During this time, the target muscles remain preserved as their associated nerve is not divided until the axons are in proximity. When the second stage is undertaken to hook up the distal end of the graft, the AIN has been "injured" for the first time. Therefore, the associated Wallerian degeneration and release of neurotrophic factors is initiated, boosting the regeneration of the axons that should have reached the distal graft by this time. This overall strategy reduces denervation time, minimizing atrophy and (in our hands) providing

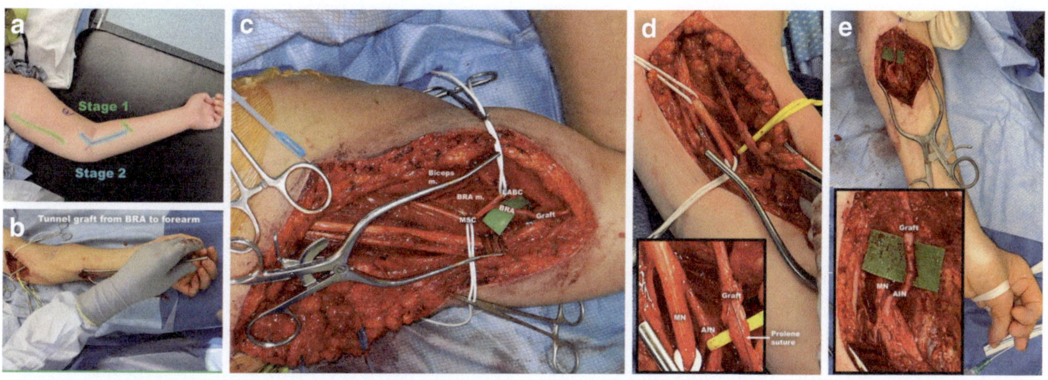

Fig. 25.4 Brachialis to AIN transfer. (**a**) The incisions for each stage are demonstrated. Stage 1 shows the proximal incision to access the BRA branch and the smaller distal incision to pass the tunneler. Stage 2 incision is the volar approach shown previously to access the MN and tunneled graft. (**b**) A metal tunneling device is used to pass the graft between the distal and proximal incisions. (**c**) The proximal incision is used to access the MCN nerve which terminates as a motor branch to the BRA and the most terminal branch continues to the forearm as the LABC. The coaptation to the graft to the BRA branch is shown. This incision was extended proximal to the axilla for a concurrent axillary to radial nerve transfer for triceps reanimation. The MABC can be harvested from this incision to provide the required graft. (**d**) Stage 2 volar exposure is used to first access the graft at the distal aspect of the incision within the subcutaneous tissue. The Prolene suture left behind at the original surgery helps confirm the identity of the nerve graft. (**e**) A tensionless coaptation of the graft to the AIN is performed, and no postoperative immobilization is required. Distal (D), proximal (P)

a more robust result. This strategy may be less ideal for a brachial plexus injury where time is of the essence.

25.9.1 Two-Stage Grafted Approach

The brachialis muscle (C5, musculocutaneous nerve) is one of three muscles responsible for elbow flexion, in addition to the biceps muscle (C5, musculocutaneous nerve), and brachioradialis (C5/6, radial nerve). In the presence of fully functioning biceps and BR muscles, patients rarely notice a deficit with elbow flexion after harvesting the brachialis nerve. This nerve transfer is less synergistic than the previously discussed transfers, but it is the only option in many patients. Pairing movements for motor re-education to close the hand—namely, flexing the elbow—tends to be less intuitive than the others. It is, however, a reasonable alternative in some cases where higher injuries have occurred, and only C5 and higher innervated nerves are available as donors [5, 7, 16], and we have many successful cases where this transfer has provided a strong grasp.

Technical aspects: When using a graft, the nerve transfer is completed in two stages as described above.

Stage 1: The brachialis nerve is identified through a medial arm incision in the interval between the anterior and posterior compartments of the arm, at the level of the mid-humerus (Fig. 25.4A). The interval between the biceps and brachialis muscles is developed, and the musculocutaneous nerve is identified within this space. At the mid humerus level, the nerve typically bifurcates into the lateral antebrachial cutaneous (LABC) nerve and the brachialis nerve. The LABC passes over the brachialis muscle and heads laterally to eventually emerge on the lateral side of the biceps tendon. The brachialis nerve stays more medial but then quickly spreads out into a few branches to cover the surface of the brachialis muscle. In cases in which the brachioradialis is quite strong, concern for downgrading elbow flexion is typically not a concern. In higher injuries where this muscle is not present, we recommend extending the incision more proximally to access the biceps branch to directly stimulate this branch and ensure that it provides strong elbow flexion on its own. The brachialis branch is harvested at the site where it begins to branch and it is divided there (Fig. 25.4c). In cases where loss of elbow flexion is a concern, we occasionally take the additional step of crushing the brachialis branch just distal to the site of intended division using a hemostat to create a recoverable conduction block and then stimulate the proximal musculocutaneous nerve again to confirm that the elbow flexion is still adequate. If so, the brachialis branch is divided without concern for downgrading elbow function.

The graft: When using the MABC nerve as a graft, we take the incision quite proximally and follow the nerve into the axilla and divide it as high as is safe within the distal brachial plexus. This will often include the medial brachial cutaneous nerve which can then be peeled away from the MABC as it is typically too short to be included. The nerve is then followed distally until close to the elbow, where it gives off multiple branches. It is best to harvest prior to this branching. This graft is usually about 18–20 cm long. The graft is reversed in orientation with the larger branching end being repaired to the brachialis (which is also branching), usually for a nice size match. The thin proximal end is then made available for the thinner AIN distally, and this is what is tunneled into the forearm. We use a shunt tunneler (as is used when passing the peritoneal tube during placement of a ventriculoperitoneal shunt) and pass this from our arm incision into the forearm in the subcutaneous layer (Fig. 25.4b). A stab incision is made and the tunneler is passed through this within the mid volar forearm. We typically use a 6-0 proline suture which is sutured to the former proximal end of the graft (now oriented distally) and run in the connective tissue of the epineurium to mark the graft. This allows us to easily identify the nerve months in the future at the second stage operation. A snap is attached to the tied end of the proline, and a suction is attached to the tunneler proximally. The graft is fed into the tunneler with saline irrigation and typically the nerve will feed nicely. The tunneler is then pulled through, and the former distal end of the graft is now positioned by the brachialis nerve. Once this is completed, the nerve coaptation is undertaken at this level (as described above) and all incisions are closed.

Stage 2: This stage is undertaken 4–9 months later, after axonal regeneration through the graft is expected to have reached the distal graft. A volar forearm incision is made as discussed previously for the other transfers. The stab incision from passing the graft can be incorporated into the incision. Care should be taken during the opening to avoid damaging the tunneled nerve graft from the brachialis. A nerve with associated 6-0 Prolene suture is usually easy to find (Fig. 25.4d). It is lifted and dissected proximally, and then the graft is wrapped in a wet gauze, while the rest of the AIN dissection is undertaken. The nerve is usually distinct in that it will not have a cuff of fatty tissue and not look like a normal nerve. If that is found, it is usually a branch of the LABC and not the graft. The repair is undertaken where the best size match is identified and not much proximal dissection of the AIN is required. This repair is typically very tension free and will generally require no post-op immobilization (Fig. 25.4e).

25.9.2 Single-Stage Approach

In cases which are time sensitive, such as a lower BPI, we often favor a single-stage operation and exclusion of a graft to decrease regenerative time from donor to target muscle [7, 16].

Technical aspects: In this case a large incision combining both of the incisions described above are used. We connect the incisions for a single-stage approach by crossing the elbow flexion crease with a Bruner's-type zigzag. The AIN is accessed through the distal half of the incision as described previously. This nerve is then very carefully neurolyzed as proximally as possible. This is a tedious undertaking and, done properly, will likely take a couple hours. In some cases, the anatomy is favorable and this can be done all the way to the level of the brachialis branch. In most cases, however, there is branching within the median nerve where fascicles are both joining and emerging from the AIN fascicle just after passing the antecubital fossa. A few of these connections can be divided without severely compromising the operation, but at times we cannot effectively reach the brachialis nerve because of these connections and a gap remains precluding an easy reach to the brachialis branch with the elbow in full extension. This is then addressed by flexing the elbow to overcome the gap. Other surgeons will interpose a short nerve graft in these cases. When a graft is avoided, the repair is performed with the elbow flexed at 90°, and the patient is immobilized is elbow flexion brace for 6–12 weeks, with 2 weeks at 90° and progressive extension over the following month or two until the elbow rests in full extension once again.

The single-incision, single-stage approach requires extensive proximal neurolysis of the AIN along the MN, well above the level of the antecubital fossa to get as close to the brachialis nerve as possible. For the donor nerve, the brachialis branch, it is equally as important to get as distal as possible on the nerve as it dives into the muscle, in order provide as much length as possible for the nerves to reach each other for a tensionless coaptation. Unfortunately, the more proximal the AIN dissection, the smaller the caliber. Similarly, the more distal the brachialis dissection, the larger its caliber. This can make the repair quite challenging and compromise the success of this transfer [6, 7, 17]. Therefore, even when the lengths achieved appear ideal, we will often cut away both ends until a better size match is achieved. That is why elbow flexion is often preferred by our team to allow a more proximal site of repair on the brachialis nerve for a technically more favorable coaptation when a single-stage operation is required.

25.10 Other Transfers

While other transfers can be considered to recover AIN function, these are often only available in special cases. For example, FCU (ulnar nerve) or FCR (MN) can both be used as a donor for AIN, but most cases that eliminate AIN function also eliminate these options or provide better alterative solutions (e.g., side to side tenodesis of FDPs is ulnar nerve is intact). Other donors may not be available if they are already being utilized for higher priority transfers, or in cases where a high cervical spine injury precludes the use of other donors, as described in the "Brachialis to AIN" section above. Given the recent influx of interest in distal peripheral nerve transfers, especially to restore function in SCI, new transfers may arise in the coming years, making a regular review of the nerve literature important for the ongoing education of any nerve reconstructive surgeon.

25.11 Special Consideration: BR to AIN

While several authors have described a BR (C5/6, RN) to AIN transfer [7, 18], this has not been a transfer that we have employed. Technically we have not found that this is not an easier reach than to the BRA transfer described above, nor do we believe that it has benefits not afforded by the BRA. Contrary to the BRA, it makes an excellent tendon transfer for several targets while maintaining its elbow flexion assistance. Typically, we will complete all of our nerve transfers for hand function, and then, once the final result is achieved, the BR is used to optimize the function achieved. For example, weak thumb flexion undergoes a BR to FPL transfer, a weak thumb extensor undergoes a BR to EPL transfer. BR can augment inadequate wrist extension to ECRB tendon transfer. We have even used BR for an opponensplasty. And the list goes on.

25.12 Adjunct Reconstructive Considerations

As alluded to above, a combination of nerve and tendon transfers is typically the best method to achieve the desired functional goal for hand reanimation, including procedures to optimize hand positioning [2, 19]. In our C5 patients, we typically perform a SUP to PIN to restore finger extension and a two-stage graft approach for BRA-AIN form grasp and pinch. Following reinnervation, a BR to FPL tendon transfer and a thumb carpometacarpal fusion may be performed. The thumb interphalangeal (IP) joint is another consideration in these cases. Strong reanimation of FPL function, whether by nerve or tendon transfer, can result in a thumb that folds into the palm or that simply misses its target on the side of the first metacarpal for an effective pinch. Straightening the IP joint makes a pinch much easier to perform and holds the thumb in a more functional position. This is either done with a split FPL to EPL tendon transfer or via a thumb IP fusion. Additionally, when there is no hand intrinsic musculature tone, MCP hyperextension will result and the hand becomes clawed. We often perform a volar plate advancement (House anticlaw correction may also be used) to correct this clawing of the digits and to provide better extension of the IP joints [20].

25.13 Chapter Summary

The importance of this chapter is that it illustrates the variety of nerve transfer options available for reanimation of AIN/hand grip and pinch for the reconstructive peripheral nerve surgeon. The four most common donor nerves are discussed in detail here, with others available as well. While there is limited data available comparing these various AIN transfer outcomes thus far, it is worth noting the common tenants for successful nerve transfers still apply, namely, patient factors (young age, earlier surgery), surgical factors (proximity to the target muscle, size match of donor and recipient nerves, axon count, primary axon type), and synergy between the function of the target muscle compared to the recipient muscle for retraining, and finally consideration of the source nerve for flexion versus the source nerve for finger extension in the rehabilitation plans. Surgical consideration may also vary from patient to patient depending on individual anatomy and injury type, as well as the patient's injury level, which would dictate available nerve donors. The use of nerve transfers, while providing potential physiologic functional restoration, need not be the only part of the reconstructive plan. Augmentation with tendon transfers, joint fusions, etc. can enhance the patient's functional outcomes. As always though, the choice in surgical approach should be dictated by (1) the entire reconstructive plan for the patient and (2) the patient's priorities for functional restoration, not simply for anatomic reconstruction.

References

1. Anderson KD. Targeting recovery: priorities of the spinal cord-injured population. J Neurotrauma. 2004;21(10):1371–83.
2. Bazarek S, Brown JM. The evolution of nerve transfers for spinal cord injury. Exp Neurol. 2020;333:113426.
3. Sammer DM, Chung KC. Tendon transfers: part II. Transfers for ulnar nerve palsy and median nerve palsy. Plast Reconstr Surg. 2009;124(3):212e–21e.
4. Hentz VR. Tendon transfers after peripheral nerve injuries: my preferred techniques. J Hand Surg Eur. 2019;44(8):775–84.
5. van Zyl N, Hill B, Cooper C, Hahn J, Galea MP. Expanding traditional tendon-based techniques with nerve transfers for the restoration of upper limb function in tetraplegia: a prospective case series. Lancet. 2019;394(10198):565–75.
6. Javeed S, Dibble CF, Greenberg JK, Zhang JK, Khalifeh JM, Park Y, et al. Upper limb nerve transfer surgery in patients with tetraplegia. JAMA Netw Open. 2022;5(11):e2243890.
7. Bertelli JA, Ghizoni MF. Nerve transfers for restoration of finger flexion in patients with tetraplegia. J Neurosurg Spine. 2017;26(1):55–61.
8. Zlotolow DA, Kripke LA, Kozin SH. Current concepts in elbow extension reconstruction for the tetraplegic patient. J Am Acad Orthop Surg. 2023;31(5):221–8.
9. Brown JM, Mackinnon SE. Nerve transfers in the forearm and hand. Hand Clin. 2008;24(4):319–40. v
10. Bertelli JA, Patel N, Soldado F, Duarte ECW. Patterns of median nerve branching in the cubital fossa: implications for nerve transfers to restore motor function in a paralyzed upper limb. J Neurosurg. 2021;135(5):1524–33.
11. Matavelli FC, Gobbi L, Dos Santos MPS, Caetano EB, Vieira LA, de Andrade RA. Transfer of the radial nerve branches for the treatment of the anterior interosseous nerve lesion: an anatomical study. Acta Ortop Bras. 2019;27(6):298–303.
12. Ziaziaris WA, Ahadi MS, Gill AJ, Ledgard JP. The anatomy of nerve transfers used in tetraplegic hand reconstruction. J Hand Surg Am 2022;47(11):1121 e1- e6.
13. Bazarek S, Sten M, Nin D, Brown JM. Supinator to posterior interosseous nerve transfer for restoration of finger extension. Oper Neurosurg (Hagerstown). 2021;21(5):E408–E13.
14. Bertelli JA, Mendes Lehm VL, Tacca CP, Winkelmann Duarte EC, Ghizoni MF, Duarte H. Transfer of the distal terminal motor branch of the extensor carpi radialis brevis to the nerve of the flexor pollicis longus: an anatomic study and clinical application in a tetraplegic patient. Neurosurgery. 2012;70(4):1011–6. discussion 6.
15. Bazarek S, Sten M, Thum J, Mandeville R, Magee G, Brown JM. Supinator to posterior interosseous nerve transfer for recovery of hand opening in the tetraplegic patient: a case series. Neurosurgery. 2023; https://doi.org/10.1227/neu.0000000000002819.
16. Ray WZ, Yarbrough CK, Yee A, Mackinnon SE. Clinical outcomes following brachialis to anterior interosseous nerve transfers. J Neurosurg. 2012;117(3):604–9.
17. Brown JM. Nerve transfers in tetraplegia I: background and technique. Surg Neurol Int. 2011;2:121.
18. Garcia-Lopez A, Sebastian P, Martinez F, Perea D. Transfer of the nerve to the brachioradialis muscle to the anterior interosseous nerve for treatment for lower brachial plexus lesions: case report. J Hand Surg Am. 2011;36(3):394–7.
19. Titolo P, Fusini F, Arrigoni C, Isoardo G, Conforti L, Artiaco S, et al. Combining nerve and tendon transfers in tetraplegia: a proposal of a new surgical strategy based on literature review. Eur J Orthop Surg Traumatol. 2019;29(3):521–30.
20. Friden J, House J, Keith M, Schibli S, van Zyl N. Improving hand function after spinal cord injury. J Hand Surg Eur. 2022;47(1):105–16.

26 Nerve Transfers for Ulnar Nerve Injury

Benjamin A. Plog, Vivek P. Gupta, Fernando Guedes, and Wilson Z. Ray

26.1 Introduction

Brachial plexus injuries are a uniquely debilitating group of traumatic lesions secondary to the motor and sensory neurological deficits and pain symptoms they can cause [7, 8]. Ulnar nerve lesions, as well as pan-plexus (C5-T1) or lower trunk (C8-T1) lesions, which lead to ulnar dysfunction due to their upstream position, are particularly debilitating due to loss of wrist flexion, flexion of the fourth and fifth digits, finger abduction and adduction, finger pinch, and dorsoulnar hand sensation [17]. Traumatic lesions of the ulnar nerve can lead to a reduction in grasp and pinch strength up to 77% [12, 17]. This combined with a loss of protective sensation [7, 8] limit activities of daily living (ADLs) such as eating, personal hygiene, and toileting, as well as instrumental activities of daily living (IADLs) required for activities such as maintaining a home, meal preparation, and occupational activities that lead to a rich and full life. Consequently, there is much excitement surrounding recent advancements in the treatment of these lesions afforded by nerve transfers leading to improved motor and sensory function and reduced pain. Historically, while nerve transfers for restoration of elbow and shoulder function have seen the most success, and transfers to restore hand function have had less positive outcomes, more recent data suggests transfers to the ulnar nerve can provide clinically meaningful motor and prehensile sensory improvement [17, 21].

The incidence of all types of brachial plexus injuries has a high degree of variability depending on country, for example, with rates of 0.58 cases/100,000/year in the UK and 1.75 cases/100,000/year in Brazil [10]. Among all types of brachial plexus injuries, the pooled prevalence of closed injuries was 93% [10]. In the USA, the incidence of closed brachial plexus injuries ranges from 0.64 to 3.9/100,000/year [10]. When breaking this down further into the segment of plexus injuries that affect ulnar nerve function, pan-plexus injuries represent approximately 30–46% of all brachial plexus injuries, and isolated lower trunk lesion are even more rare, representing 3–7% of all brachial plexus injuries [8]. Biomechanically, lower plexus lesions typically arise when the arm is pulled into abduction and extension, whereas complete lesions often occur in the presence of severe forces with multiple different vectors [10]. Ulnar nerve injuries specifically represent the most common major peripheral nerve injury of the upper extremity requiring hospital admission [23]. Brachial plexus injuries in general have a male pooled prevalence of 93% and 7% for females for a 13.3:1 male to female ratio [10].

B. A. Plog · V. P. Gupta · F. Guedes · W. Z. Ray (✉)
Department of Neurological Surgery, Washington University in St. Louis, St. Louis, MO, USA
e-mail: bplog@wustl.edu; vivek.gupta@wustl.edu; rayz@wustl.edu

F. Guedes et al. (eds.), *Nerve Transfers for Brachial Plexus Reconstruction after Trauma*,
https://doi.org/10.1007/978-3-031-92445-3_26

Further, this disease process tends to disproportionately affect the young with a mean age ranging from 23 to 34 years [10]. By far the dominant etiology of brachial plexus injuries is motorcycle accidents with a prevalence of 67% [10].

Pathophysiologically, brachial plexus and peripheral nerve (e.g., ulnar) injuries can be categorized based on open vs closed mechanisms. Open injuries include gunshot wounds and lacerations. Laceration can often be accompanied by a fracture of the humerus or concomitant soft tissue injury such as damage to large blood vessels [10, 20]. Laceration can also be iatrogenic in the setting of axillary plexus block, resection of neck tumors, or operation on large blood vessels [10, 20]. Closed injuries can result from nerve compression, traction/stretch, or combination of both [7, 8, 10, 20]. At the most extreme, traction forces can lead to root avulsion [20]. As a result of the presence of the cervical fascia, cervical roots are better protected against tractional forces than the C8 and T1 roots, which are prone to avulsion leading to an ulnar palsy [20]. This is relevant for surgical planning, as lesions proximal to the dorsal root ganglion (DRG), or preganglionic, often carry a worse surgical prognosis than postganglionic lesions due to the absence of a proximal nerve stump for grafting [7, 8, 20]. Similarly, high ulnar nerve lesions tend to carry a worse prognosis due to the long distance over which reinnervation must occur to the target muscle group [17]. This may explain why historical attempts at reversing deficits in hand function resulting from ulnar injury have failed.

26.2 Preoperative Assessment

The assessment of the patient presenting with a suspected ulnar nerve injury begins with a thorough history and physical examination. Motor function evaluation should first include a qualitative assessment of muscle bulk throughout the affected extremity. Muscle atrophy can be graded visually as mild, moderate, or severe [15]. It should be noted here, however, that following a traumatic peripheral nerve injury, there is a sudden loss of motor function to a given muscle or group of muscles, but muscular atrophy will take weeks to develop following denervation and therefore assessment of muscle bulk does not always perfectly correlate with motor performance [15]. Further, as more than one muscle will often contribute to a particular movement, it is critical to assess individual muscles to best characterize the specific peripheral nerve injured [15]. Individual muscles should be tested and graded in a standardized fashion, such as with the British Medical Research Council grading system [7, 8] to allow comparison between examiners and over time. In this grading paradigm, muscular strength is assigned a value of 0 to 5. 0 indicates no muscular contraction: 1 a flicker of contraction, 2 represents movement with gravity removed, 3 is movement against gravity, 4 is full range of motion against resistance, and 5 signifies normal muscle strength [7, 8, 15]. In patients specifically with ulnar nerve injury, the lateral key pinch can be used to assess strength of the intrinsic hand musculature [15]. Notably, patients with ulnar nerve injury may attempt to generate increased pinch force through contraction of the flexor pollicis longus, leading to flexion of the interphalangeal joint of the thumb (Froment sign). There also may be simultaneous extension of the metacarpophalangeal joint of the thumb (Jeanne sign) [15].

Ulnar nerve distribution sensation in the hand should be evaluated over the palmar aspect of the medial fourth digit and the entirety of the fifth digit. A number of different sensory modalities can be evaluated including light moving touch, pressure, vibration, and two-point discrimination. To interrogate light moving touch, the ten test has been validated with the Semmes-Weinstein monofilaments and when compared to other tests was found to be most sensitive [15]. This is performed by applying a light moving stimulus to a contralateral unaffected digit, which is assigned a normal sensation score of 10/10. This same light moving stimulus is then applied to the digit to be tested and the patient assigns a score of 0 (no sensation) to 10 (identical sensation as contralateral side) [15]. Following nerve injury, return of innervation of quickly adapting vibratory sense receptors often precedes perception of light touch [15]. Vibratory sense can be qualitatively evaluated with a low-frequency tuning fork applied, for example, to the tip of the fifth digit for ulnar nerve injury, which if sensed by the patient indicates a positive response [15]. For interrogation of slowly adapting pressure sense receptors, Semmes-Weinstein monofilaments are used to incrementally apply force with the smallest monofilament that can be detected by the patient representing the pressure threshold [15]. Finally, two-point discrimination can be used to help determine the quantity of innervated sensory receptors. This task is performed by applying two probes to the digit pulp with minimal pressure and asking the patient the number of probes present. Increasingly sensitive two-point discrimination is indicated by smaller distances between probes at which the patient is still able to determine the correct number of probes present [15]. Formal grading of sensory function is less well defined than that for motor function. Highet put forth a system assigning a grade of S0 for no sensation and S4 for normal sensation [2]. This system was later modified by Zachary and Holmes to include a component of two-point discrimination [4].

In conjunction with a thorough physical examination, electrodiagnostic testing can aid in localization of the injured nerve or nerves, the location of the injury along the course of the nerve, and assessment of recovery of sensory and motor function over time. Sensory nerve action potentials (SNAPs) can be used to localize the lesion to a pre- vs postganglionic site. If there is a sensory deficit but preserved SNAPs, this indicates that signal is getting between the sensory end organ and the sensory cell body in the dorsal root ganglion, and consequently the injury is determined to be preganglionic. Conversely, if there is a sensory deficit and absence of SNAPs, this suggests a disruption of the signal traveling from the sensory end organ back to the sensory cell body and thus a postganglionic injury [8]. Electromyography (EMG) can be used to predict injury severity; however, clinically meaningful data typically cannot be collected earlier than 3–4 weeks following injury, and many centers wait at least 6–12 weeks to make an initial assessment with EMG [8]. The presence or absence of motor unit action potentials during the recruitment phase of EMG can be followed serially over time to assess for the spontaneous return of muscular innervation; however, if function has not returned by 3 months, this tends to suggest a higher-grade axontometic injury and poorer prognosis [8]. In these scenarios, EMG can also be used to help identify potential donors for nerve transfer [8].

Specialized advanced neuroimaging studies also play an important role in the diagnosis, prognostication, and preoperative planning for the traumatic peripheral nerve injured patient. CT myelogram is the gold standard study for diagnosis of a root level injury such as avulsion [7, 8]. The presence of a pseudomeningocele at 3–4 weeks following injury is highly suggestive of a root avulsion [7, 8]. CT is of more limited utility in diagnosing postganglionic injuries. A more recent technique, magnetic resonance neurography, is capable of providing high resolution images down to the level of the fascicle and can identify neuromas, perineural scar, and pathologic fluid shifts and can help discern acute from chronic denervation [8]. Finally, ultrasound offers superior spatial resolution to MRI, which can be particularly useful when imaging smaller caliber nerves and injury at the level of individual fascicles [8]. Ultrasound also allows for real-time imaging of blood flow within adjacent vasculature, which is helpful for assessing for concomitant vascular injury or perfusion to a potential donor nerve [8].

The preoperative assessment of patients with suspected peripheral nerve injuries, such as to the ulnar nerve, is not complete without a thorough history and work up for associated injuries. Among patients with a traumatic brachial plexus injury, the most common associated injury is fracture of the upper extremity (55%) follow by spinal cord injury (43%) [10]. Consequently, there should be adequate imaging with either X-ray or CT of the cervical spine, upper extremity, and chest to rule out bony fracture of the spine, humerus, clavicle, and ribs, as well as scapulothoracic trauma [7, 8, 20]. Additionally, given the risk for associated soft tissue injury, vascular imaging of the upper extremity and neck should be considered when deemed clinically appropriate [7, 8, 20].

26.3 Timing of Surgical Intervention

Once the diagnosis of a brachial plexus or peripheral nerve injury has been made, the decision surrounding operative timing is based both on the mechanism of injury as well as the degree of spontaneous recovery of function of the injured nerve. Open injuries due to laceration or high velocity projectiles should be explored within 72 hours due to lower likelihood of spontaneous recovery and the fact that these injuries may be more amenable to direct repair [8]. Low velocity projectile injuries may be more associated with a transient neurapraxia rather than a permanent deficit and can be observed for a period of time to determine the need for intervention [8]. Root avulsion, while a closed injury, should undergo earlier intervention rather than observation given the low likelihood of spontaneous recovery [8, 20]. Generally speaking, closed injuries that do not involve root avulsion benefit from observation with serial EMG to determine the degree of spontaneous recovery. As previously mentioned, the earliest that EMG can provide clinically meaningful data is 3–4 weeks following injury, but in practice most centers wait a minimum of 6–12 weeks prior to obtaining a baseline EMG. If adequate spontaneous recovery is not seen by 3 months from the time of injury, surgical intervention should be considered [8]. For motor nerve transfers, our group advocates exploration and nerve transfer within 6 months, and no later than 12 months from the time of injury, as beyond this period denervation-related fibrosis of target muscles decreases the efficacy of the nerve transfer [17].

26.4 General Principles and Indications for Nerve Transfers

A variety of techniques have been employed in isolation and combination for reanimation of the upper extremity following brachial plexus or peripheral nerve injury including plexus exploration, primary nerve repair, nerve grafting, free functional muscle transfer, tendon transfer, arthrodesis, and amputation. These latter procedures, in particular muscle and tendon transfers, are less than ideal as they disrupt the normal biomechanics of the muscle unit, which should be preserved whenever possible [21]. Primary nerve repair remains the gold standard against which all other procedures are compared; however, there are often scenarios where the likelihood of neurologic recovery after repair is low, in which nerve transfers have seen an emerging role. These scenarios include delayed presentation after injury, proximal injury such as root avulsion or high ulnar nerve injury, large neuromas-in-continuity, significant scarring at the primary injury site, unclear injury site, injury at the level of the cell body, and injury at multiple locations along the course of the nerve [21]. Further, in situations such as that of a lower trunk injury, exploration can pose significant risk of causing iatrogenic vascular or pleural injuries [8]. Additionally, secondary to the long distances over which reinnervation must occur, grafting is also suboptimal for high, proximal injuries [17]. Consequently, nerve transfers have emerged as a tool for converting a proximal injury into a distal injury [17]. It is the redundancy of innervation of mixed peripheral nerves of the upper extremity that make this a viable therapeutic option [21]. While there has been much success using nerve transfers for the reanimation of the shoulder and elbow, consensus historically has been that the restoration of hand function secondary to high ulnar, pan-plexus, or lower trunk injuries is much more challenging [21]. This paradigm shifted, however, in 1991 when the terminal branch of the anterior interosseous nerve was first transferred to the deep motor branch of the ulnar nerve with good clinical results [16, 21].

There are several criteria that have been created for successful motor and sensory nerve transfers. For motor nerve transfers, these include that the donor nerve is geographically close to the target muscle, the donor nerve is redundant, the donor nerve contains purely motor fibers (as opposed to mixed motor and sensory), the donor nerve carries a large number of axons, the donor nerve innervates a synergistic muscle to the target muscle, and that motor reeducation will improve patient function [21]. Similarly, for sensory nerve transfers, criteria include that the donor nerve is near the target sensory nerve, the donor nerve is redundant, that the denervated distal donor nerve can be repaired end-to-side to adjacent sensory nerve or a sensory nerve that will be innervated, and finally that sensory reeducation improves patient function [21].

26.5 Anatomy of the Ulnar Nerve and Potential Donor Nerves

26.5.1 Anatomy of the Ulnar Nerve

The ulnar nerve is an upper extremity peripheral nerve and terminal branch of the brachial plexus that originates from the medial cord of the brachial plexus. It predominantly contains nerve fibers from the C8 and T1 spinal roots, though may also variably contain a small contribution from the C7 spinal root. After the medial cord splits into the median nerve and ulnar nerve, the ulnar nerve courses medial to the brachial artery alongside the median nerve. The ulnar nerve continues along this course through the upper arm until it reaches the elbow, where it then deviates posteriorly and passes through the retroepicondylar groove. After this, it courses underneath an aponeurosis between the flexor carpi ulnaris (FCU) tendon attachments; this structure is also known as Osborne's ligament, and the area beneath it through which the ulnar nerve passes is called the cubital tunnel. The nerve travels through the FCU and innervates both the FCU and the flexor digitorum profundus (FDP) via small motor branches. Two sensory branches, the palmar and dorsal ulnar cutaneous branches, break off from the ulnar nerve in the forearm after this point. The palmar ulnar cutaneous branch provides hypothenar skin sensory innervation, and the dorsal ulnar cutaneous courses medially and posteriorly to innervate the skin of the medial hand, medial portion of the fourth digit, and entirety of the fifth digit (Fig. 26.1).

The remainder of the ulnar nerve continues distally through Guyon's canal, bordered by the pisiform bone and the hook of the hamate bone. The nerve divides within the canal into the superficial sensory branch, which innervates the palmar aspects of the medial portion of the fourth digit and the entirety of the fifth digit, and the deep palmar motor branch, which innervates the hypothenar muscles, the adductor pollicis, one head of the flexor pollicis brevis, the third and fourth lumbricals, and multiple intraosseous muscles [14, 23] (Fig. 26.1 **inset**).

26.5.2 Ulnar Nerve Injury Patterns and Deficits

Ulnar nerve injury can be classified into two major groups: high injuries and low injuries. High injuries occur proximal to the takeoff of the motor branches to forearm muscles and affect the entirety of ulnar nerve function. Low injuries occur distal to the takeoff of the motor branches to the FCU and FDP. The result is sensory loss in the palmar aspect of the medial hand and loss of motor function in the interossei, ulnar lumbricals, the hypothenar muscles, the adductor pollicis, and deep head of the flexor pollicis brevis, but sparing of the aforementioned forearm muscles [23].

Sensory deficits from ulnar neuropathy are limited to the medial aspect of the wrist and hand, as the ulnar nerve does not contribute significantly to sensory innervation of the upper arm or forearm. Ulnar neuropathy at the elbow has the potential to cause sensory deficits in all the inner-

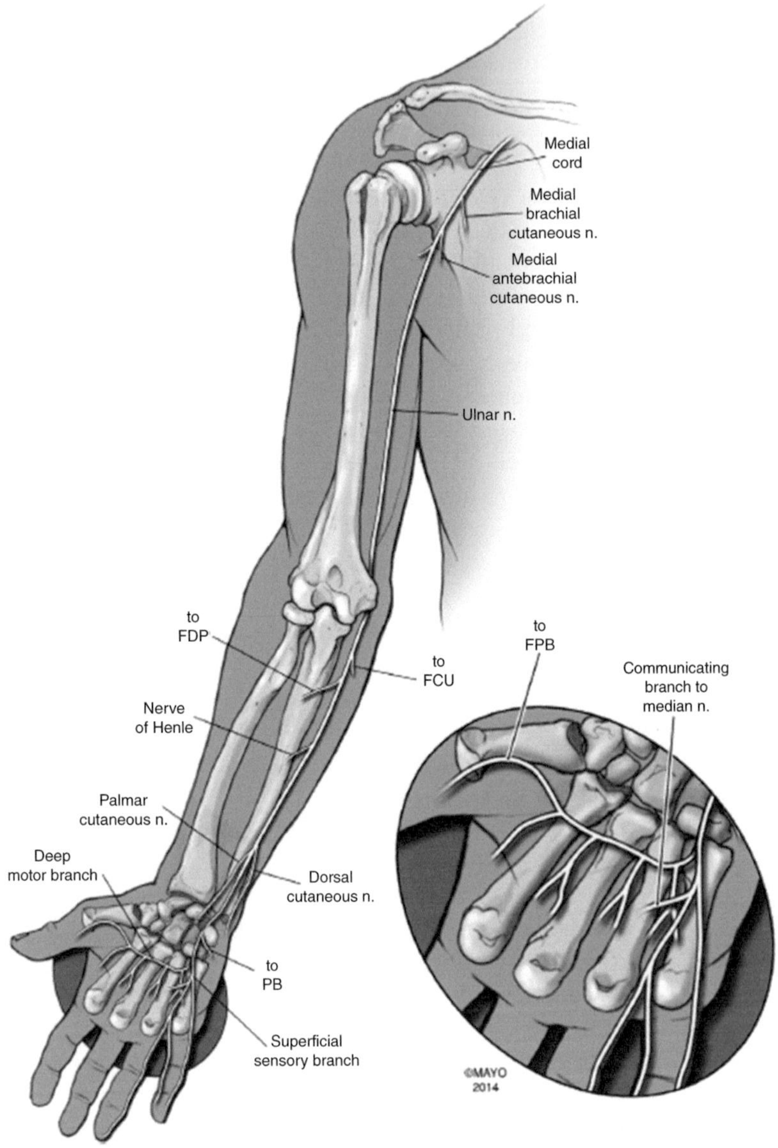

Fig. 26.1 Anatomy of the ulnar nerve after its origin from the medial cord of the brachial plexus. Abbreviations: *FCU* flexor carpi ulnaris, *FDP* flexor digitorum profundus, *PB* palmaris brevis, *FPB* flexor pollicis brevis. (Adapted from Woo et al. [23])

vated distributions, while neuropathy at the wrist typically affects the medial aspect of the fourth digit and the entirety of the fifth digit.

Motor deficits follow from decreased function of the specific muscles that the ulnar nerve innervates. Possible deficits including clawing of the fourth and fifth digits, Froment's sign (compensatory flexion of the flexor pollicis longus and thus the interphalangeal joint of the thumb when asked to pinch a flat item that is trying to be removed forcibly from the grip), and Wartenburg's sign (persistent abduction of the fifth digit). The benediction sign can also be present in ulnar neuropathy, though careful examination is required to distinguish it from a similar sign that can be seen in median nerve neuropathy. In ulnar neuropathy, the benediction sign can be seen with attempted extension of all fingers. Due to impaired ulnar nerve function, the metacarpophalangeal (MCP) joints of the fourth and fifth digits will be in extension, while the proximal and distal interphalangeal joints (PIP and DIP, respectively) will be in flexion [5, 6].

26.5.3 Anterior Interosseous Nerve Anatomy and Function

The anterior interosseous nerve (AIN) is a motor nerve that branches off of the median nerve in the forearm between the two heads of the pronator teres just distal to the elbow. It runs concurrently with the anterior interosseous artery [1]. The AIN innervates the flexor pollicis longus, pronator quadratus, and the radial half of the FDP. The function of the AIN can be tested by asking a patient to form the "OK" sign, creating a circular ring with their thumb and forefinger by flexing the interphalangeal joint of the thumb and the distal interphalangeal joint of the forefinger [1, 3].

26.5.4 Posterior Interosseous Nerve Anatomy and Function

The posterior interosseous nerve (PIN) is a predominantly motor nerve that branches off the radial nerve. The radial nerve divides into deep and superficial branches distal to the elbow. The deep branch of the radial nerve courses through the heads of the supinator and then emerges underneath it, becoming the PIN. The PIN innervates the dorsal forearm, specifically nearly all of the muscles of the posterior compartment of the forearm with the notable exceptions of the brachioradialis muscle and the extensor carpi radialis longus, which are innervated directly by the radial nerve itself [11, 22]. The PIN also supplies proprioception from the wrist joint via a terminal branch [19].

26.6 Nerve Transfer Options

26.6.1 Median Nerve: Anterior Interosseous Nerve Branch to Pronator Quadratus

Median nerve branches have been the primary focus as donors for restoration of ulnar nerve function, but additional possible donors also include radial, musculocutaneous, and ulnar branches [17]. The oldest, and perhaps still the most promising, motor nerve transfer involves the anterior interosseous nerve branch for the pronator quadratus from the median nerve to the deep branch of the ulnar nerve [15]. This procedure is typically performed through an extended carpal tunnel release incision. A zigzag incision crosses the wrist crease and continues proximally to include the distal one-third of the volar forearm in the midline (Fig. 26.2). The dissection then proceeds by opening Guyon canal and retracting the ulnar neurovascular bundle in the ulnar direction. The leading edge of the hypothenar muscle group is then identified adjacent to the hook of the hamate and incised. The deep motor branch of the ulnar nerve can then be visualized arising from the radial and deep surface of the ulnar nerve. This motor branch can then be either physically neurolyzed from the remainder of the ulnar nerve, or simply visually traced proximally. By avoiding physical neurolysis whenever possible, this prevents disruption of the vasculature supplying the nerve and consequent scarring. The motor branch is traced 4–6 cm proximal to the most proximal aspect of the pronator quadratus muscle, and a vessel loop is placed around the nerve for later identification. Next, the median nerve and the superficial and deep finger flexors are retracted radially to identify the pronator quadratus lying over the distal radioulnar joint. At the proximal edge of the muscle, the anterior interosseous nerve will be lying on the ulnar

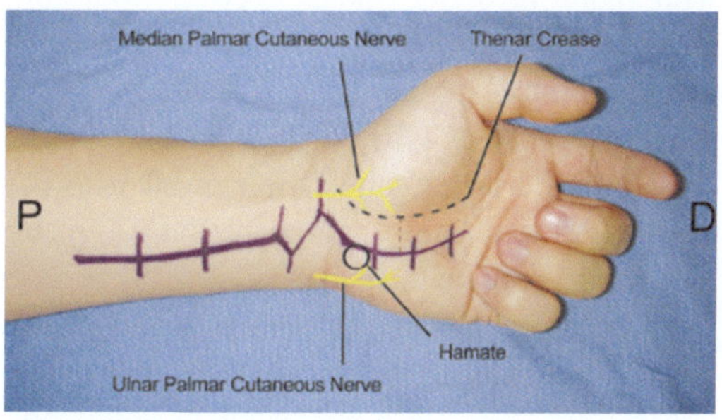

Fig. 26.2 Taleisnik incision for the exposure of relevant anatomy for anterior interosseous nerve to ulnar nerve transfer in a patient's left hand. This type of incision spares the palmar cutaneous branch of the median and ulnar nerves. Abbreviations: *P* proximal, *D* distal. (Adapted from Brown et al. [3])

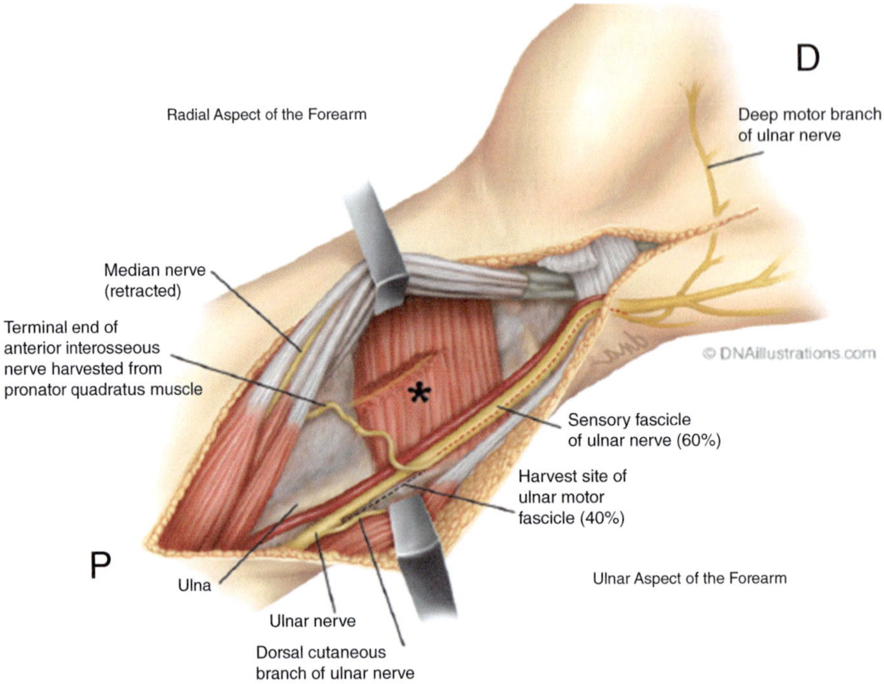

Fig. 26.3 Dissection through the pronator quadratus of the left hand to obtain maximal length of the anterior interosseous nerve, which is then cut and transferred to the ulnar nerve motor fascicle. Abbreviations: *AIN* anterior interosseous nerve, *P* proximal, *D* distal. (Adapted from Brown et al. [3])

aspect of the neurovascular bundle. The muscle is then divided, and the nerve is followed into the muscle to mobilize an additional 0.7–1.5 cm of nerve before arborization. The anterior interosseous nerve is then divided distally followed by the deep motor branch of the ulnar nerve being divided proximally [21] (Fig. 26.3). End-to-end coaptation can be employed for low ulnar injuries with more favorable motor recovery outlook; however, end-to-side coaptation is frequently utilized for high ulnar injuries to increase the transferred axon counts [17]. Finally, prior to wound closure, the transfer should be viewed with the arm in full supination and pronation to ensure minimal tension on the nerve construct [21].

The drawback of this transfer is twofold: first, the nerves innervate antagonistic muscle groups, and second, there is a mismatch in donor and recipient size [21]. Interestingly, though the pronator quadratus branch has approximately 25% less axons than the ulnar nerve, multiple studies have been able to demonstrate good return of ulnar function without loss of pronation strength [17]. At 18 months of follow-up, Barbour and colleagues and Novak and Mackinnon were able to demonstrate a sixfold increase in pinch strength and a sevenfold increase in grip strength [17]. Further, in five separate studies, a motor score of at least 4 (from a baseline of 0) was achieved in 60–100% of patients [17].

26.6.2 Radial Nerve: Posterior Interosseous Nerve Branches

High ulnar nerve injuries can also be treated with radial nerve donor branches. Specifically, branches of the posterior interosseous nerve to the extensor indicis, abductor pollicis longus, and extensor pollicis brevis can be utilized [17]. These branches are identified distal to the supinator muscle deep to the wrist extensors. It should be noted that when posterior interosseous branch donors are used, there will often be a transient loss of extension of the metacarpophalangeal joint of the index finger, but this will return over time as the extensor digitorum communis takes over this function [17]. There is less available literature to evaluate outcomes following posterior interosseous to ulnar nerve transfers; however, there is at least a single promising study demonstrating return of antigravity motor function from a baseline of 0 [17].

26.7 Postoperative Care

Postoperatively, patients are placed in a dorsal or volar splint with the wrist in a neutral position and the elbow and fingers free. The splint is typically continued for a total of 7 days. Depending on the necessity for concomitant tendon transfers, splinting may be continued for up to 4 weeks. Following this, the patient can begin work with occupational therapy performing both passive and active range of motion exercises. Notably, the patient will begin reeducation exercises where they will attempt to contract both the donor muscle and the reinnervated muscle at the same time. This will encourage cortical remapping, which will ultimately determine the patient's final functional outcome [21].

26.8 Future Directions and Donor Possibilities

Although the AIN and to a lesser extent the PIN are the two candidates for nerve transfer in ulnar nerve injury that have been described and validated in the literature, there exist other possible donor nerves that have been used for other injuries that may represent candidates for future investigation. The thoracodorsal nerve is a nerve that originates from the posterior cord of the brachial plexus and is composed of fibers from C6 through C8. It provides the sole motor innervation to the latissimus dorsi muscle. While it has not been described as a candidate for use in ulnar nerve injuries, it has been described as a donor nerve to the musculocutaneous and axillary nerve in cases of upper brachial plexus injuries [18]. There are several advantages to using the thoracodorsal nerve in these cases including it being a voluntary motor nerve that only innervates a single muscle and having high number of motor axons. Loss of function of the internal rotation and shoulder abduction provided by the latissimus dorsi does not have a significant impact on function. However, it may not be a viable target if the C7 nerve root is not spared in the trauma [9, 18]. Other candidates including the spinal accessory nerve, intercostal nerves, and phrenic nerve have been described [13] particularly as donors to help improve elbow flexion in patients with C5 and C6 injuries, but their candidacy for ulnar nerve transfers has not yet been fully evaluated given the improvement in overall function that restoring elbow flexion confers compared to the benefits of improving ulnar nerve mediated function.

References

1. Aljawder A, Faqi MK, Mohamed A, Alkhalifa F. Anterior interosseous nerve syndrome diagnosis and intraoperative findings: a case report. Int J Surg Case Rep. 2016;21:44–7. https://doi.org/10.1016/j.ijscr.2016.02.021.
2. Birch R, Bonney G, Wynn Parry C. Surgical disorders of the peripheral nerves. London: Churchill Livingstone; 1998.
3. Brown JM, Yee A, MacKinnon SE. Distal median to ulnar nerve transfers to restore ulnar motor and sensory function within the hand: technical nuances. Neurosurgery. 2009;65:966–77.
4. Dellon A. Evaluation of sensibility and re-education of sensation in the hand. Baltimore: Williams & Wilkins; 1981.
5. Dy CJ, Mackinnon SE. Ulnar neuropathy: evaluation and management. Curr Rev Musculoskelet Med. 2016;9:178–84.
6. Futterman B. Analysis of the papal benediction sign: the ulnar neuropathy of St. Peter. Clin Anat. 2015;28:696–701.
7. Giuffre JL, Kakar S, Bishop AT, Spinner RJ, Shin AY. Current concepts of the treatment of adult brachial plexus injuries. J Hand Surg Am. 2010;35:678–88. https://doi.org/10.1016/j.jhsa.2010.01.021.
8. Hill JR, Lanier ST, Brogan DM, Dy CJ. Management of Adult Brachial Plexus Injuries. J Hand Surg Am. 2021;46:778–88.
9. Janes LE, Crowe C, Shah N, Sasson D, Ko JH. Alternative nerve transfer for shoulder function: thoracodorsal and medial triceps to anterior axillary nerve. Plast Reconstr Surg - Glob Open. 2022;10:E4614.

10. Kaiser R, Waldauf P, Ullas G, Krajcová A. Epidemiology, etiology, and types of severe adult brachial plexus injuries requiring surgical repair: systematic review and meta-analysis. Neurosurg Rev. 2020;43:443–52.
11. Kim DH, Murovic JA, Kim YY, Kline DG. Surgical treatment and outcomes in 45 cases of posterior interosseous nerve entrapments and injuries. J Neurosurg. 2006;104:766–77.
12. Kozin SH, Porter S, Clark P, Thoder JJ. The contribution of the intrinsic muscles to grip and pinch strength. J Hand Surg Am. 1999;24:64–72.
13. Lee YH, Lu JCY, Wong A, Chang TNJ, Chuang DCC. The evolution of the reconstructive strategy for elbow flexion for acute C5, C6 brachial plexus injuries over two decades. J Reconstr Microsurg. 2022;40:3–8.
14. Lleva JMC, Munakomi S, Chang K-V. Ulnar neuropathy, in StatPearls. Treasure Island: StatPearls Publishing; 2023.
15. Novak CB. Evaluation of the patient with nerve injury or nerve compression. In: Mackinnon S, editor. Nerve surgery. 1st ed. New York: Thieme; 2015. p. 41–58.
16. Novak CB, MacKinnon SE. Distal anterior interosseous nerve transfer to the deep motor branch of the ulnar nerve for reconstruction of high ulnar nerve injuries. J Reconstr Microsurg. 2002;18:459–63.
17. Ray WZ, Chang J, Hawasli A, Wilson TJ, Yang L. Motor nerve transfers: a comprehensive review. Neurosurgery. 2015;78:1–25.
18. Samardzic MM, Grujicic DM, Rasulic LG, Milicic BR. The use of thoracodorsal nerve transfer in restoration of irreparable C5 and C6 spinal nerve lesions. Br J Plast Surg. 2005;58:541–6.
19. Strohl AB, Zelouf DS. Ulnar tunnel syndrome, radial tunnel syndrome, anterior interosseous nerve syndrome, and pronator syndrome. J Am Acad Orthop Surg. 2017;25:e1–e10.
20. Tung TH, Moore AM. Brachial Plexus Injuries. In: Mackinnon S, editor. Nerve surgery. 1st ed. New York: Thieme; 2015. p. 391–467.
21. Weber R, Davidge K. Nerve transfers for the forearm and hand. In: Mackinnon S, editor. Nerve surgery. 1st ed. New York: Thieme; 2015. p. 101–56.
22. Wolf JM, Patel R, Ghosh K. Radial tunnel syndrome: review and best evidence. J Am Acad Orthop Surg Publish Ah. 2023;31:813–9.
23. Woo A, Bakri K, Moran SL. Management of ulnar nerve injuries. J Hand Surg Am. 2015;40:173–81. https://doi.org/10.1016/j.jhsa.2014.04.038.

Nerve Transfers for Wrist, Finger, and Thumb Extension

27

Kitty Y. Wu and Amy M. Moore

27.1 Radial Nerve Anatomy

The radial nerve is one of two terminal branches of the posterior cord, receiving contributions from C5 to T1. Lying posterior to the axillary artery, it courses through the triangular space bordered by the long and lateral heads of the triceps and teres major muscles. The nerve then travels within the spiral groove, providing innervation to the triceps muscles, before piercing the lateral intermuscular septum to enter the anterior compartment of the arm. Proximal to the elbow, the radial nerve gives branches to the brachialis, brachioradialis (BR), anconeus, and extensor carpi radialis longus (ECRL). Within the forearm, the radial nerve divides into the superficial radial nerve and the posterior interosseous nerve (PIN). The superficial radial nerve emerges between the BR and ECRL tendons distally at Wartenberg's point, providing sensory innervation to the dorsal radial hand and thumb. The PIN travels deep to the supinator muscle before dividing further at its distal edge. The PIN bifurcates into a superficial branch (SBPIN) innervating the extensor digitorum communis (EDC), extensor digiti quinti (EDQ), and extensor carpi ulnaris (ECU) and a deep branch (DBPIN) innervating abductor pollicis longus (APL), extensor pollicis longus (EPL), extensor pollicis brevis (EPB), and extensor indicis proprius (EIP).

27.2 Radial Nerve Injury

The radial nerve is most commonly injured as a result of humerus fractures [1–3], but can also be affected by direct blunt or sharp trauma, compressive neuropathy, tumor infiltration, brachial neuritis, brachial plexus injuries, and iatrogenic etiologies [4–7]. Radial nerve injuries are functionally debilitating and result in the loss of wrist, finger, and thumb extension. More proximal injuries can also cause triceps weakness and the additional loss of elbow extension. While radial nerve paralysis does not directly affect the long finger and thumb flexors, grip strength is weakened due to the loss of wrist extension and the tenodesis effect. With the wrist held in passive flexion, the long finger flexors are biomechanically disadvantaged and produce an ineffective grip.

Depending on the mechanism, level of injury, timing of presentation, and patient goals, numerous reconstruction options are available including direct nerve repair, nerve grafting, nerve transfers, and tendon transfers. Primary repair, when possible, can provide good recovery

K. Y. Wu
Division of Plastic Surgery, Mayo Clinic, Rochester, MN, USA
e-mail: Wu.Kitty@mayo.edu

A. M. Moore (✉)
Department of Plastic and Reconstructive Surgery, The Ohio State University, Columbus, OH, USA
e-mail: Amy.M.Moore@osumc.edu

F. Guedes et al. (eds.), *Nerve Transfers for Brachial Plexus Reconstruction after Trauma*,
https://doi.org/10.1007/978-3-031-92445-3_27

especially with more distal injuries that are closer to the target muscle [8]. In patients presenting with a larger zone of injury, nerve grafting may be required; however, results have been variable depending on the timing of presentation, level of injury, and required length of grafts [9, 10]. Tendon transfers for radial nerve injuries are reliable, provide good results in long-term follow-up, and can be performed even in patients presenting in a delayed fashion many years after injury [11]. However, the potential disadvantages include the altered biomechanics with rerouting of muscles/tendons, prolonged postoperative immobilization, required rehabilitation and relearning of tendon transfers, and the lack of independent finger extension. Nerve transfers, in carefully selected patients, have emerged as an elegant alternative reconstructive option to restore radial nerve function.

27.3 Nerve Transfers

Nerve transfers utilize expendable and redundant motor branches to reconstruct more critical missing functions. Recovery can be optimized with faster times to reinnervation by using a normal donor motor nerve or fascicle that is close to the target muscles' motor end plates. Nerve transfers can often be performed outside of the zone of injury, avoiding dissection within a scarred bed. Compared to tendon transfers, they also do not alter the resting length, tension, or biomechanics of the involved muscles. However, unlike tendon transfers which function immediately once the tenorrhaphy is healed, nerve transfers have a requisite postoperative period of reinnervation before expected functional return. In patients with radial nerve injuries, nerve transfers provide the possibility of more independent and dextrous finger and thumb extension.

27.3.1 Patient Selection

The recovery of useful motor function from a nerve transfer is dependent on regenerating axons reaching and reinnervating the target muscle within a critical time window. Prolonged muscle denervation, greater than 18 months, results in irreversible degenerative changes at the neuromuscular junction. While open and sharp nerve injuries should be explored at the time of injury, closed injuries can be managed conservatively for a period of time to monitor for spontaneous recovery. Initial electrodiagnostic studies (EDX) performed at 6 weeks allows for Wallerian degeneration to occur and helps to establish a baseline, determine the degree of injury (neurapraxic, axonotmetic, neurometric), and potential for recovery. The appearance of motor unit action potentials (MUAPs) and nascent units at 3–4 months postinjury is a positive prognostic sign [12]. Conversely, fibrillation potentials and positive sharp waves portend a poorer prognosis. Reinnervation is expected in a "step-wise" fashion in the triceps, brachioradialis, ECRL, and ECRB, depending on the level of injury. This can be followed clinically and with EDX at a predictable rate of nerve growth at 1 mm a day and 1 inch per month [13]. The optimal time window for operative decision-making is between 4 and 6 months [2, 14, 15]. This allows for adequate time to monitor for intrinsic recovery, while balancing the ability to intervene in a timely fashion to optimize functional recovery.

Shared decision-making with the patient regarding reconstructive options should be based on their timing of presentation, occupational demands, functional goals, and ability to participate in postoperative rehabilitation. While nerve transfers ideally would be performed within 4–6 months of injury, tendon transfers can be offered even years later. Nerve transfers allow the ability for independent finger extension, while tendon transfers typically utilize a single donor to all finger extensors, resulting in composite finger extension. Another consideration is that tendon transfer options (PT, FDS, FCR) cannot not be used if the same motor branches were previously utilized as a donor for nerve transfer. The exception is PL, if present, which can be neurolyzed from the FCR motor branch and therefore preserved as a possible salvage tendon transfer option for thumb reconstruction.

27.3.2 Wrist and Finger Extension

Expendable branches of the median nerve are typically selected to reconstruct wrist and finger extension. The proximity of the median nerve to the radial nerve in the forearm allows for direct nerve coaptation without the need for interpositional nerve grafts. In patients with intact median nerve function, the two flexor digitorum superficialis (FDS), flexor carpi radialis (FCR), and palmaris longis (PL) branches are possible donor options for nerve transfer [16]. Earlier permutations of these nerve transfers involved transferring the stronger FCR branch to the ECRB; however, this was difficult for patients to relearn given the directly antagonistic actions of wrist flexion and wrist extension [12]. Instead, synergistic nerve transfers such as the FDS/PL to ECRB and FCR to PIN are preferred. This takes advantage of the synergistic tenodesis actions of wrist extension with finger flexion and wrist flexion with finger extension, which facilitates the ease of relearning these nerve transfers.

In patients with only one FDS motor branch, the PT or distal AIN motor branch to the pronator quadratus (PQ) are other possible donor options for wrist extension [17]. The PQ motor branch from the AIN is dissected distally from the proximal border of the PQ muscle to the proximal limit of the PT muscles. This is then transected distally and passed proximally under the PT to allow for primary coaptation to the ECRB motor branch. If the median nerve is also injured or unavailable as a donor option, transfer of the flexor carpi ulnaris (FCU) fascicles from the ulnar nerve to the PIN has been described [18].

In addition to the above nerve transfers, a PT to ECRB end-to-side tendon transfer can be performed at the same time, acting as an "internal brace" for wrist extension, while waiting for the ECRB reinnervation from the nerve transfer. Despite typically having two motor branches, the PT should either be used as a donor for either nerve or tendon transfer, and not both. This decision is often made intraoperatively, depending on the number of FDS nerve branches.

27.3.3 Surgical Technique: FCR to PIN, FDS to ECRB

This procedure is performed with the patient under general anesthesia, with an upper arm tourniquet. Long-acting muscle paralytic agents are avoided to allow for intraoperative stimulation. A single curvilinear incision in the proximal forearm can be used to expose both the donor median nerve branches and recipient radial nerve branches. In the superficial dissection above fascia, care is taken to protect the lateral antebrachial cutaneous (LABC) branches, which course with the cephalic vein (Fig. 27.1).

The lacertus fibrosis is released, and the forearm fascia is incised to allow for dissection of the radial vascular bundle running between the PT and BR muscles. The median nerve can then be found deep and ulnar to the radial neurovascular bundle and then traced distally to identify possible donor branches. Pronator teres step-lengthening can be performed at this stage but is usually not needed. If a PT to ECRB tendon transfer is planned, then harvesting of the PT with a periosteal extension is performed. This step, along with release of the FDS fibrous arch, allows for adequate distal exposure of the median nerve for safe dissection and identification of possible donor branches.

The anatomy of the median nerve and its branches at this level are consistent, except for possible variations in the FCR motor branch [19]. At the antecubital fossa, the first branch is to the PT, lying on the superficial surface of the median nerve, with a second more distal branch innervating the deep head. The larger-caliber AIN branches from the radial aspect of the median nerve. From the ulnar side, branches to the FCR, FDS, and PL can be identified (Fig. 27.2).

The FCR motor branch can arise either with the PL branch (35% of cases), more distally with the AIN motor branch (35% of cases), or less frequently with the distal branch of the deep head of PT [19]. Most commonly, the two FDS branches are usually more distal than the FCR [20, 21]; however in 40% of cases, there may be a single FDS branch [19]. Should this be the case, a decision can be made to preserve the FDS motor

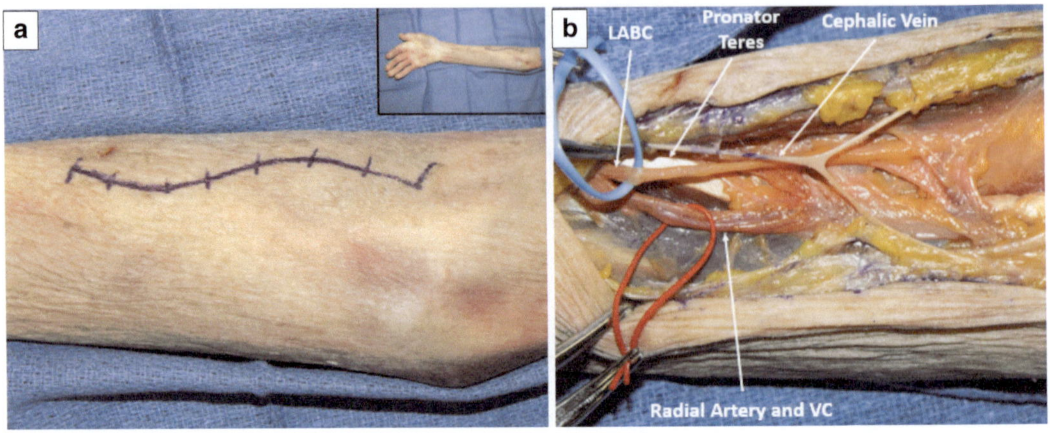

Fig. 27.1 Surgical exposure and superficial dissection. (**a**) Curvilinear incision in the proximal radial forearm. (**b**) Superficial dissection above the fascia demonstrating close relationship between the lateral antebrachial cutaneous (LABC) nerve and the cephalic vein. The radial artery and two venae comitantes course just medial to the pronator teres tendon. Distal: left, proximal: right

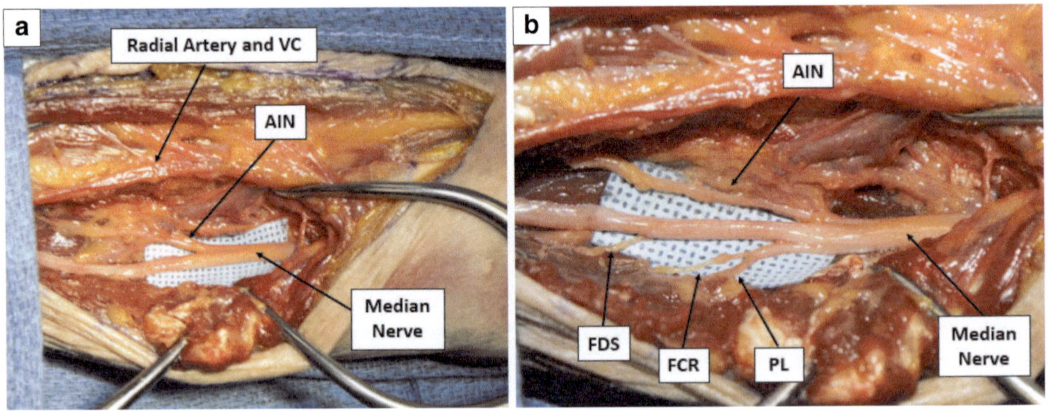

Fig. 27.2 Median nerve dissection. (**a**) The median nerve can be identified with dissection medial to the radial neurovascular bundle. The anterior interosseous nerve (AIN) branch is large caliber and the only branch along the radial side of the median nerve. (**b**) Along the ulnar side, motor branches to the PL and FCR, which often share a common trunk, and FDS are seen. This specimen has only one FDS motor branch, which is found in up to 40% of cases. Distal: left, proximal: right

branch and instead utilize the PT motor branch as an alternative donor option to restore wrist extension [22]. Intraoperative electrical stimulation should be used to confirm both the potential donor motor branches and to ensure that the critical branches are protected. Depending on the time required for this initial dissection, the tourniquet may need to be let down to allow for transient tourniquet-induced paralysis to abate. Typically, internal neurolysis is not required for donor identification, except for separation of the FCR and PL motor branches. The allows preservation of the PL innervation for use as a possible tendon transfer option for thumb extension if required as a salvage option.

Next, the radial nerve recipient branches should be identified with dissection on the radial side of the radial vessels. The superficial radial nerve can be identified on the deep surface of the brachioradialis muscle. Tracing this proximally will allow for identification of the ECRB motor and main trunk of the PIN. The vascular leash of Henry, comprised of the radial recurrent vessels, may need to be ligated for full exposure. The PIN should be followed distally as it dives under the leading edge of the supinator muscle, which can be released (Fig. 27.3a). The supinator motor branch can be excluded from the nerve transfer as an intact biceps muscle will provide adequate supination strength. Using the mantra "donor distal, recipient proximal," the recipient motor branches should be traced well proximal to the elbow crease to all for tension free primary nerve coaptation. The ECRB and PIN branches are transected proximally and transposed ulnarly toward the donor nerves, which are transected as distally as possible within the muscle bellies. The nerve coaptation from FDS to ECRB and FCR to PIN is then performed with 9-0 nylon sutures using meticulous microsurgical technique (Fig. 27.3b). After wound closure, the patient is immobilized in a posterior elbow splint for 1 week.

27.3.4 Thumb Extension

In addition to the nerve transfers for wrist and finger extension, the distal anterior interosseus nerve (DAIN) can be transferred to the deep branch of the posterior interosseus nerve (DBPIN) for thumb reconstruction [23]. In the posterior forearm, the PIN divides into a superficial branch (SBPIN) which innervates the EDC, ECU, and EDQ and a deep branch (DBPIN) which innervates the APL, EPB, EPL, and EIP.

Septocutaneous perforators from the posterior interosseous artery (PIA) can be used to help identify the interval between the ECRB and EDC. Once this interval is opened, the PIN can be identified within a fat stripe between the APL and supinator muscles. This can be traced proximally to identify the PIA coursing adjacent to the nerve and then dissected distally to identify the DBPIN. The DAIN can either be dissected through this same incision by incising through the interosseous membrane or through a separate anterior incision in the volar forearm. Adhering

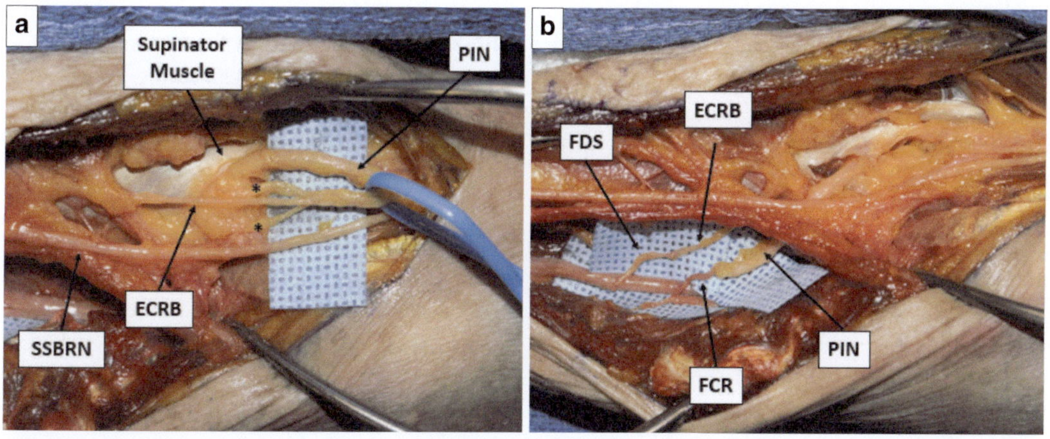

Fig. 27.3 Radial nerve dissection and nerve transfer. (**a**) Branches of the radial nerve in the proximal forearm. Following the superficial sensory branch of the radial nerve (SSBRN) from a distal to proximal direction will allow for identification of the posterior interosseous nerve (PIN), which then courses distally under the leading edge of the supinator muscle. Ulnar to this, the extensor carpi radialis brevis (ECRB) motor branch and two motor branches to the supinator muscle (*, asterix) can be found. (**b**) Nerve transfer of the FCR to PIN and FDS to ECRB can be performed following the mantra "donor distal, recipient proximal." The recipient PIN and ECRB motor branches can be passed deep to radial artery. Of note, this illustrates the most common set of median nerve-based transfers; however, typically if there was only one FDS motor branch, then the AIN motor branch to the pronator quadratus or pronator teres motor branch can be used as a donor instead. Distal: left, proximal: right

to the same adage of "donor distal, recipient proximal," the AIN is traced as distally as possible into the pronator quadratus muscle before division, while the DBPIN is cut as proximally as possible. The DAIN is brought proximally toward the DBPIN, which is brought distally to allow for primary coaptation.

27.4 Outcomes

First described by Lowe et al. in 2002, median nerve-based nerve transfers have been used for reconstruction in both patients with isolated radial nerve palsy and with brachial plexus injuries [16, 24]. Ray et al. reviewed 19 patients with radial nerve injuries undergoing median nerve based nerve transfers at a mean of 5.7 months postinjury. At a minimum of 1-year follow-up, 18 patients had Medical Research Council (MRC) ≥ 4 wrist extension, and 12 patients had ≥ MRC 4 finger and thumb extension. The one patient with a poor outcome and M0 wrist extension underwent an FCR to ECRB nerve transfer [25]. This patient's recovery was thought to be hindered by the antagonistic nature of this transfer and the associated difficulty in motor reeducation. Half of the patients in this series also underwent simultaneous PT to ECRB tendon transfers for wrist extension and therefore difficult to separate the individual contributions of the nerve versus tendon transfer on wrist extension strength. Comparable results of six patients undergoing PT to ECRL and FCR to PIN nerve transfers were reported by Garcia-Lopez et al. where all patients achieved ≥M4 wrist extension and four of six patients had ≥M4 finger and thumb extension [26].

Bertelli compared the outcomes of his patients with radial nerve lesions undergoing nerve transfer (AIN to ECRB and FCR to PIN) within 12 months of injury to those with tendon transfers (PT to ECRB, FCU to EDC, PL to EPL) greater than 12 months from injury [27]. Both tendon and nerve transfer options for wrist extension were reliable, with all patients in both groups achieving M4 strength. However, the nerve transfer group demonstrated improved wrist extension and flexion range of motion (67° and 66°, respectively) compared to the tendon transfer group (35° and 37°). Furthermore, almost 70% of patients with tendon transfers had limitations in passive wrist flexion, and five patients had permanent radial wrist deviation, neither of which were observed in the nerve transfer group. Other than two patients in each group, the majority of patients in both the nerve and tendon transfer group achieved M4 finger extension. However, 86% of patients in the nerve transfer group achieved M4 finger extension with the wrist either in neutral or an extended position, while this was possible in only 54% of tendon transfer patients. Nerve and tendon transfer options for restoration of thumb extension were similarly less predictable. Only one patient in each group recovered full motion at the thumb carpometacarpal (CMC), metacarpal-phalangeal (MCP), and interphalangeal (IP) joints and two patients in each group had failed reconstruction. Similar to the differences between achievable wrist range of motion following tendon and nerve transfers, full CMC joint was observed in 79% of nerve transfer and only 31% of tendon transfer patients. Both groups, however, had a 30° extension lag, poor EPL recovery, and failure of achieving full MCP extension. Bertelli hypothesized the lower number of nerve fibers in the donor FCR as compared to the PIN as a possible explanation for poor recovery [28]. This led to the addition of the DAIN to DBPIN nerve transfer to augment thumb function. In five patients that underwent this nerve transfer, all achieved full CMC range of motion [23]. Two patients achieved full MCP range of motion, while the other three had a residual 15–20° lag at the MCP joint. All patients were able to regain independent thumb and finger extension.

Patterson et al. also presented their comparison of a single institution's outcomes from nerve versus tendon transfers for isolated radial nerve palsy [29]. In this review of 30 patients with tendon transfers with mean 45-week follow-up and 16 patients with nerve transfers with mean 105-week follow-up, both groups had improvements in grip and pinch strength. Nerve transfers, however, had greater recovery of grip strength

(14.7 kg preoperatively to 56.1 kg postoperatively) compared to tendon transfers (25.5 kg preoperatively to 34.4 kg postoperatively). Of note, 15 of 16 patients in the nerve transfer group underwent concomitant PT to ECRB tendon transfer to augment wrist extension. Among patients undergoing tendon transfers with recorded strength measurements, 7 of 7 had ≥M4 wrist extension and 2 of 2 had ≥M4 finger and thumb extension. In comparison to patients with recorded measurements following nerve transfers, 11 of 13 had ≥M4 wrist extension and 7 of 11 had ≥M4 finger and thumb extension. Both groups had similar improvements in disabilities of the arm, shoulder, and hand and quality of life scores.

A 2018 systematic review comparing tendon and nerve transfers for radial nerve palsy, which included 16 studies, demonstrated equivalent outcomes between the two techniques. Among the studies reporting motor outcomes, 93% of tendon transfers and 96% of nerve transfer patients achieved ≥M3 wrist extension. Ninety-one percent of tendon transfer patients achieved ≥M4 wrist extension. A more recent systematic review in 2023 comparing 339 tendon transfer and 64 nerve transfer patients concluded that tendon transfers were the most reliable method for reconstruction [30]. A "good outcome" was considered ≥M4 strength, >6 on the Bincaz scale, > 3 on the Louisiana State University Health System scale, antigravity strength on the Haas scale, or "very good/good" on the Zachary scale [30]. Comparative analysis demonstrated a good outcome in 82% of tendon transfer and 59% of nerve transfer patients. Poor outcomes were seen in 9% of tendon transfer and 13% of nerve transfer patients. In subgroup analysis, both nerve and tendon transfers had superior results for restoring wrist extension compared to finger and thumb extension. Considering the outcomes of wrist extension alone, 71% of nerve transfer and 96% of tendon transfer patients had a good outcome. The disparity between the conclusions of the two systematic reviews may be reflective of the consideration of predominantly wrist extension outcomes in the first review and wrist, finger, and thumb outcomes in the latter. Also the definition of a "good outcome" in the second review includes multiple different rating scales and outcome measures. Therefore, although "good outcomes" were compared between nerve and tendon transfer patients, different specific outcome measures were being compared amongst the studies. While the performance of nerve transfers for radial nerve palsy needs to be fully explored in a larger patient population with longer follow-up, the results from multiple groups thus far highly encouraging.

27.5 Conclusions

Tendon transfers for radial nerve palsy have withstood the test of time as a reliable reconstructive option; however, there is a growing literature to support the use of nerve transfers as an exciting alternative option. For patients that present early following injury, nerve transfers may provide the opportunity for improved wrist range of motion, full finger extension with wrist extension, and independent finger function. Ultimately, the decision to pursue either tendon transfers or nerve transfers, or a combination, should be tailored to help the patient best achieve their functional goals.

References

1. Mast JW, Spiegel PG, Harvey JP Jr, Harrison C. Fractures of the humeral shaft: a retrospective study of 240 adult fractures. Clin Orthop Relat Res. 1975;112:254–62.
2. Ring D, Chin K, Jupiter JB. Radial nerve palsy associated with high-energy humeral shaft fractures. J Hand Surg Am. 2004;29(1):144–7. https://doi.org/10.1016/j.jhsa.2003.09.013.
3. Ekholm R, Adami J, Tidermark J, Hansson K, Tornkvist H, Ponzer S. Fractures of the shaft of the humerus. An epidemiological study of 401 fractures. J Bone Joint Surg Br. 2006;88(11):1469–73. https://doi.org/10.1302/0301-620X.88B11.17634.
4. Kim DH, Kam AC, Chandika P, Tiel RL, Kline DG. Surgical management and outcome in patients with radial nerve lesions. J Neurosurg. 2001;95(4):573–83. https://doi.org/10.3171/jns.2001.95.4.0573.
5. Kim DH, Cho YJ, Tiel RL, Kline DG. Outcomes of surgery in 1019 brachial plexus lesions treated at

Louisiana State University Health Sciences Center. J Neurosurg. 2003;98(5):1005–16. https://doi.org/10.3171/jns.2003.98.5.1005.

6. Wu KY, Cook DJ, Amrami KK, Spinner RJ. Radial nerve myofibroma: a rare benign tumor with perineural infiltration. Illustrative case. J Neurosurg Case Lessons. 2023;5(19) https://doi.org/10.3171/CASE23115.
7. Midha R. Epidemiology of brachial plexus injuries in a multitrauma population. Neurosurgery. 1997;40(6):1182–8.; discussion 1188–9. https://doi.org/10.1097/00006123-199706000-00014.
8. Ljungquist KL, Martineau P, Allan C. Radial nerve injuries. J Hand Surg Am. 2015;40(1):166–72. https://doi.org/10.1016/j.jhsa.2014.05.010.
9. Bertelli JA, Ghizoni MF. Results of nerve grafting in radial nerve injuries occurring proximal to the humerus, including those within the posterior cord. J Neurosurg. 2016;2016(1):179–85. https://doi.org/10.3171/2014.12.JNS141944.test.
10. Zhu S, Lei GW, Pang Z, Gao ZR, Shen YD, Xu WD. Outcomes and prognostic factors for nerve grafting following high radial nerve injury. J Hand Surg Eur. 2023;48(8):747–54. https://doi.org/10.1177/17531934221147651.
11. Ropars M, Dreano T, Siret P, Belot N, Langlais F. Long-term results of tendon transfers in radial and posterior interosseous nerve paralysis. J Hand Surg Br. 2006;31(5):502–6. https://doi.org/10.1016/j.jhsb.2006.05.020.
12. Mackinnon SE. Nerve transfers for the forearm and hand. Nerve Surgery. Thieme; 2015.
13. Seddon HJ, Medawar PB, Smith H. Rate of regeneration of peripheral nerves in man. J Physiol. 1943;102(2):191–215. https://doi.org/10.1113/jphysiol.1943.sp004027.
14. Foster RJ, Swiontkowski MF, Bach AW, Sack JT. Radial nerve palsy caused by open humeral shaft fractures. J Hand Surg Am. 1993;18(1):121–4. https://doi.org/10.1016/0363-5023(93)90255-2.
15. Niver GE, Ilyas AM. Management of radial nerve palsy following fractures of the humerus. Orthop Clin North Am. 2013;44(3):419–24. https://doi.org/10.1016/j.ocl.2013.03.012.
16. Lowe JB 3rd, Tung TR, Mackinnon SE. New surgical option for radial nerve paralysis. Plast Reconstr Surg. 2002;110(3):836–43. https://doi.org/10.1097/00006534-200209010-00019.
17. Bertelli JA, Tacca CP, Winkelmann Duarte EC, Ghizoni MF, Duarte H. Transfer of the pronator quadratus motor branch for wrist extension reconstruction in brachial plexus palsy. Plast Reconstr Surg. 2012;130(6):1269–78. https://doi.org/10.1097/PRS.0b013e31826d16cf.
18. Weber RVMS. Upper extremity nerve transfers. In: Slutsky DJHV, editor. Peripheral nerve surgery: practice applications in the upper extremity. Churchill Livingstone: Elsevier; 2006.
19. Bertelli JA, Patel N, Soldado F, Duarte ECW. Patterns of median nerve branching in the cubital fossa: implications for nerve transfers to restore motor function in a paralyzed upper limb. J Neurosurg. 2021;135(5):1524–33. https://doi.org/10.3171/2020.9.Jns202742.
20. Mackinnon SE, Roque B, Tung TH. Median to radial nerve transfer for treatment of radial nerve palsy. Case report. J Neurosurg. 2007;107(3):666–71. https://doi.org/10.3171/JNS-07/09/0666.
21. Brown JM, Tung TH, Mackinnon SE. Median to radial nerve transfer to restore wrist and finger extension: technical nuances. Neurosurgery. 2010;66(3 Suppl Operative):75–83.; discussion 83. https://doi.org/10.1227/01.NEU.0000354364.13224.C8.
22. Tian J, Leng M, Wang K, Huang Q. Pronator teres nerve branch transfer to the extensor carpi radialis brevis nerve branch for wrist extension reconstruction in proximal radial nerve injury following humeral shaft fractures. BMC Musculoskelet Disord. 2022;23(1):980. https://doi.org/10.1186/s12891-022-05950-1.
23. Bertelli JA, Nehete S, Winkelmann Duarte EC, Ghizoni MF. Transfer of the Distal Anterior Interosseous Nerve for Thumb Motion Reconstruction in Radial Nerve Paralysis. J Hand Surg Am. 2020;45(9):877 e1–10. https://doi.org/10.1016/j.jhsa.2020.02.011.
24. Ukrit A, Leechavengvongs S, Malungpaishrope K, Uerpairojkit C, Chongthammakun S, Witoonchart K. Nerve transfer for wrist extension using nerve to flexor digitorum superficialis in cervical 5, 6, and 7 root avulsions: anatomic study and report of two cases. J Hand Surg Am. 2009;34(9):1659–66. https://doi.org/10.1016/j.jhsa.2009.07.004.
25. Ray WZ, Mackinnon SE. Clinical outcomes following median to radial nerve transfers. J Hand Surg Am. 2011;36(2):201–8. https://doi.org/10.1016/j.jhsa.2010.09.034.
26. Garcia-Lopez A, Navarro R, Martinez F, Rojas A. Nerve transfers from branches to the flexor carpi radialis and pronator teres to reconstruct the radial nerve. J Hand Surg Am. 2014;39(1):50–6. https://doi.org/10.1016/j.jhsa.2013.10.011.
27. Bertelli JA. Nerve versus tendon transfer for radial nerve paralysis reconstruction. J Hand Surg Am. 2020;45(5):418–26. https://doi.org/10.1016/j.jhsa.2019.12.009.
28. Sukegawa K, Suzuki T, Ogawa Y, Kobayashi T, Matsuura Y, Kuniyoshi K. A Cadaver Study of Median-to-Radial Nerve Transfer for Radial Nerve Injuries. J Hand Surg Am. 2016;41(1):20–6. https://doi.org/10.1016/j.jhsa.2015.10.015.
29. Patterson JMM, Russo SA, El-Haj M, Novak CB, Mackinnon SE. Radial nerve palsy: nerve transfer versus tendon transfer to restore function. Hand (N Y). 2022;17(6):1082–9. https://doi.org/10.1177/1558944720988126.
30. Jain NS, Barr ML, Kim D, Jones NF. Tendon transfers, nerve grafts, and nerve transfers for isolated radial nerve palsy: a systematic review and analysis. Hand (N Y). 2023:15589447221150516. https://doi.org/10.1177/15589447221150516.

28 Sensory Nerve Transfers for Nerve Injuries

Sami Ramadan, Shayoni Nag, and Amy M. Moore

28.1 Introduction

Nerve injuries affecting the upper limb can be functionally devastating. They predominantly occur as a result of trauma, but other etiologies exist including cancer, benign tumors, and iatrogenic causes. Complete functional recovery, despite surgical intervention, is relatively rare, and thus nerve injuries have a significant socioeconomic impact [1, 2].

Nerve injuries can occur anywhere along the upper extremity from the brachial plexus at the neck to the digital nerve in the hand. They are graded according to the level of injury (supraclavicular or infraclavicular), type of injury (avulsion, traction/stretch or rupture), and degree of injury (neurapraxia, axonotmesis or neurotmesis). These factors determine the severity of injury and resulting deficits. Deficits can include loss of motor function, sensation, and sympathetic/autonomic regulation.

Reconstructive efforts have been focused, for the most part, on motor deficits. With the advancement of nerve transfers and the increased understanding of intraneural topography, improvements in functional motor outcomes compared to nerve grafting have been observed [3]. Less focus has been on sensory restoration, and nerve transfers for the restoration of sensation have not advanced as fast as their motor counterparts. In this chapter, we will review the principles of nerve transfers in the setting of sensory deficits and highlight the available nerve transfers that can be used for restoration of sensation.

28.2 Principles of Nerve Transfers

Nerve transfers consist of transferring an expendable or redundant donor nerve to a recipient nerve for either motor or sensory restoration [3, 4]. The benefits of nerve transfers are that it can occur closer to the target organ (muscle or skin) than the original nerve injury. Given the slow rate of nerve regeneration, i.e., 1 mm/day, nerve transfers closer to the target effectively reduce the regeneration time needed for nerve recovery. Nerve transfers also avoid the need for nerve grafting and the potential of loss of axons across two coaptation sites. The ability to perform an end-to-end coaptation is that the donor nerve is harvested "distally" and the recipient "proximally" to allow for a tension-free repair. Lastly, nerve transfers can often be performed in a non-traumatized field closer to the target organ and away from the primary nerve injury. This provides an improved regenerative environment for the nerve repair.

S. Ramadan · S. Nag · A. M. Moore (✉)
The Ohio State University Wexner Medical Center, Department of Plastic and Reconstructive Surgery, Columbus, OH, USA
e-mail: Sami.Ramadan@osumc.edu; Shayoni.Nag@osumc.edu; amy.m.moore@osumc.edu

F. Guedes et al. (eds.), *Nerve Transfers for Brachial Plexus Reconstruction after Trauma*,
https://doi.org/10.1007/978-3-031-92445-3_28

For both motor and sensory nerve transfers, *timing* of the intervention after the nerve injury is important. It is well understood that motor endplates in muscle have a finite life span of about 12–18 months after injury after which irreparable neuromuscular loss occurs [3]. For this reason, and taking account slow nerve regeneration speeds, surgical interventions with nerve repair or grafting for proximal injuries resulted in less than ideal functional outcomes. Motor transfers therefore need to be planned and undertaken relatively early—ideally within 6 months of injury—to account for these factors.

Conversely, sensory nerve transfers may not be subject to the same time-constraints. Sensory end organs are thought to have a higher denervation tolerance potentially allowing for delayed sensory nerve transfers in cases of failure or inadequate reinnervation with alternative treatments [3, 5]. However, the ideal sensory reinnervation window is poorly understood. It is posited that early reinnervation, though not an absolute requirement, may result in better outcomes [6].

28.2.1 Nerve Transfers Vs Nerve Grafting and Primary Repair

In recent years, nerve transfers have superseded nerve grafts and direct nerve repairs for the management of motor loss in proximal brachial plexus injuries. This phenomenon has not universally been applied to sensory loss. Restoring continuity to a nerve is thought to modulate the pain response associated with nerve injuries [5]. Repairing or grafting a sensory nerve at the site of injury may address the neuropathic pain that can occur in these patients. For this reason, and the lack of defined time constraints, primary nerve repairs and grafting are currently the preferred treatments for sensory nerve injuries.

There are, however, limitations to using nerve grafts. Factors such as reinnervation distance; nerve gap length; mechanism of injury (with inability to determine quality of remaining nerve), as well as age; and, as mentioned earlier, time from injury may all impact recovery [3–5]. Longer nerve grafts have been found to result in poorer outcomes, and, particularly in motor transfers, the type of graft used (motor vs sensory nerves) can affect recovery [3, 7]. For these reasons, nerve transfers are presently often used when grafting, and primary repair are not available or as salvage procedures.

28.2.2 Sensory Nerve Transfers

Sensation is a critical tool in the interaction with our environment and, some argue, the most important hand function. Our hands provide tactile feedback, proprioception for fine control and the ability to detect—and therefore withdraw—from noxious and potentially harmful stimuli [8, 9]. Thus, the focus of sensory reinnervation attempts have been on restoring critical sensation to the hand.

The hand has established critical sensory areas. The ulnar border of the hand innervated by the ulnar nerve, as well as the thumb and index finger pinch areas innervated by the median nerve, are considered priorities [3, 5, 8]. The former area is key for nociceptive withdrawals, and the latter is more important for the functional use of the hand. Re-establishing protective sensation to the limb, although difficult, can also be beneficial in pan-plexus injuries with resulting trophic ulceration and poor skin quality due to autonomic dysfunction.

The first successful description of a sensory nerve transfer was reported in 1921 and involved the transfer of the superficial radial nerve to a distal branch of the median nerve [10]. Since then, a number of sensory transfers have been described in the literature with variable outcomes. The numbers are low compared to motor nerve transfers and the heterogeneity in outcome measurement limit the ability to reach meaningful conclusions regarding their use and indications [5].

Sensory nerve transfers, like their motor counterparts, are preferably performed in an end-to-

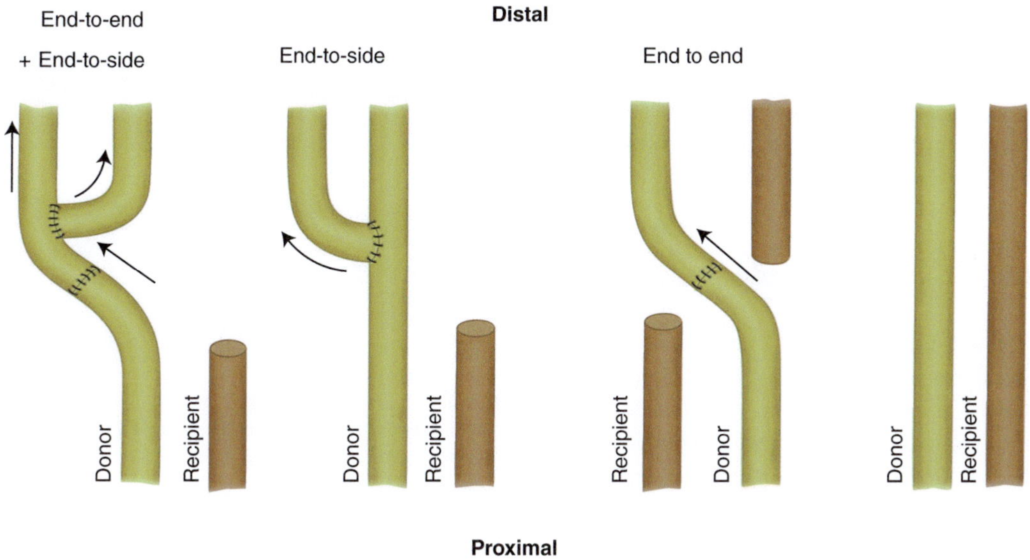

Fig. 28.1 Types of sensory nerve transfers. Green indicates live and reinnervated nerve and arrows describe direction of nerve regeneration. End-to-end transfer is preferred to restore sensation in critical area. End-to-side can be used in conjunction with end-to-end transfer to restore a degree of protective sensation in the donor area

end fashion; however, they can also be transferred end-to-side although this results in limited sensory recovery [3, 11]. An end-to-side transfer involves suturing the proximal end of the recipient nerve to the side of an intact donor nerve. This can be done alone or in addition to an end-to-end transfer. An additional end-to-side transfer could be performed to potentially restore protective sensation to the donor nerve as a backfill. Thus, after the donor nerve is transected and transferred in an end-to-end fashion, the distal end of the donor nerve can be connected in an end-to-side fashion to the recipient nerve. This is done to re-establish some protective sensation in the donor nerve territory (Fig. 28.1).

Another factor affecting outcomes includes the proximity of nerve transfers; distal nerve transfers seem to fare better than proximal transfers in the reported literature [5]. In general, sensory transfers have been described as proximal, distal, and very distal, indicating the axilla/arm, forearm, and hand, respectively [12]. Common sensory transfers are described from distal to proximal in the following section.

28.3 Sensory Nerve Transfers

28.3.1 Median Nerve Territory Sensory Loss

Sensation in the median nerve territory is affected in upper trunk injuries of the brachial plexus or, more commonly, in high or low median nerve injuries. Despite adequate repair or grafting, there is often suboptimal recovery due to the long reinnervation distance. This sensory loss affects the first webspace, thumb, index and middle fingers, particularly on the volar aspect. In our experience, this sensory loss is relatively well-tolerated in upper trunk injuries, but more bothersome in isolated median nerve injuries. Patients can suffer from ulceration and injury to the affected fingertips.

28.3.1.1 Ulnar (Fourth Webspace) to Median (First Webspace) Nerve Transfer: Very Distal

The ulnar nerve, arising from the lower trunk, remains intact upper trunk or direct median nerve injuries and is available for nerve transfers. The branch to the fourth webspace is purely sensory and considered noncritical. It can be transferred to the sensory branch to the first webspace, thereby innervating the thumb and radial border of the index finger [6, 13–15].

28.3.2 Surgical Procedure

A distal palmar volar Bruner incision in the fourth webspace is made, and the common digital nerve is identified along with its branches to the ulnar aspect of the ring finger and radial aspect of the ring finger. A second incision is made in the midpalm, distal to the carpal tunnel. The sensory branch of the median nerve to the first webspace is identified and traced to its bifurcation to the thumb and radial aspect of the index finger (Fig. 28.2). The fourth webspace nerve is divided distal to its bifurcation and tunneled subcutaneously to the first webspace incision. The two donor nerve ends are coapted under the microscope to the two recipients without any tension (Fig. 28.3).

Alternatively, incisions extending into the finger and isolating proper digital nerves to the ulnar aspect of the ring finger or radial aspect of the little finger have been described [6]. The proper digital nerve can be used individually and transferred to the thumb or index as needed.

28.3.2.1 Radial Sensory (Thumb and Index) to Median (First Webspace) Nerve Transfer: Very Distal

In the upper trunk brachial plexus and isolated median nerve injuries, the radial nerve function remains intact and can be used as a donor nerve. The dorsal sensory radial nerve branches of the index finger and thumb can be transferred to the median-innervated first webspace recipients with minimal to no donor site morbidity [12].

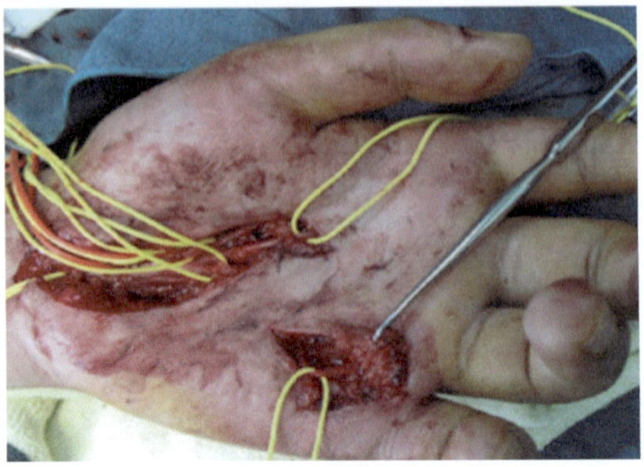

Fig. 28.2 Incision 1 is a distal palmar volar incision in the fourth webspace. Incision 2 in midpalm to expose the donor and recipient nerves. (Source: Emamhadi and Andalib [13])

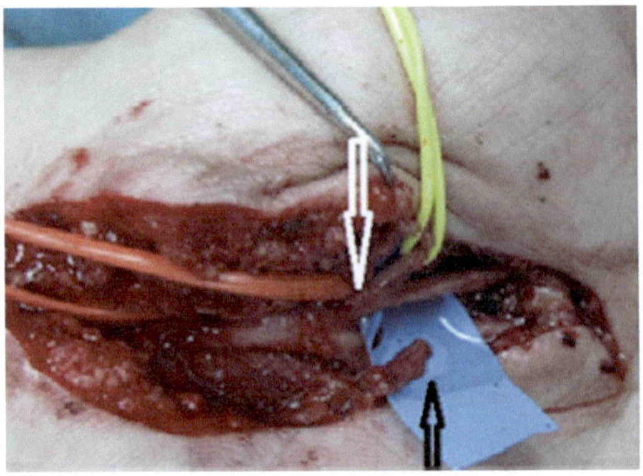

Fig. 28.3 The fourth webspace nerve is tunneled subcutaneously to the first webspace incision, and the donor's nerve is coapted to the recipient nerve. (Source: Emamhadi and Andalib [14])

28.3.3 Surgical Procedure

After a detailed preoperative evaluation of dorsal sensory boundaries to the thumb and index, V-shaped incisions are made on the dorso-radial aspect of the index finger and on the dorso-ulnar aspect of the thumb [12]. It is important to ensure the incisions are within sensate territories identified on exam. Through these incisions, the dorsal radial nerves and the volar median nerves are

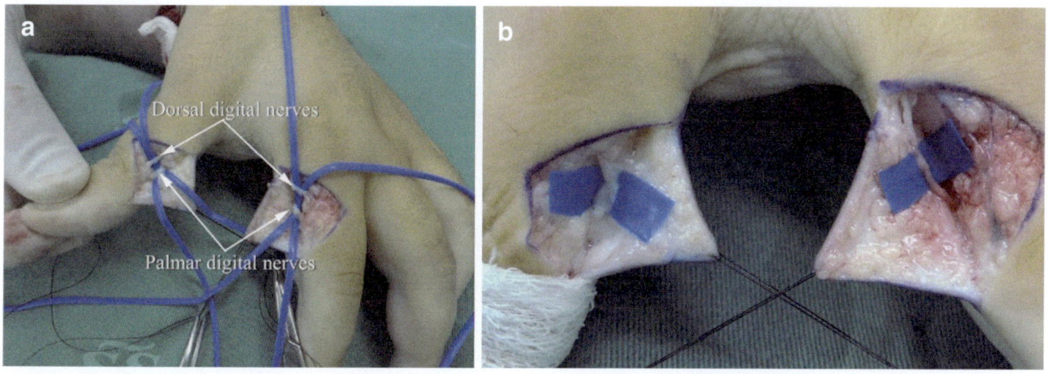

Fig. 28.4 (**a**) View of the dissection of dorsal and palmar nerves in the proximal phalanx of the thumb and index finger. (**b**) Intraoperative view of the coaptation site. The donor nerve is sectioned distally, whereas the recipient is sectioned more proximally to allow for redundancy of the nerve stumps. (Source: Bertelli and Ghizoni [12])

identified. The distal radial nerve branches are transected distally and the median nerve branches are transected proximally. The branches are sutured under the microscope without any tension (Fig. 28.4).

28.3.3.1 Dorsal Cutaneous Branch of the Ulnar Nerve to the Branches of the Median Nerve: Distal

The use of the dorsal cutaneous branch of the ulnar nerve in the forearm for nerve transfer to the median nerve is an option for sensory restoration of the hand [12, 16]. In this transfer, the dorsal cutaneous branch of the ulnar nerve is transferred end-to-end to the first webspace branch of the median nerve to restore critical radial thumb and first web space sensation.

Restoration of donor site sensation, i.e., "noncritical sensation," can be performed by an end-to-side coaptation of the distal dorsal cutaneous branch of the ulnar nerve (non-transferred end) to the side of the intact superficial sensory branch of the ulnar nerve. This will provide some protective sensation to the dorsal hand. The use of an end-to-side coaptation of the distal third webspace fascicles of the median nerve to restore noncritical sensation has also been described [17].

28.3.4 Surgical Procedure

A curvilinear incision is made in the distal forearm to expose both the ulnar and median nerves. A carpal tunnel release is also performed to confirm the first webspace fascicular topography and to release any distal nerve entrapment. The dorsal cutaneous ulnar branch of the ulnar nerve is identified on the most ulnar aspect of the ulnar nerve. Neurolysis of this branch is performed distally as it travels dorsally onto the dorsal hand. The first webspace nerve branches are identified distally in the hand, and the first webspace nerve branch is separated from the thenar motor fascicle. The recipient first webspace nerve branch is transected proximally in the forearm and brought toward the dorsal cutaneous nerve branch. The dorsal cutaneous nerve is transected in the distal forearm, and the nerve transfer is performed in an end-to-end fashion for critical sensation restoration. For noncritical sensation, i.e., restoring protective sensation to the donor site, the remaining distal dorsal cutaneous branch at the distal forearm (and the third web space fascicle, if desired) can be coapted to the intact sensory component of the ulnar nerve in an end-to-side fashion (Fig. 28.5) [17].

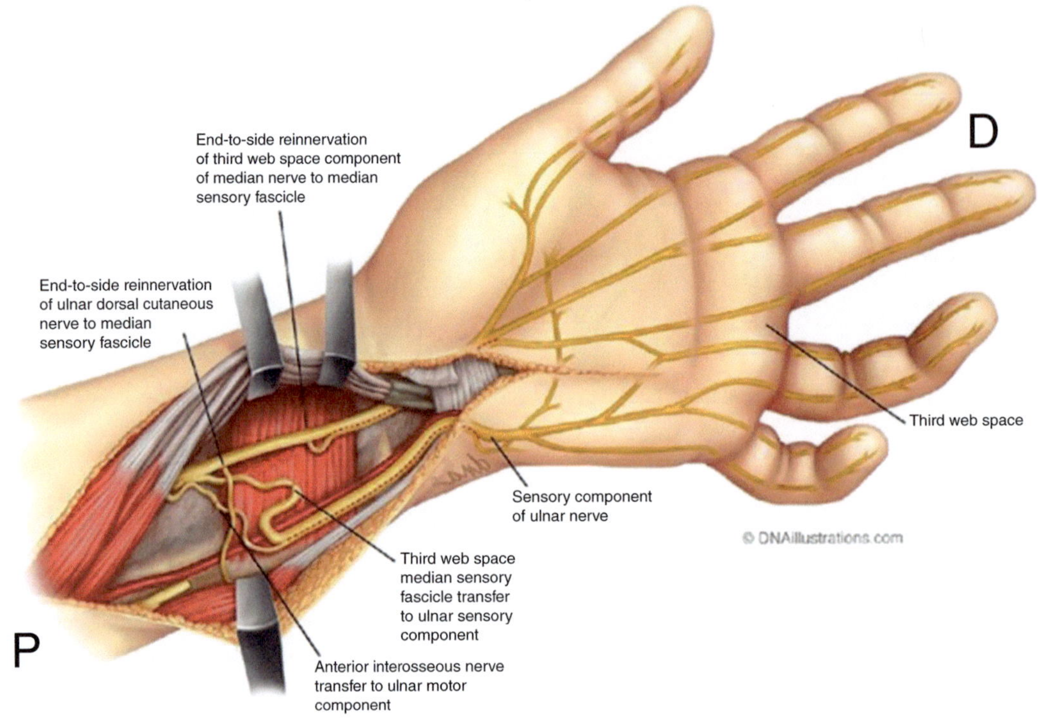

Fig. 28.5 End-to-side reinnervation of dorsal branch of ulnar nerve to median sensory nerve fascicle. Orientation: left hand, proximal (P) and distal (D). (Source: Brown et al. [17])

28.3.4.1 Superficial Radial Nerve to Median Nerve: Distal

The radial nerve can be used as a nerve transfer in cases where the ulnar nerve is not available [18]. There are documented reports—and it is our experience—that the radial nerve can be symptomatic at the donor site [18]. This donor site pain can be problematic and difficult to manage. Thus, we do not recommend this transfer.

28.3.5 Ulnar Nerve Territory Sensory Loss

The ulnar nerve is predominantly innervated by the C8 and T1 nerve roots and arises from the medial cord. There are three terminal branches of the ulnar nerve: the dorsal cutaneous sensory branch, the motor branch, and the sensory branch that extends into the hand. The sensory loss in ulnar nerve injuries thus involves the medial/ulnar aspect of the palm, the entirety of the small finger and part of the ring finger, and the dorso-ulnar aspect of the hand. The ulnar aspect of the small finger is considered a critical sensory area and helps with nociceptive withdrawal from pain if in contact with a noxious stimuli. Reinnervation of the sensory branch of the ulnar nerve traveling into the hand is the target of sensory nerve transfers.

28.3.5.1 Median (Third Webspace) to the Ulnar Sensory Branch Nerve Transfer: Very Distal or Distal

The third web space branch of the median nerve is considered noncritical sensation and can be neurolyzed from distally in the hand to proximally in the forearm. The restoration of critical ulnar nerve sensation can be performed with an end-to-end coaptation to the main sensory branch ulnar nerve in the either the palm, wrist, or distal forearm. The distal forearm is preferred site for this nerve transfer when the median nerve is the donor as it can restore critical sensation to the ulnar hand, small finger, and the ulnar half of the ring finger [17].

28.3.6 Surgical Procedure

A curvilinear incision in the distal forearm is made for adequate exposure of the median and ulnar nerves. A carpal tunnel and Guyon canal release is performed distally into the hand to expose the nerves and their terminal branches. In the forearm, the third web space fascicles of the median nerve can be identified as the median nerve's most superficial and ulnar-laying fascicles. Microforceps can also be used to define a natural plane separating the third webspace fascicle from the rest of the nerve. However, identifying the branch distally in the hand and neurolyzing it proximally is also an option. The sensory branch of the ulnar nerve is identified distally in the hand and separated from the motor component which dives deep under the hypothenar musculature. A plane is developed between the motor and sensory fascicular groups of the ulnar nerve at Guyon's canal and followed proximally. Complete neurolysis of these two branches is not necessary as long as the knowledge and the topography is confirmed distally. The third webspace donor is transected distally and transferred in an end-to-end fashion to the sensory component of the ulnar nerve (Fig. 28.6).

28.3.6.1 Palmar Cutaneous Branch of Median Nerve to the Ulnar Nerve (Sensory Branch of Ulnar Nerve or Ulnar Digital Nerve of the Fifth Finger): Very Distal or Distal

The palmar cutaneous nerve of the median has been described as a donor nerve to restore sensation on the ulnar side of the hand in lower plexus injuries [19, 20]. The palmar cutaneous branch of the median nerve is not thought to be "critical sensation" and can be transferred to the ulnar digital nerve of the small finger or to the sensory branch of the ulnar nerve in the palm or distal forearm, respectively [19, 20].

28.3.7 Surgical Procedure

To expose the ulnar nerve at the level of the wrist and access Guyon's canal, a longitudinal incision in the palm is made in line with the ulnar aspect of the ring finger. The incision is carried across the wrist in a zigzag manner, extending longitudinally onto the forearm. The ulnar and median nerves are identified in the distal forearm. The palmar cutaneous branch of the median nerve is identified on the radial aspect of the median nerve about 5–6 cm proximal to the wrist crease. The nerve branch is transected distally and brought over to the ulnar nerve. The sensory branch of the ulnar nerve is then separated from motor branch

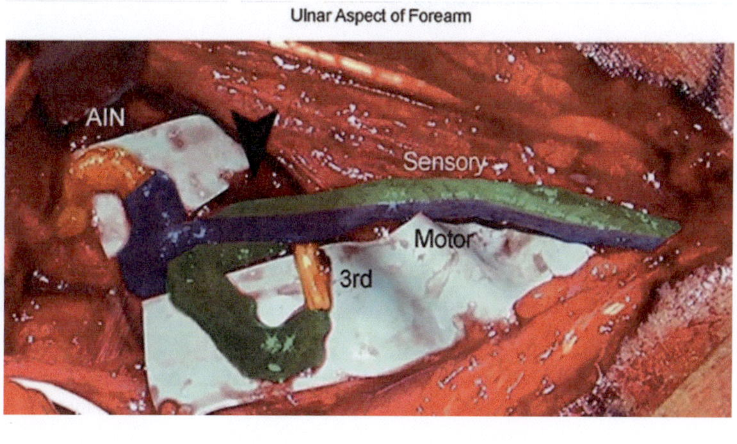

Fig. 28.6 Motor: AIN of median nerve (yellow) transferred to deep motor fascicle of the ulnar (blue). Sensory: Third webspace fascicle of median (yellow) transferred to sensory fascicle of the ulnar (green). (Source: Brown et al. [17])

and transected proximally. A tension free end-to-end coaptation is performed under the microscope (Fig. 28.7).

28.3.7.1 Superficial Branch of the Radial Nerve to the Sensory Branch of the Ulnar Nerve: Distal

In the setting of lower root brachial plexus injuries, the superficial radial nerve can be transferred to the sensory branch of the ulnar nerve. [21, 22] As mentioned above with the median nerve, we do not recommend this transfer in isolated ulnar nerve injuries given the potential donor site morbidity and neuropathic pain that can occur with harvesting the radial sensory nerve.

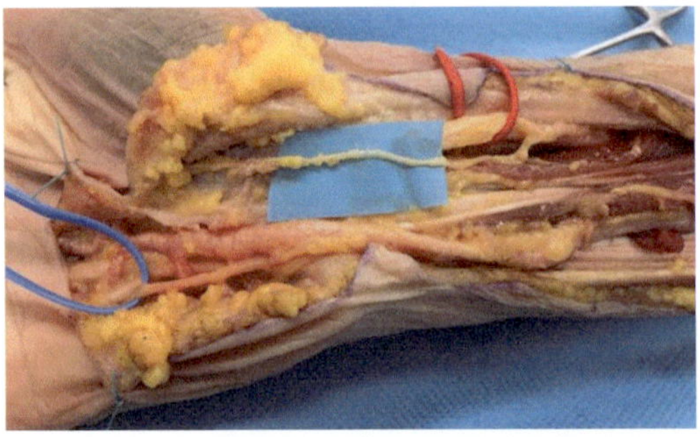

Fig. 28.7 Release of the palmar cutaneous branch of the median nerve. Blue loop isolates the sensory branch of the ulnar nerve. Red loop identifies the median nerve, and the palmar cutaneous branch was released as far as possible. (Source: Nguyễn et al. [20])

28.3.8 Surgical Procedure

An S-shaped incision starting at the radial styloid is made to expose the brachioradialis tendon and identify the superficial radial nerve. The radial nerve is neurolyzed distally into its multiple terminal branches. The most radial branch can be isolated and transferred to the ulnar nerve. A second incision is made on the ulnar side of the wrist and extended across the wrist in a zigzag fashion. A Guyon's canal is performed and the sensory branch of the ulnar nerve is identified. The radial branch of superficial radial nerve is transected distally then subcutaneously tunneled volarly to the ulnar sensory branch and coapted in an end-to-end fashion (Fig. 28.8).

28.3.9 Proximal Nerve Transfers in the Setting of Complete Brachial Plexus Injury

When treating proximal injuries including complete brachial plexus injuries, motor reconstruction has been the priority. However, a significant aspect of function relates to sensation, and this should be taken into consideration when embarking on functional reconstruction of the extremity. The intercostal nerves, intercostobrachial nerve, and supraclavicular nerve as well as CC7 have all been described as donors for sensory restoration [23–26].

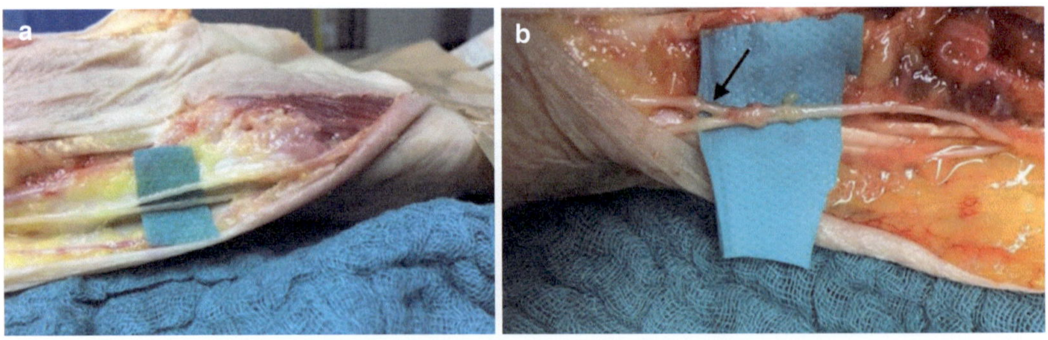

Fig. 28.8 (**a**) The superficial radial nerve (SRN). The superficial radial nerve (SRN) gives two subdivisions. (**b**) The superficial branch of the radial nerve (SBRN). The most radial one gives a little thenar branch and the dorsal radial collateral nerve for the thumb (black arrow) or SBRN. (Source: Nguyễn et al. [20])

Hattori et al. presented long-term results involving 17 patients who underwent sensory reconstruction of the hand using intercostal nerve transfer to either the median or ulnar nerve. Their findings indicated a lack of consensus on the choice of recipient nerve. In a prior series by Hattori and colleagues, the ulnar nerve was used because of its size matching to donor intercostal nerves compared to the median nerve. However, in more recent studies, the median nerve has been preferred due to its wider sensory cutaneous distribution of the hand [23, 27]. Foroni et al. showed that the intercostobrachial nerve (ICBN) can be used as a for the lateral cord and resulted in better localization of sensory stimuli than other sensory transfers. They posited that this could be due to the proximity of the ICBN to the median nerve within the cerebral homunculus [26].

28.4 Challenges with Sensory Nerve Transfers

28.4.1 Morbidity

The idea of using expendable nerves as donors for more critical functions is an elegant solution to a complex problem. This concept, however, is perhaps more naturally suited to address the loss of motor function compared to sensory loss. Indeed, in successful motor nerve transfers, there is a potential to gain "something for nothing"; there should be no downgrade of the muscle innervated by the donor fascicle or, if completely denervated, the loss of a specific muscle should not impact overall function (e.g., pronator quadratus denervation compensated by functioning pronator teres). These principles unfortunately do not directly apply to sensory nerve transfers.

In sensory nerve transfers, sensation from a noncritical area is sacrificed in an attempt to restore sensation to a more critical area. There are a few potential downsides to this approach. First, there is a potential risk of irreversible loss of sensation in the donor area without the gain of sensation in the intended area. Secondly, and more devastating, the risk of creating a problematic donor site with cold intolerance, symptomatic neuroma or triggering neuropathic pain needs to be considered [5, 28]. The potential to make things worse needs to be understood by all parties involved. The decision to proceed with sensory nerve transfers remains a surgeon's preference as there is little in the literature to act as a definitive guide.

28.4.2 Measurement of Outcomes

A current limitation in the sensory nerve literature is the lack of good quality data on sensory nerve transfers. Most published studies are small case series, and there is significant heterogeneity in the reporting of outcomes. There is no accepted standardized way of measuring sensation, and, as a result, drawing meaningful conclusions becomes a difficult exercise. Without the ability to define quantitative and qualitative sensory recovery, counselling of patients and surgeons alike remains a challenge.

Moving forward, the need for standardization is key to determining the success or failure of sensory transfers [29]. It is also important to what constitutes a "useful" sensory recovery. Currently, there are multiple tools to measure sensory outcomes. The Medical Research Council (MRC) classification has been criticized for its subjective latitude leading to interobserver discrepancies. The Highet-Zachary scale and other modifications of the MRC classification such as the one proposed by Mackinnon and Dellon have been used to add granularity to these results but have led to heterogenous outcomes [29, 30]. The addition of different pain scaled and Patient Reported Outcome Measures also contribute to this heterogeneity. Attempts at standardizing reporting in sensory testing to reduce bias have been proposed but need to be widely adopted to effect a meaningful change [29].

28.5 Sensory Reeducation

The idea that sensory reeducation significantly improves outcomes in nerve injuries has been accepted for many years. Initially implemented following nerve repairs by Parry [31], and later popularized by Dellon [32], the establishment of a sensory reeducation program, in addition to a motor one, was demonstrated to significantly improve functional outcomes in affected patients. Indeed, this led Dellon to state that "failure to demonstrate improved end results following nerve repair is less a failure of the surgeon to achieve fascicular alignment as it is a failure of the patient to realize the potential given to him at surgery." These concepts are now also being applied in the field of nerve transfers where similar challenges are observed.

The sensory reeducation is divided into two phases and is started once early signs of reinnervation occur at the distal target. The early phase aims to reeducate sensory perceptions such as static touch versus moving touch. It also deals with localization of sensory signals and tries to eliminate misperception and misdirection of touch. This is particularly relevant to the field of sensory nerve transfers as patients initially feel the sensation arising from the newly innervated area as emanating from the donor territory.

The late phase starts when the early phase goals of static and moving-touch discrimination are achieved. The aim of the late phase is the recovery of tactile gnosis and object recognition to achieve functional sensitivity in the affected areas [32].

It is thought that sensory reeducation may enable central reorganization, the so-called plasticity which enable the patient to intuitively reinterpret the signals arising from the injured hand. This ultimately results in a much faster return to function and increases the likelihood of a successful nerve transfer.

28.6 Conclusion

Sensory nerve transfers offer the potential to regain a degree of sensation in potentially devastating injuries. The functional benefits of this are undeniable if successful, but the risk-benefit profile remains incompletely understood, and the procedure remains at the discretion of individual nerve surgeons. A recent scoping review of sensory nerve transfers in the upper limb concluded that distal nerve transfers are more likely to succeed than proximal ones, but the authors determined that more research is needed before meaningful conclusions regarding their implementation can be drawn [5]. The review commented on the heterogeneity of outcome measures, paucity of data involving small patient series, and lack of standardization as challenges in the current literary landscape.

Our belief is that the restoration of sensation via nerve transfers is a promising field which we should continue to advance. Our current practice integrates these transfers when primary anatomical repair fails as a salvage procedure or if primary repair is not an option. Moving forward, there is a need for standardization of assessment and reporting of data. Larger studies also need to be conducted before this treatment modality will be widely adopted.

References

1. Midha R. Epidemiology of brachial plexus injuries in a multitrauma population. Neurosurgery. 1997;40(6):1182–8.; discussion 1188-1189. https://doi.org/10.1097/00006123-199706000-00014.
2. Kaiser R, Waldauf P, Ullas G, Krajcová A. Epidemiology, etiology, and types of severe adult brachial plexus injuries requiring surgical repair: systematic review and meta-analysis. Neurosurg Rev. 2020;43(2):443–52. https://doi.org/10.1007/s10143-018-1009-2.
3. Mackinnon SE, Colbert SH. Nerve transfers in the hand and upper extremity surgery. Tech Hand Up Extrem Surg. 2008;12(1):20–33. https://doi.org/10.1097/BTH.0b013e31812714f3.
4. Moore AM, Franco M, Tung TH. Motor and sensory nerve transfers in the forearm and hand. Plast Reconstr Surg. 2014;134(4):721–30. https://doi.org/10.1097/PRS.0000000000000509.
5. Duraku LS, Hundepool CA, Moore AM, et al. Sensory nerve transfers in the upper limb after peripheral nerve injury: a scoping review. J Hand Surg Eur Vol. Published online November 21, 2023. 2023; https://doi.org/10.1177/17531934231205546.
6. Stocks GW, Cobb T, Lewis RC. Transfer of sensibility in the hand: a new method to restore sensibility in ulnar nerve palsy with use of microsurgical digital nerve translocation. J Hand Surg. 1991;16(2):219–26. https://doi.org/10.1016/S0363-5023(10)80100-5.
7. Sallam AA, El-Deeb MS, Imam MA. Nerve transfer versus nerve graft for reconstruction of high ulnar

nerve injuries. J Hand Surg. 2017;42(4):265–73. https://doi.org/10.1016/j.jhsa.2017.01.027.
8. Graczyk EL, Gill A, Tyler DJ, Resnik LJ. The benefits of sensation on the experience of a hand: A qualitative case series. Pazzaglia M, ed. PLOS ONE. 2019;14(1):e0211469. https://doi.org/10.1371/journal.pone.0211469.
9. Axelrod FB, Gold-von SG. Hereditary sensory and autonomic neuropathies: types II, III, and IV. Orphanet J Rare Dis. 2007;2:39. https://doi.org/10.1186/1750-1172-2-39.
10. Harris RI. The treatment of irreparable nerve injuries. Can Med Assoc J. 1921;11(11):833–41.
11. Hendry JM, Head LK. Alternative nerve Coaptations. Hand Clin. 2024;40(3):369–77. https://doi.org/10.1016/j.hcl.2024.03.002.
12. Bertelli JA, Ghizoni MF. Very distal sensory nerve transfers in high median nerve lesions. J Hand Surg. 2011;36(3):387–93. https://doi.org/10.1016/j.jhsa.2010.11.049.
13. Emamhadi M, Andalib S. Successful recovery of sensation loss in upper brachial plexus injuries. Acta Neurochir. 2018;160(10):2019–23. https://doi.org/10.1007/s00701-018-3648-z.
14. Özkan T, Özer K, Gülgönen A. Restoration of sensibility in irreparable ulnar and median nerve lesions with use of sensory nerve transfer: long-term follow-up of 20 cases. J Hand Surg. 2001;26(1):44–51. https://doi.org/10.1053/jhsu.2001.20156.
15. Ducic I, Dellon AL, Bogue DP. Radial sensory neurotization of the thumb and index finger for Prehension after proximal median and ulnar nerve injuries. J Reconstr Microsurg. 2006;22(02):073–8. https://doi.org/10.1055/s-2006-932500.
16. Brunelli GA. Sensory nerves transfers. J Hand Surg. 2004;29(6):557–62. https://doi.org/10.1016/J.JHSB.2004.06.005.
17. Brown JM, Yee A, Mackinnon SE. Distal median to ulnar nerve transfers to restore ulnar motor and sensory function within the hand: technical nuances. Neurosurgery. 2009;65(5):966–78. https://doi.org/10.1227/01.NEU.0000358951.64043.73.
18. Rodriguez-Lorenzo A, Söfteland MB, Audolfsson T. Acute transfer of superficial radial nerve to the medial nerve: case report. Ann Plast Surg. 2012;69(5):547–9. https://doi.org/10.1097/SAP.0b013e318248b60d.
19. Bertelli JA. Distal sensory nerve transfers in lower-type injuries of the brachial plexus. J Hand Surg. 2012;37(6):1194–9. https://doi.org/10.1016/j.jhsa.2012.02.047.
20. Nguyễn MV, Pierrart J, Crenn V. Sensory neurotization of the ulnar nerve, surgical techniques and functional outcomes: a review. J Clin Med. 2022;11(7):1903. https://doi.org/10.3390/jcm11071903.
21. Wu F, Ng CY. Sensory nerve transfer for lower roots brachial plexus injury: superficial radial nerve to the dorsal cutaneous branch and the superficial branch of the ulnar nerve. J Hand Microsurg. 2019;11(3):178–80. https://doi.org/10.1055/s-0039-1685545.
22. Xu B, Dong Z, Zhang CG, Gu YD. Transfer of the radial branch of the superficial radial nerve to the sensory branch of the ulnar nerve for sensory restoration after C7-T1 brachial plexus injury. J Plast Reconstr Aesthet Surg. 2016;69(3):318–22. https://doi.org/10.1016/j.bjps.2015.10.043.
23. Hattori Y, Doi K, Sakamoto S, Yukata K. Sensory recovery of the hand with intercostal nerve transfer following complete avulsion of the brachial plexus. Plast Reconstr Surg. 2009;123(1):276–83. https://doi.org/10.1097/PRS.0b013e31819348a7.
24. Terzis JK, Kokkalis ZT, Kostopoulos E. Contralateral C7 transfer in adult plexopathies. Hand Clin. 2008;24(4):389–400. https://doi.org/10.1016/j.hcl.2008.04.003.
25. Ihara K, Doi K, Sakai K, Kuwata N, Kawai S. Restoration of sensibility in the hand after complete brachial plexus injury. J Hand Surg. 1996;21(3):381–6. https://doi.org/10.1016/S0363-5023(96)80348-0.
26. Foroni L, Siqueira MG, Martins RS, Heise CO, Sterman Neto H, Imamura AY. Good sensory recovery of the hand in brachial plexus surgery using the intercostobrachial nerve as the donor. Arq Neuropsiquiatr. 2017;75(11):796–800. https://doi.org/10.1590/0004-282x20170148.
27. Hattori Y. Intercostal nerve transfer for sensory reconstruction of the hand following complete avulsion of the brachial plexus. In: Shin AY, Pulos N, editors. Operative brachial plexus surgery. Springer; 2021. p. 403–5. https://doi.org/10.1007/978-3-030-69517-0_36.
28. Leechavengvongs S, Ngamlamiat K, Malungpaishrope K, Uerpairotkit C, Witoonchart K, Kulkittiya S. End-to-side radial sensory to median nerve transfer to restore sensation and relieve pain in C5 and C6 nerve root avulsion. J Hand Surg. 2011;36(2):209–15. https://doi.org/10.1016/j.jhsa.2010.10.009.
29. Hooper G, Ruettermann M. Reporting numerical values for sensory testing. J Hand Surg Eur. 2022;47(11):1178–80. https://doi.org/10.1177/17531934221132666.
30. Wang Y, Sunitha M, Chung KC. How to measure outcomes of peripheral nerve surgery. Hand Clin. 2013;29(3):349–61. https://doi.org/10.1016/j.hcl.2013.04.004.
31. Wynn Parry CB. Rehabilitation of the Hand/ C. B. Wynn Parry. Assist. By. 4. ed., reprint. Butterworths; 1986.
32. Dellon AL. Evaluation of sensibility and re-education of sensation in the hand. Williams & Wilkins; 1981.

Part V

Distal Nerve Transfers

29 The Contralateral C7 Transfer

Christian Heinen and Thomas Kretschmer

29.1 Introduction

Few techniques in nerve surgery have been as controversially discussed as the contralateral C7 transfer (CC7). Since its introduction for brachial plexus surgery by Yu-dong Gu [1], numerous papers have been published on surgical techniques, variations, results, and outcomes—important and in contrast to many other nerve transfers: donor site morbidity has been assessed. There are regional differences in the perception and use of CC7 [2]. Some important plexus surgery groups abandoned the technique [3]. To others the contralateral C7 transfer not only is an important treatment option, but they even expanded its use. It not only can be applied after pure nerve lesions but also serves as an axon donor for free muscle transfers, or as a means to improve function and spasticity after central lesions.

The idea for this transfer derived from a clinical observation: In C7-only lesions (quite rare), patients were able to recover almost normal function without any reconstruction [1] after an initial sensorimotor impairment. Studying the specific microanatomy and contribution of each root/spinal nerve to the respective nerves and patterns of muscle innervation in more detail revealed that C7 despite its dominant extensor function shares a substantial overlap with the neighboring roots C6 and T1 [2]. This extensive functional overlap can also be seen and used as "spare add-on" to function minimizing potential loss if C7 were disconnected. This contrasts with other roots/spinal nerves that are more "exclusive" in their functional supply. These findings were supported by intraoperative electrophysiological stimulation studies [3, 4].

After an experimental study in an animal model, with reconfirming results, Gu's group came up with the basic principle that a healthy contralateral C7 root can be used as an axon donor and driver for the lesioned contralateral plexus. The satisfying experimental setting encouraged Gu to apply the CC7 transfer for the first time in humans.

On August 26, 1986, the first CC7 was performed on a patient [5].

In 1989 the first results were published in China reporting on already n = 50 cases with a follow-up of 1–2 years and an effective rate of 70% [6]. Ever since, a plethora of reports on techniques, variations, indications, and results have been published. The application spectrum of the CC7 subsequently grew over the years. Also, the

C. Heinen (✉)
Neuro-, Spine and Nerve Surgery, Christliches Krankenhaus Quakenbrück, Quakenbrück, Germany
e-mail: c.heinen@ckq-gmbh.de

T. Kretschmer
Department of Neurosurgery & Neurorestoration, Neurosurgical Intensive Care, Neurooncological Center (DKG), Skull Base Center (GSB), Paralysis Center, Klinikum Klagenfurt, Austria
e-mail: THOMASHRETSCHMER@KABEG.AT

F. Guedes et al. (eds.), *Nerve Transfers for Brachial Plexus Reconstruction after Trauma*,
https://doi.org/10.1007/978-3-031-92445-3_29

awareness for the most appropriate functional aims. More recently the evolving and commercially available bioelectrical orthoses for BPI patients open yet another door in the use of the CC7 transfer for patients deprived of good ipsilateral reconstructive nerve options: electromyographic orthoses can detect and amplify very weak muscle signals on the injured extremity. These amplified signals can drive implemented motors of the attached orthosis, and thus move the natural joint, e.g., to flex the elbow, or close and open the hand. By simple programming measures, the elbow, finger, and hand joints can thus be moved voluntarily tuned control, after a feedback learning interval.

In a more recent attempt, CC7 was introduced in the treatment of central lesions like hemiparesis due to stroke [7, 8], transgressing its application to the treatment of pure nerve lesions.

The following will elucidate pertinent anatomy, indications, surgical techniques, outcomes, and donor site morbidity, as well as involved risks and critique on its overall usefulness.

29.2 Anatomical Considerations

The whole brachial plexus C5-Th1 contains 85.000–166.000 myelinated fibers, of which alone 18.000–40.000 myelinated fibers belong to C7 [2], according to Xu and Gu 27,213 ± 5417[x]. Thus, by sheer number of axons, C7 is a very powerful axon donor.

The C7 root contains motor and sensory fibers. In general, more motor fibers are located in the posterior root division, and more sensory fibers in the anterior division. The ulnar portion of the anterior division of C7/the medial trunk contains predominantly sympathetic and sensory fibers, whereas the radial portion of the anterior division consists mainly of motor fibers. The posterior division of C7/medial trunk is even richer in both sensory and motor fibers. At the same time, it contains less sympathetic fibers [3].

The contributions to the radial portion of the median nerve and the pectoral nerve mostly derive from the anterior division of C7. The posterior division contains the supplies for the radial nerve (more radially located) and the ulnar nerve (more ulnar-caudal) [9].

To a certain degree, we can also test and reconfirm individual motor supply patterns intraoperatively by fascicular root or plexus element stimulation and EMG recording (see below) [10–12]. An overlap in a single muscle's innervation can thus be reconfirmed: serially stimulate neighboring roots/fascicles while recording from same muscle (method developed by the authors and published [12]).

The sensory area covered by C7 is mainly the index finger (74%), the middle finger (58%) and the thumb (28%), the ring finger (20%), and little finger (2%) [13].

As observed by Gu, patients with C7 lesions often recover function in a short period of time or do not display severe impairments at all. The underlying anatomical basis being that C7 supplies muscles that share significant co-supply with the neighboring spinal nerves. In comparison to the other brachial plexus roots, C7 appears to have no autonomous, or exclusive muscle territory for innervation but acts as safeguard supply [3, 14]. In other words, predominantly C7-innervated muscles share cross-innervation from upper or lower trunk elements. This enables functional compensation in the case of C7 disconnection.

The long thoracic nerve is the most proximal C7 branch. Meticulous dissection and protection of the nerve is mandatory when accessing the healthy side [37].

29.3 Indication

To some degree all ipsilateral nerve transfers put the physiological function of the donor at risk. But none of them can potentially harm the healthy side at the plexus level. A serious CC7 transfer complication due to a non-recognized innervation anomaly or pronounced innervation variation could lead to a drop hand or other functional deficits on the healthy hand and extremity. New onset neuropathic pain is also conceivable. In wheelchair-bound paraplegics, a severe triceps and extensor deficit is a severe loss of function diminishing independency further.

The indication for this procedure is thoroughly evaluated and discussed with the patient and his family. Apart from the involved procedural risk, the anticipated reinnervation time of over 9–12 months for functional results will be considerably longer. First results might appear only after 9–12 months.

Surgeons using this transfer are well aware of these risks, counsel the patient accordingly, and implement safety measures into their surgical routine prior to sacrificing/cutting the donor (e.g., intraoperative electrophysiology).

CC7 was introduced for patients with complete avulsions of the affected side and little or no choice of ipsilateral axon donors as mentioned in the other chapters.

In incomplete lesions, the ipsilateral motor axon donors (accessory nerve/ intercostal nerves/ phrenic nerve) are limited and mainly used to provide shoulder and elbow flexion. However, completely avulsed patients' hand and finger flexors and extensors as well as elbow extensors lack additional axon donors and might therefore not be reconnected unless a contralateral donor is used. After a more widespread use of CC7 for these indications, another potential merit of the procedure emerged: It is also useful for protective sensory reinnervation of the hand; to a certain degree, it can be used simultaneously for both, motor and sensory reinnervation. Being aware of the predominant topographical arrangement of fibers within the C7 spinal nerve and middle trunks is a prerequisite for such sophisticated sensorimotor rerouting.

Ipsilateral sensory axon donors are sparse and basically consist of the intercostal nerves and the cervical plexus. CC7 offers sensory fibers that can be used, too.

After decades of brachial plexus surgery experience, also reconstruction for partial motor and sensory hand function in adult flail arm patients turned into an objective increasingly pursued by many "plexus groups."

CC7 offers both modalities [3, 13, 15]. In the course, indications for CC7 were subsequently adapted, and now also comprise patients with incomplete lesions to enhance reconstructive strategies by enlarging the number of axon donors.

Gu makes a point that CC7 should not be used when the patient has associated injury in the contralateral upper limb or around the shoulder.

Besides the question of inherent harvesting and rerouting risk and justification for that, the question of plasticity and donor site independent use of the reconnected sensory area or muscle group remains ("co-contraction" issue).

29.4 Complete or Partial Use of CC7 as a Donor

The issue of the partial or complete application of CC7 revolves around the risk for the donor site (less if partial root taken), selective choice of predominant fibers (motor vs sensory), and maximum number of sprouting axons (whole root). So, some authors favor the partial use to avoid donor site morbidities; others advocate the use of the complete CC7 to supply the affected limb with more myelinated fibers [16, 17].

In terms of brain plasticity, it may be easier to reeducate the patients if the complete CC7 is harvested and thus becoming a pure contralateral spinal nerve.

Eventually, it is a matter of chosen reconstructive scheme, the individual needs and readiness of the patient to be exposed to a risk of losing healthy side function that leads to the decision between the partial vs complete use of the CC7.

29.5 Rewiring Strategies and the Choice of Recipient

The concept of rewiring needs to be meticulously planned and verified intraoperatively by electrophysiology. The patient and surgeon should also be prepared to abandon the procedure if intraoperative testing of the healthy side that reveals to be not enough or insecure cross-innervation from the neighboring roots. Highly selective stimulation probes that prevent current spread help in the stimulation test.

Knowing the intraneural topography at different levels of the C7 spinal nerve/medial trunk and its divisions is crucial to avoid donor site morbidities (Fig. 29.1).

Moreover, specific functions can be coaptated and thus targeted to the affected side [9].

The rewiring pattern needs to be clear during surgery: the patient needs to know which original function or sensation on the healthy side will now be connected to which "new" function.

This is crucial for successful reeducation and facilitating brain plasticity in relearning the function via the contralateral side using specific movements of the healthy side.

One could, for example, use the pectoral major portion of the ventromedial healthy C7 to reinnervate hand and finger flexion in the affected side via the median nerve.

Thus, the patient needs to learn that adduction of the healthy arm will lead to a grasp on the affected side. The same applies when using the healthy triceps portion/wrist extensors, etc. portion of the posterior division [18].

For sensory reeducation it is similar. Patients need to learn to properly localize sensory input from the healthy to the affected side.

In patients with severe muscle trauma and complete lesions or late referral and highly degenerated ipsilateral muscles, CC7 can serve as an axon donor for the free muscle transfers.

The recent commercial availability of myoelectric strap-on orthoses widens reconstructive strategies even more.

These devices can detect tiny, nonfunctional EMG signals of voluntary contraction in the reinnervated muscles. The detected voluntary signals are amplified and used to activate inbuilt motors of the orthosis which then initiates a joint movement: in principle elbow flexion/extension ± grasp. This opens a path to use even minor reinnervation for function: even if reached reinnervation is considered to be not useful (e.g., M1–M2), this can be translated/amplified into function. Thus, the role of CC7 in patients with no ipsilateral axon donors might be revised by some authors.

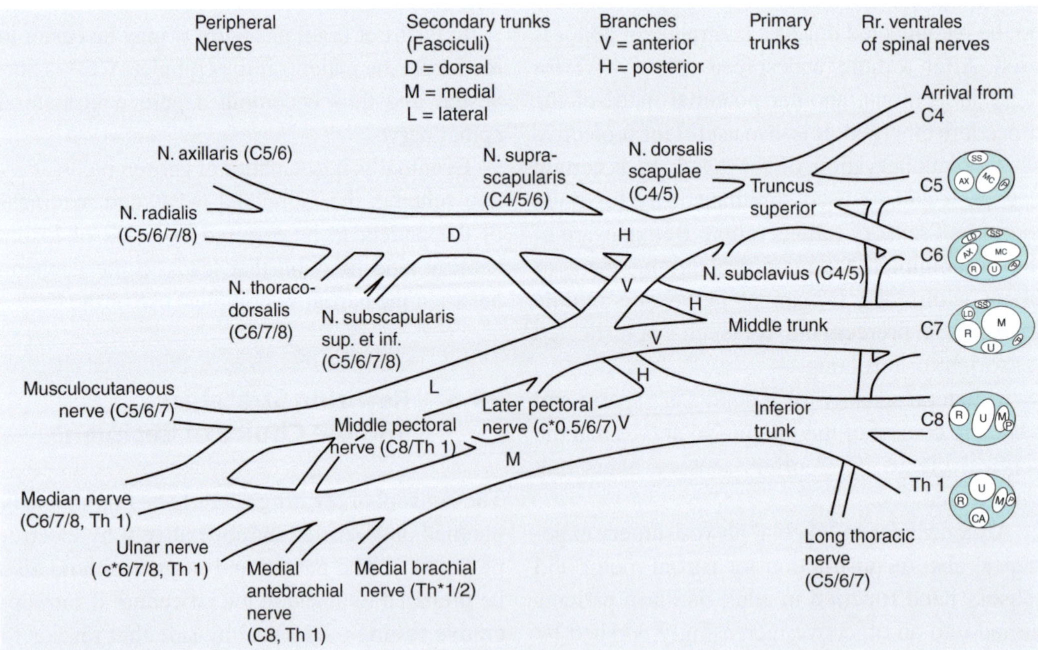

Fig. 29.1 Intraneural functional topography. (Reproduced with permission from http://link.springer.com/10.1007/978-3-642-36895-0)

29.6 Rewiring Strategies

29.6.1 Surgical Considerations

29.6.1.1 Positioning and Draping

The positioning and draping of the patient are time-consuming and need to warrant optimal access to the surgical site, optimal access for the anesthesiologists, and optimal conditions for intra-OP electrophysiology.

As potentially a large area of the skin is exposed for many hours, preparations need to be taken to prevent hypothermia.

Usually, the patient is in prone position with the head slightly rotated to the affected side enabling the exposition of the healthy supraclavicular plexus.

In single-staged CC7 procedures, the patient needs to be accessible supra- and infraclavicularly, at the upper/forearm, and legs on both sides. In multiple transfers (e.g., intercostals/accessory/triceps branch transfer, etc.), the respective regions are incorporated as well.

There are multi-staged approaches, too.

In a first surgery, the ipsilateral reconstruction is carried as far as possible, applying all tools with an individually tailored combination of autologous repair and nerve transfers.

If consented with the patient to perform a CC7 in the future, the grafts on the ipsilateral affected side can already be coaptated.

In preparation for a second stage CC7, these grafts are marked and positioned subcutaneously at the clavicular level of the healthy side. In the second surgery, they are easily located and sutured to the donor C7.

Some groups use the vascularized ulnar nerve of the affected side as a graft. In a first stage, the graft is coaptated to the healthy donor plexus and its distal end transferred to the affected side. Then after a defined period, the coaptation on the affected side is performed [6].

In the case of using the CC7 as an axon donor for a free functional muscle transfer (FFMT), some groups perform multi-staged surgeries. Stage 1 is to connect the CC7 with the graft, bringing the latter then to the site of the future FFMT.

After the calculated time of nerve growth through the graft has passed, a biopsy from the distal graft tip reconfirms reinnervation. Only then, the FFMT is connected (personal communication M. Becker/F. Lassner).

Since in vascular/cardiac/thoracic surgery draping of multiple extremities is routine, it is worthwhile to have a look in their OR and ask the nurses.

U-shaped drapes or extremity drapes can be useful.

29.7 Surgical Approach Donor Site

The surgical approach to the C7 donor site follows the usual supraclavicular plexus approach.

An incision parallel to the clavicle reaches to the lateral margin of the sternocleidomastoid muscle (SCM). After the dissection of the platysma, the SCM margin is visualized, the fascia opened, and the omohyoid muscle identified and mobilized cranially. The deep fascia is opened, and the anterior scalene muscle with the phrenic nerve is dissected.

Stepwise the upper trunk with its C5 and C6 contributions, C7 and medial trunk, and C8/ Th1 and inferior trunk are visualized. It is important to depict the entire supraclavicular plexus to minimize chances for incorrect identification. In addition it is necessary to thoroughly test the individual innervation pattern of the plexus by electrophysiological exam in order to rule out a very dominant C7 innervation pattern of the extensors with a lack of sufficient cross-innervation.

CC7/medial trunk are identified proximally and then followed distally to its divisions.

It is important to check for intermingling tributaries of the upper and lower trunk into the anterior and posterior division. **This is to ensure that the disconnection of C7/middle trunk will not be at the level of the lateral or posterior cord.** Otherwise, the patients have a high risk of significant functional impairments as the cross-innervation of the other spinal nerves will be damaged.

Figure 29.2 with intra-OP photo with stimulation.

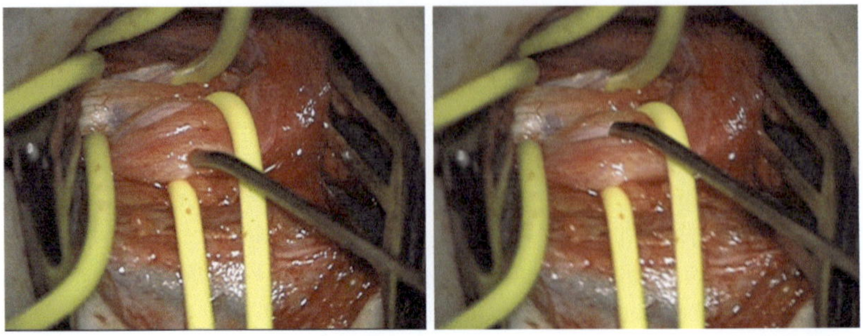

Fig. 29.2 Intra-op stimulation healthy C7

29.8 Surgical Approach to Recipient Site

The recipient site approach is dependent on targeted nerves and chosen CC7 route. In previously operated, multi-staged patients entry point and dissection avert already established coaptations.

To some extent imaging such as MR-neurography or ultrasound might help to locate coaptation sites and identify rerouted connections. Ultimately meticulous and careful dissection is necessary to avoid damage to established rewiring routes.

A targeted coaptation to specific muscle branches or sensory portions of the recipient nerves may enable better reeducation of the patients.

29.9 Intraoperative Monitoring

Intraoperative monitoring is decisive in CC7.

Direct stimulation can be used or slightly more sophisticated its combination with intra-OP EMG [19]. Several settings and techniques have been described [3, 12]. It not only provides qualitative information but also objectifies in a quantitative way the actual input of the individual spinal nerves/trunks.

Aside from ruling out possible loss of function, it also facilitates decision-making in complete versus partial use of the CC7.

In the case of a middle trunk-posterior division dominated triceps or wrist extension, only the anterior division might be used.

For some time, Millesi used a ligation of the donor CC7 in a first surgery to simulate C7 outage. If the patients did not suffer from significant functional loss, the main surgery was carried out during the same hospital stay [20]. However, ligature, if loose enough, might not simulate complete loss, and if too tight might already create a substantial lesion. To our knowledge this routine is not followed by other groups.

29.10 Graft

As substantial graft length might be needed, usually both legs are prepared for sural and saphenous nerve, sometimes also sensory branches of the superficial and/or deep peroneal nerve.

On the affected arm, medial and lateral cutaneous antebrachial nerve and/or superficial radial nerve can serve as grafts. Some authors use intercostals, too. However, given their potential as axon donors, we prefer to use them to reconstruct and not as grafts.

The role of the (vascularized) ulnar nerve of the affected side as a graft has been published and evaluated in numerous papers.

In rats, the vascularized ulnar nerve graft showed superior results [21]. However, in patients, there was no evidence for its superiority or advantage. Some authors even target the affected ulnar nerve to reinnervate intrinsic hand function and regain protective sensory function in the ulnar portion of the hand [22].

Once the grafts are harvested and the principal route is defined, the challenge is to tunnel functionally assigned grafts to the other side without losing this assignment on the way to the targets. Markings by different sutures, the use of color pens or different tubes to separate grafts for their respective functions, may be helpful.

We recommend to first put all grafts in place and to recheck their assignment and then to coapt them accordingly in one go.

29.11 Choice of Route-Direct Vs Interposed Graft

A large variety of routes have been described. Purely subcutaneous positioning of the grafts starting supraclavicular on the healthy side was the initial route described by Gu in the first surgeries. The grafts are then brought to the infraclavicular space or upper arm to be connected to the recipient nerves.

This route requires long grafts which are routed superficially across the chest or neck; thus they are susceptible to trauma or compression. Graft length as such is an issue. Another issue can be the generation of hematomas along the subcutaneous tunnel as dissection is carried out blind. So far, no laceration of larger vessels, the lung or lymphatic tissue has been reported.

Therefore, new, shorter routes across the neck and modifications were investigated.

The main concept is to shorten the distance using anatomical spaces such as the prespinal retropharyngeal area [23, 24]. Even end-to-end coaptations to the upper or lower trunk of the affected side were reported to be feasible with this technique.

The complication rates in using prespinal modifications reached over 5% including laceration of the vertebral artery and esophagus, brainstem thrombosis, hoarseness, and pain while swallowing due to mechanical irritation of the CC7. Some authors even developed a transspinal and retrospinal route [25].

To shorten the distance even more and to enable direct coaptation without interposing grafts, some authors proposed a shortening of the affected arm [26].

29.12 Outcomes

For an account of outcomes both, functional results on the recipient site and donor site morbidity should be considered. The overall result of this technique is the combination of both.

Since the method was developed in China, most of the published series are from China or the Asian countries.

Gu et al. reported on a group of patients with a follow-up of at least 2 years—an overall motor recovery of at least M3 of 50–80% and a sensory recovery of at least S3 more than 60%. They found differences depending on the nerves targeted.

The musculocutaneous nerve seems to be the most successful motor target [27].

In a meta-analysis Li et al. included a total of $n = 754$ patients. The authors confirmed these target nerve-depending results. A strength of M3-M4 was found in 75% ($n = 113/151$) of the patients for elbow flexion, 50% ($n = 38/75$) for elbow and wrist extension, 49% for wrist flexion ($n = 136/281$), and 43% for finger flexion ($n = 188/451$) [28].

Fifty-six percent ($n = 133/239$) of the patients regained sensory function level S3 in the median nerve territory [1].

Most of the included studies dealt with patients from China ($n = 351/754$ patients), followed by Taiwan ($n = 118/754$), Thailand ($n = 117/754$), and the USA ($n = 104/754$). Most of the patients had total brachial plexus (avulsion) injuries ($n = 566/754$).

In the meta-analysis the main technique used was a complete CC7 donor with subcutaneous graft positioning. The main graft was the ulnar nerve of the affected side according to the Gu technique.

Wang et al. published their series of $n = 116$ patients using the prespinal route with similar results. In 2012 the results of CC7 prespinal to the upper trunk in $n = 41$ patients were presented. After 48 months, M3+ was found for biceps in 85.4%, deltoid in 82.9%, and major pectoral in 92.7%. If the suprascapular nerve on the affected side was additionally addressed via ipsilateral accessory or phrenic nerve, the results of shoulder abduction seemed to fare even better [29].

In a second study in 2013, the same authors performed direct coaptation of the CC7 to the lower trunk of the affected side in $n = 75$ patients. They yielded at least M3 in 60% in elbow flexion, 64% finger flexion, 53% thumb flexion, and 72% wrist flexion after 57-month follow-up. $N = 35/75$ patients additionally received an arm shortening of 3–4.5 cm to facilitate direct coaptation. No differences in functional recovery were observed between the patients with and without shortening; no persistent complications were found [30].

Liu et al. reported on their experience with $n = 51$ patients using the Gu method in global plexus avulsions. Follow-up was 4.2 years. For motor recovery 57.7% "effective rate" (M3 or more) was yielded for wrist flexion via median nerve only (group 1), 45.5% when CC7 was used for both median and biceps branch (group 2), and 36.4% when CC7 was used for median nerve, biceps, and triceps branch (group 3). Sensory recovery showed very similar results to the motor in the three groups. Elbow flexion was significantly better in group 2. Temporary sensory problems on the donor site were the only complication reported in their series [16].

In the US population, Terzis et al. and Sammer et al. shared their experiences.

In 2008 Terzis described their results in $n = 56$ patients also using a selective use of CC7 with a follow-up of 6.1 years.

M3+ or greater was achieved in 20% ($n = 2/10$) for deltoid, 52 ($n = 12/23$) for biceps, 52% ($n = 5/21$) for triceps, and 34% ($n10/29$) for wrist and finger flexion, whereas only 20% ($n = 2/10$) for finger and wrist extension. Patients reached S2 or greater in 76% ($n = 22/26$) after median nerve coaptation. Again, no persistent donor deficits were detected. Young age and early referral were significantly positive for the outcome [31].

In 2012, in a paper on elbow extension reconstruction, the same group proposed intercostal nerves and CC7 (posterior division) as preferable axon donors. In a total of $n = 156$ patients, $n = 23$ received CC7. $N = 5/23$ regained M3+ or greater; the mean MRC was 2.66 [32].

Partially confirming these promising results of Terzis, Hierner et al. reported their observations in a small group of $n = 10$ patients. Although the study's title contains "partial CC7," it is not explained exactly which part of CC7 was used. In $n = 4$ patient the median nerve was addressed, in n = 6 MCN. $N = 5/6$ reached M3 or greater for elbow flexion, with $n = 3/6$ having an independent motion. However, only $n = 1/4$ patient in the median nerve group developed what the authors called "primitive grip pattern" without further elucidating this [17].

Another US group published a paper in 2012 on $n = 55$ patients who underwent hemi-CC7 transfers targeting different nerves. Hemi-CC7 was defined using mostly the C7 portion for the pectoral major muscle and sparing the wrist and finger extensors. Of these, $n = 28$ patients were included with a mean follow-up of at least 27 months. $N = 11$ patients received CC7 to axillary nerve (AN) and suprascapular nerve (SSC), $n = 2$ to AN only, $n = 14$ to median nerve (MN) only, and n = 1 MN and musculocutaneous nerve (MCN). Both pedicled vascularized and non-vascularized grafts were used.

The results were not comparable to the Chinese literature and the Terzis group. In the MN and/or MCN group, only $n = 3/15$ gained positive EMG signs leading to a maximum of M2 in $n = 1/15$ patients, $n = 2/15$ with M1, and $n = 12/15$ with no motor function at all. In the AN and/or SSC group, $n = 12/13$ showed EMG reinnervation; however, only $n = 3/13$ yielded M3 or more [33]. Again, no persistent donor site deficits were detected.

Waikakul et al. from Thailand described similar results in 1999 for anterior division of CC7 to median nerve in $n = 96$ patient with total root avulsions. Ipsilateral phrenic nerve was used for shoulder abduction and accessory nerve for MCN. The authors state poor results in forearm and hand muscles; only 20–30% yielded significant function. For sensory function in the hand, encouraging recovery was observed [34]. After at least 3 years of follow-up, no persistent donor site deficit was observed. No significant differences between vascularized and nonvascularized grafts were found.

In a talk in 2010, Millesi reported on his experience on a total of $n = 20$ patients; of these $n = 10$ were included. $N = 8/10$ yielded reinnervation of the forearm muscles with grasp function in $n = 6$. No persistent deficit was observed (personal communication).

Not only general motor and sensory results were published. Shulin et al. selectively used the ulnar nerve (UN) for the posterior CC7 division and the medial cutaneous antebrachial nerve (MCAN) for the anterior CC7 division in a total of $n = 16$ patients. The UN was then coapted to the affected MN, whereas the MACN was connected to the affected MCN. 68.75% reached M3 or better for elbow flexion and 43.75% M3 or greater for wrist and finger flexion. 68.75% gained at least S2 in the median nerve territory. However, only $n = 6$ patients achieved independent motion for elbow flexion and $n = 1$ for wrist and finger flexion [35].

Regarding complications and donor site deficits, Yang analyzed the literature in a systematic review and presented results. A total of $n = 904$ patients were included, of which $n = 668/897$ (74%) developed sensory alterations after CC7. Of these, $n = 618/633$ (98%) completely recovered to normal within a mean time of 3 months. $N = 118/592$ (20%) showed motor deficits postop. $N = 107/1177$ (91%) regained normal function within 6 months. $N = 19/904$ patients suffered from long-term donor site morbidities. The authors observed that the use of the complete CC7 was associated with more donor site morbidity than the partial use [36]. As mentioned above, the prespinal route bears a higher risk than across the chest the subcutaneous positioning of grafts. This needs to be discussed with the patients in advance [24] (personal communication Becker/Lassner/Chapter 5.3. "Kontralaterale Transfers" in "Nervenchirurgie" Kretschmer [37]).

29.13 Brain Plasticity

Cerebral plasticity is known to play a key role in reeducation and relearning of function after nerve transfers [38].

Gu stated in 2011 that "usually independent movement" can be achieved once M3 is reached by the reinnervated muscles. They observed that the patients needed a period of 5 years for that [39].

Interestingly, fMRI studies revealed activation of similar cortex regions on both ipsilateral and contralateral cortex in patients after CC7 [40].

Tie Li found a difference in the recovery of hand extrinsic (represented by flexor digitorum FD muscle innervation) and hand intrinsic (represented by abductor pollicis brevis APB muscle) motor function. Using fMRI and TMS, different developments were observed for FD and ABP. Whereas FD was represented in the bilateral, APB was only found in the ipsilateral motor cortex. They concluded that depending on the movement and muscles involved, the patients might undergo different types of plasticity [41].

Yu et al. investigated patients after CC7 by fMRI in resting state. After CC7 the interhemispheric connectivity for the M1 area was increased compared to healthy controls. The authors interpreted this as a sign of synchronization following functional reorganization between the two hemispheres. However, the connectivity between the supplementary motor areas showed a reduction [42].

In glucose-PET, Ma et al. demonstrated in a small patient sample that the cerebral glucose metabolism positively correlated in corpus callosum, premotor cortex, and precuneus with the reinnervation of the affected hand after CC7 [43].

In 2021 a paper on rats was published by Guo et al. They examined the impact of a partial vs complete use of the CC7 on cortical plasticity. In all groups they avulsed the complete left brachial plexus. Then different treatments were applied. Group 1 was treated according to the Gu protocol with a complete use of CC7 and a vascularized ulnar nerve graft to the ipsilateral median nerve. In Group 2 the complete CC7 was transected, with the posterior division being coaptated via ulnar nerve graft to the ipsilateral median nerve. The anterior division was coaptated to the contralateral pectoralis major muscle with a graft. In Group 3, only the posterior division was coaptated via ulnar nerve graft to the ipsilateral median nerve. The control Group 4 received just a plain avulsion of the left brachial plexus. Different markers were applied to the primary motor cortex analysis serving as indicators for cortical reorganization (BDNF/TNF-alpha/IL-6/miR132/134). Interestingly, they found differences in the distribution of the markers after different surgical techniques. **The rate of induced microglia as an index for cortical reorganization was the highest in Group 1 (complete CC7 dissection and grafting) and Group 2 (complete CC7 dissection, posterior division only transfer).** This may even explain the seemingly better results for complete CC7 in humans [44].

Patients after CC7 still perceive the sensory stimuli in the donor side limb. They demonstrated that the sensory input of the affected hand was mainly located in cortical area S1 and vastly overlapped with the area of the non-affected limb. This could be an explanation why patients not only have problems with independent motor function but also with sensory perception [45].

Socolovsky and Malessy clinically examined their patients for volitional and independent control after ipsilateral nerve transfers for elbow and shoulder function. However, no CC7 was included in this population. In the paper, a classification of volitional control based on the plasticity grading level was introduced. They could show that in general, only 20% of their patients reached a completely independent movement. This led to the conclusion that brain plasticity might be succumbed to limitations [46].

29.14 Conclusions

CC7 is a viable option in treating severe brachial plexus lesions when ipsilateral donors are lacking or are few. The choice of complete or partial use, the choice of route, recipient, and grafts used remain a highly individual one. It incorporates a tailored approach and thorough counseling and discussion with the patient. After surgery, an intensive and long-term reeducation and training is mandatory to achieve the best results possible.

It is an additional tool in the armamentarium when dealing with such a devastating trauma as a brachial plexus lesion.

Upcoming techniques, enhancing the CC7 with free functional muscle transfer, and the use of myoelectric orthoses might add indications for brachial plexus patients. Despite its inherent controversy, its potential for functional reconstruction after stroke/cerebral hemorrhages might open a whole new spectrum of CC7 applications.

References

1. Yang G, Chang KWC, Chung KC. A systematic review of contralateral C7 transfer for the treatment of traumatic brachial plexus injury. Plast Reconstr Surg. 2015;136:794–809.
2. Bonnel F. Microscopic anatomy of the adult human brachial plexus: an anatomical and histological basis for microsurgery. Microsurgery. 1984;5:107–18.
3. Gu Y. Functional motor innervation of brachial plexus roots. An intraoperative electrophysiological study. J Hand Surg: J Br Soc Surg Hand. 1997;22:258–60.
4. Gu Y, Shen L. Electrophysiological changes after severance of the C7 nerve root. J Hand Surg: J Br Soc Surg Hand. 1994;19:69–71.
5. Gu Y-D. Contralateral C7 root transfer over the last 20 years in China. Chin Med J. 2007;120:1123–6.
6. Gu YD. Cervical nerve root transfer from the healthy side in the treatment of brachial plexus root avulsion. Zhonghua Yi Xue Za Zhi. 1989;69:563-5–38.
7. Alawieh AM, Yong NA, Boulis NM. Contralateral C7 nerve transfer for stroke recovery: new frontier for peripheral nerve surgery. J Clin Med. 2021;10:3344.
8. Zheng M-X, et al. Trial of contralateral seventh cervical nerve transfer for spastic arm paralysis. New Engl J Med. 2017;378:22–34.
9. Sinha S, Prasad GL, Lalwani S. A cadaveric microanatomical study of the fascicular topography of the brachial plexus. J Neurosurg. 2016;125:355–62.
10. Chuang DC, Cheng SL, Wei FC, Wu CL, Ho YS. Clinical evaluation of C7 spinal nerve transection: 21 patients with at least 2 years' follow-up. Br J Plast Surg. 1998;51:285–90.
11. Bai Y, et al. Contralateral C7 nerve transfer in the treatment of upper-extremity paralysis: a review of anatomical basis, surgical approaches, and neurobiological mechanisms. Rev Neurosci. 2022;33:491–514.
12. Dengler NF, et al. Super-selective cervical nerve root stimulation in contralateral C7 transfer: an

intraoperative study. Clin Neurophysiol: Off J Int Feder Clin Neurophysiol. 2017;128:2384–91.
13. Gu Y. Distribution of the sensory endings of the C7 nerve root and its clinic significance. J Hand Surg: J Br Soc Surg Hand. 1994;19:67–8.
14. Wang G-B, et al. Contralateral C7 to C7 nerve root transfer in reconstruction for treatment of total brachial plexus palsy: anatomical basis and preliminary clinical results. J Neurosurg Spine. 2018;29:491–9.
15. Lu W, Xu J-G, Wang D-P, Gu Y-D. Microanatomical study on the functional origin and direction of the thoracodorsal nerve from the trunks of brachial plexus. Clin Anat. 2008;21:509–13.
16. Liu Y, et al. Outcome of contralateral C7 transfers to different recipient nerves after global brachial plexus avulsion. Brain Behav. 2018;8:e01174.
17. Hierner R, Berger AK. How to improve the results of peripheral nerve surgery. Acta Neurochir Suppl. 2007;100:33–5.
18. Terzis JK, Kokkalis ZT. Selective contralateral C7 transfer in posttraumatic brachial plexus injuries: a report of 56 cases. Plast Reconstr Surg. 2009;123:927–38.
19. Lu W, Xu J, Wang D. Intraoperative decision making by electrophysiological detection of the origin of thoracodorsal nerve in the C7 nerve root transfer procedure. J Reconstr Microsurg. 2010;27:001–4.
20. Millesi H. Die Chirurgie traumatischer Plexus brachialis-Läsionen (Aus persönlicher Sicht des Jahres 2003). Handchir Mikrochir P. 2004;36:29–36.
21. Chen L, Gu Y-D. An experimental study of contralateral C7 root transfer with vascularized nerve grafting to treat brachial plexus root avulsion. J Hand Surg Br Eur. 1994;19:60–6.
22. Chen X, et al. Modified contralateral C7 transfer to restore ulnar nerve function without sacrificing median nerve recovery: an experimental study. J Hand Surg Eur. 2023;175319342311701:731. https://doi.org/10.1177/17531934231170103.
23. Mcguiness CN, Kay SPJ. The prespinal route in contralateral C7 nerve root transfer for brachial plexus avulsion injuries. J Hand Surg. 2002;27:159–60.
24. Li W, et al. Complications of contralateral C-7 transfer through the modified prespinal route for repairing brachial plexus root avulsion injury: a retrospective study of 425 patients. J Neurosurg. 2015;122:1421–8.
25. Du H, Gao X, Chen Z, Guo K, Li M. A new approach for contralateral C7 nerve transfer via retrospinal route. Hand Surg Rehab. 2022;41:171–5.
26. Yu Z, Sui S, Yu S, Huang Y, Sheng J. Contralateral Normal C7 nerve transfer after upper arm shortening for the treatment of total root avulsion of the brachial plexus: a preliminary report. Plast Reconstr Surg. 2003;111:1465–9.
27. Hu S, GU, Y. Contralateral c7 transfer for treatment of brachial plexus root avulsion. Handchirurgie, Mikrochirurgie, plastische Chirurgie : Organ der Deutschsprachigen Arbeitsgemeinschaft für Handchirurgie : Organ der Deutschsprachigen Arbeitsgemeinschaft für Mikrochirurgie der Peripheren Nerven und Gefässe : Organ der Vereinigung der Deutschen Plastischen Chirurgen. 2014;46:80–4.
28. Li W-J, et al. Contralateral C7 nerve root transfer for function recovery in adults: a meta-analysis. Chin Méd J. 2017;130:2960–8.
29. Wang S, et al. Contralateral C7 nerve root transfer to neurotize the upper trunk via a modified prespinal route in repair of brachial plexus avulsion injury. Microsurgery. 2012;32:183–8.
30. Wang S, et al. Contralateral C7 nerve transfer with direct coaptation to restore lower trunk function after traumatic brachial plexus avulsion. J Bone Jt Surg. 2013;95:821–7.
31. Terzis JK, Kokkalis ZT, Kostopoulos E. Contralateral C7 transfer in adult plexopathies. Hand Clin. 2008;24:389–400.
32. Terzis JK, Barmpitsioti A. Our experience with triceps nerve reconstruction in patients with brachial plexus injury. J Plastic Reconstr Aesth Surg. 2012;65:590–600.
33. Sammer DM, Kircher MF, Bishop AT, Spinner RJ, Shin AY. Hemi-contralateral C7 transfer in traumatic brachial plexus injuries. J Bone Jt Surg. 2012;94:131–7.
34. Waikakul S, Orapin S, Vanadurongwan V. Clinical results of contralateral C7 root neurotization to the median nerve in brachial plexus injuries with total root avulsions. J Hand Surg. 1999;24:556–60.
35. Li S, et al. Contralateral C7 transfer via both ulnar nerve and medial antebrachial cutaneous nerve to repair total brachial plexus avulsion: a preliminary report. Br J Neurosurg. 2019;33:648–54.
36. Yang G, Chang KWC, Chung KC. A systematic review of outcomes of contralateral C7 transfer for the treatment of traumatic brachial plexus injury. Plast Reconstr Surg. 2015;136:480e–9e.
37. MD, P. O. T. K. & Kretschmer, T. Nervenchirurgie. Berlin/Heidelberg: Springer; 2014. https://doi.org/10.1007/978-3-662-45894-5.
38. Socolovsky M, Malessy M, Lopez D, Guedes F, Flores L. Current concepts in plasticity and nerve transfers: relationship between surgical techniques and outcomes. Neurosurg Focus. 2017;42:E13–1.
39. Zhang C-G, Gu Y-D. Contralateral C7 nerve transfer—our experiences over past 25 years*. J Brachial Plex Peripher Nerve Inj. 2011;06:e62–5.
40. Beaulieu J-Y, et al. Cerebral plasticity in crossed C7 grafts of the brachial plexus: an fMRI study. Microsurgery. 2006;26:303–10.
41. Li T, et al. Different cerebral plasticity of intrinsic and extrinsic hand muscles after peripheral neurotization in a patient with brachial plexus injury: a TMS and fMRI study. Neurosci Lett. 2015;604:140–4.
42. Yu A, et al. Functional connectivity of motor cortical network in patients with brachial plexus avulsion injury after contralateral cervical nerve transfer: a resting-state fMRI study. 2017;1–7:247. https://doi.org/10.1007/s00234-017-1796-0.

43. Ma H, Zheng M, Lu Y, Hua X, Xu W. Cerebral plasticity after contralateral cervical nerve transfer in human by longitudinal PET evaluation. J Clin Neurosci. 2018;48:95–9.
44. Guo J, Zhao X, Lao J, Gao K. Why it is necessary to use the entire root rather than partial root when doing contralateral C7 nerve transfer: cortical plasticity also matters besides the amount of nerve fibers. Neural Plast. 2021;2021:8819380.
45. Cai Z, et al. Aberrant central plasticity underlying synchronous sensory phenomena in brachial plexus injuries after contralateral cervical seventh nerve transfer. Brain Behav. 2021;11:e02064.
46. Socolovsky M, Malessy M. Brain changes after peripheral nerve repair: limitations of neuroplasticity. J Neurosurg Sci. 2021; https://doi.org/10.23736/s0390-5616.21.05298-x.

Rare Nerve Transfers

30

C. P. G. Heinen, T. Kretschmer, and R. Schmidhammer

30.1 Platysma Motor Branch/Cervical Plexus

In cases with complete plexus lesion and affection of the accessory nerve, the platysma motor branch of the facial nerve can be used to reinnervate either the trapezius muscle or any muscle supplied by the brachial plexus. Socolovsky et al. found to arise from the cervicofacial trunk with some anatomical variants. Anastomotic rami from the transverse superficial cervical plexus were observed. Diameter-wise it seems to have a good match with the medial pectoral nerve and the triceps motor branch and teres minor branch of the axillary nerve. The rationale to use this nerve at all is that it is enabling voluntary muscle contraction. Bertelli et al. described their experience with the reconstruction of the medial pectoral nerve for shoulder adduction in $n = 13$ patients, with $n = 5$ pectoralis major M3 and $n = 4$ M4. However, in $n = 4$ patients, no reinnervation was observed and that in only $n = 5$ of this group, they were sure that reinnervation derived from the platysma motor branch [1–4].

C. P. G. Heinen (✉)
Christliches Krankenhaus Quakenbrück, Nerve-, Spine and Neurosurgery, Quakenbrück, Germany

T. Kretschmer
Department of Neurosurgery and Neurorestoration, Neurosurgical Intensive Care, Head Neurooncological Center (DKG), Skull Base Center (GSB), Paralysis Center, Klinikum Klagenfurt, Klagenfurt am Wörthersee, Austria

R. Schmidhammer
Millesi Center, Vienna, Austria

30.2 Dorsal Scapular to Suprascapular Nerve

In the rare condition of affected accessory nerve but preserved dorsal scapular nerve, the latter can be used to restore suprascapular nerve function. In our personal series (CH) of $n = 4$ patients, we could do a direct coaptation in $n = 2$ patients and $n = 2$ needed a short graft of 3 cm. Supraspinatus muscle reached M4, infraspinatus M3. In a larger series in OBPP, Augustine et al. reported an improvement of the active movement scale AMS scores by 4.1 and 4.4 points for shoulder abduction and external rotation, respectively [5].

30.3 Contralateral Nerve Transfers (Not CC7)

Besides the most prominent contralateral transfer of the healthy C7 spinal nerve, there are some other rarely used contralateral nerve transfers. Bertelli et al. described the transfer of the contralateral C4 spinal nerve to the biceps muscle via a sural nerve graft reaching M3. Becker et al. described their experience of contralateral accessory and medial pectoral nerve with reasonable

F. Guedes et al. (eds.), *Nerve Transfers for Brachial Plexus Reconstruction after Trauma*,
https://doi.org/10.1007/978-3-031-92445-3_30

outcomes [6]. There are mainly few case reports using contralateral accessory to the suprascapular nerve with M2 [7].

In our hands (RS), the use of the contralateral medial pectoral nerve to ipsilateral pronator branch of median nerve yields consistently M3.

References

1. Bertelli J. Platysma motor branch transfer in brachial plexus repair: report of the first case. J Brachial Plex Peripher Nerve Inj. 2007;2:e56–60.
2. Socolovsky MP, et al. Surgical anatomy of the platysma motor branch as a donor for transfer in brachial plexus repair. Surg Radiol Anat. 2008;30:669–74.
3. Bertelli JA, Ghizoni MF. Contralateral motor rootlets and ipsilateral nerve transfers in brachial plexus reconstruction. J Neurosurg. 2004;101:770–8.
4. Bertelli JA, Ghizoni MF. Reconstruction of complete palsies of the adult brachial plexus by root grafting using long grafts and nerve transfers to target nerves. J Hand Surg Am. 2010;35:1640–6.
5. Augustine HFM, Coroneos CJ, Choi M, Bain JR. Adjunctive dorsal scapular nerve transfer to suprascapular nerve for brachial plexus birth injuries: case series. J Hand Surg. 2019;44(902):e1–902.e9.
6. Kretschmer T. Chapter 5: Verletzungen des Plexus brachialis. In: Nervenchirurgie. Berlin: Springer; 2014. https://doi.org/10.1007/978-3-662-45894-5.
7. Zermeño-Rivera J, Gutiérrez-Amavizca BE. Contralateral spinal accessory nerve transfer: a new technique in panavulsive brachial plexus palsy. Indian J Surg. 2015;77:247–50.

Correction to: Nerve Transfers for Brachial Plexus Reconstruction after Trauma

Fernando Guedes, Christian Heinen, Lukas Rasulic, Alexander Y. Shin, and Mariano Socolovsky

Correction to:
F. Guedes et al. (eds.), *Nerve Transfers for Brachial Plexus Reconstruction after Trauma*, https://doi.org/10.1007/978-3-031-92445-3

The editor's name was inadvertently published as "Lucas Rasulic" in the original version. It has been corrected as "Lukas Rasulic" in this version.

The updated version of this book can be found at
https://doi.org/10.1007/978-3-031-92445-3

F. Guedes et al. (eds.), *Nerve Transfers for Brachial Plexus Reconstruction after Trauma*,
https://doi.org/10.1007/978-3-031-92445-3_31

MIX
Papier aus verantwortungsvollen Quellen
Paper from responsible sources
FSC® C105338

If you have any concerns about our products,
you can contact us on
ProductSafety@springernature.com

In case Publisher is established outside the EU,
the EU authorized representative is:
Springer Nature Customer Service Center GmbH
Europaplatz 3, 69115 Heidelberg, Germany

Printed by Libri Plureos GmbH
in Hamburg, Germany